Psychiatric Nursing

Psychiatric Nursing
A Therapeutic Approach

Edited by
Peggy Martin

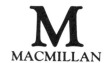

MACMILLAN

First published 1987

Published by
MACMILLAN EDUCATION LTD
Houndmills, Basingstoke, Hampshire RG21 2XS
and London
Companies and representatives
throughout the world

Typeset and designed by
Oxprint Ltd, Oxford

**Printed in Great Britain by
Scotprint Ltd., Musselburgh**

British Library Cataloguing in Publication Data
Martin, Peggy, *1939–*
Psychiatric nursing: a therapeutic approach.
1. Psychiatric nursing
I. Title
610.73'68   RC440
ISBN 0–333–43842–6

For Graham with Love

CONTRIBUTORS

Carl Dykes, RMN, is currently Charge Nurse in the Department of Child and Family Psychiatry, Children's Day Hospital, London.

Lynn Harris, BSc(Hons), RGN, RSCN, HV, is currently a clinical nurse specialist in the Guy's Support Team based at Guy's Hospital, London.

Helen Lewer, BSc(Hons), RGN, RSCN, RNT, is currently Tutor at The Nightingale School, St Thomas's Hospital, London.

Bob Payne, RGN, RMN, FETC, RCNT, is currently a nurse teacher.

Neil Vermaut, BSc, RMN, is currently Staff Nurse at Rees House Day Hospital, Croydon.

CRITICAL COMMENTERS

Dr Justus Akinsanya, PhD, BSc(Hons), STD, RNT, RGN, Orth Nurs Cert (Hons), Cert Dermatological Nursing, BTA Cert, is currently Acting Head of the Department of Nursing and Social Service, Dorset Institute of Higher Education, Poole, Dorset.

Martin Brown, RMN, RCNT, RNT, Dip N Ed, Cert Behavioural Psychotherapy, is currently Director of Nursing Services, Adult Mental Health, West Lambeth Health Authority, London.

Philip Burnard, MSc, RMN, RGN, Dip N Cert Ed, RNT, is currently Lecturer in the Nursing Studies Department at the University of Wales College of Medicine, Cardiff.

Dr P. Carr, BA, PhD, RMN, RGN, RNT, was formerly Head of Nursing Studies at Manchester Polytechnic and is currently General Secretary of the Registered Nursing Homes' Association.

Reg Everest, RMN, RGN, RNT, is currently Education Officer at The English National Board of Nursing, Midwifery and Health Visiting, London.

Helen Lewer, BSc(Hons), RGN, RSCN, RNT, is currently Tutor at The Nightingale School, St Thomas's Hospital, London.

Barbara McNulty, RGN, SCM, FRCN, is currently a bereavement counsellor working as a freelance.

David Passey, RMN, Dip Professional Studies, Cert Ed, RNT, is currently Education Officer (Mental Nursing) at The English National Board of Nursing, Midwifery and Health Visiting.

P. Tibbles, RMN, is currently Director of Nursing Services at The Bethlem Royal Hospital, Beckenham, Kent.

John Tingle, BA Law(Hons), Cert Ed, is currently Lecturer in Law at the Worcester Technical College, Deansway, Worcester.

Brian Woollatt, MBE, RGN, RMN, was formerly Senior Clinical Nurse at The Drug Dependence Clinical Research and Treatment Unit of The Bethlem Royal Hospital, Beckenham, Kent.

Contents

Foreword

The mentally ill in hospitals, in community facilities and in home services count on nurses to help them to solve their interpersonal and psychosocial problems. Meeting this expectation of patients is the purpose of psychiatric nursing practice. In order to provide useful nursing services, nurses require theoretical understanding of the common presenting problems of patients, as presented in this textbook.

The problems of mentally ill patients do not arise overnight. They consist in patterns of behaviour, evolved as adaptive response to experiences earlier in life. Individuals acquire behaviour patterns in interactions with persons who are significant to them in some way. Such interactions occur during child-rearing encounters in the home, during contacts with peers and teachers in school, in work situations and in other social institutions such as churches. Some of these patterns and behavioural acts, which are variants of a pattern, endure throughout life and serve to assure continuing growth and constructive living in the community. For the mentally ill, however, the situation is otherwise.

Persons who become mentally ill generally acquire behaviours important to them in terms of relief from anxiety and their psychosocial survival as they perceive it at a given time. These patterns of behaviour, which in earlier situations had great utility, persist and tend to become automatic, to be used without thought. This occurs, in part, because the behaviours are known, familiar and provided relief from anxiety. Such behaviours continue to be used, even though they are maladaptive in terms of continuing personal development and living in the community, for the patients are unaware that such behaviours are dysfunctional. One patient, after sustaining marked improvement in her condition, referred to her previous behaviour as her 'trapadaptation', an apt characterisation.

Maladaptive behaviours reflect lacks and gaps in the development of intellectual, interpersonal and social skills in accord with age, in-born capacities and social expectations. They prevent or limit social living within the community. Such inept behavioural patterns are replayed, recurringly, within the in-patient milieu, by patients in their interactions with other patients, nurses and other staff members of the hospital. Helping patients to recognise and to resolve these difficulties is the main challenge of nurses employed in psychiatric services.

Nurses do not change the behaviour of patients. What nurses do is to initiate, assist and support patients in their efforts to change their own behaviour. Nurses do this first by defining the nature of the problems of each patient. This requires application of the nursing process and of theory, as described in this textbook. Armed with theoretical understanding of presenting difficulties of patients, nurses then use nurse–patient interactions as opportunities to generate self-awareness in patients as a basis for patients gradually to reshape their own behaviour. Nurses also assist patients to know, to test and therefore to acquire new health-seeking behaviours as maladaptive patterns are gradually and slowly given up.

The work of nurses in psychiatric services is indeed disciplined, purposeful and difficult. It requires continuing self-study by the nurse so that patients are not used to meet the needs of the nurse. It requires theory so that the nurse's understanding of problems is guided by the best available scientific knowledge. It requires that the nurse's attention is focused on getting to know the patient as a person, so that the patient's dilemmas are appreciated while latent capacities for growth are tapped as new skills are developed. It requires that the nurse supports separateness of identity of both nurse and patient and yet uses the connectedness of the nurse–patient relationship for purposes beneficial for the patient.

Promoting changes in behaviour, in oneself and in others, is an elusive goal, limited by the available knowledge, and therefore a stimulating challenging field of work for intelligent enterprising nurses. This textbook will assist student nurses to acquire some of the basic intellectual tools with which to begin a career in this important, socially relevant and interesting component of nursing.

1986   Hildegard E. Peplau, RN, Ed D, FAAN
                                               Professor Emerita
                           Rutgers—The State University of New Jersey
                                                      USA

Preface

Psychiatric Nursing: A Therapeutic Approach centres on the skills used by psychiatric nurses in caring for patients with psychological problems in both hospital and community settings.

The book is primarily designed to help nurses to think about what they do and to clarify their roles and functions within the multi-disciplinary setting. The focus on nursing as an activity in its own right is intentional and deliberate, while recognising the importance of a wide knowledge gained from a number of different disciplines.

The book emphasises the significance of the therapeutic use of self in communicating with patients productively and in carrying out the process of nursing effectively. The first part of the book is concerned with the nurse's therapeutic approach to care as a member of a multi-disciplinary team and as an individual. The second part of the book explores the application of patient care through the use of patient profiles and the application of different nursing models and approaches to care.

Purley, 1987   P.M.

Acknowledgements

I should like to thank Elizabeth Horne, formerly Senior Editor, Macmillan Education, for inviting me to write this book, Mary Waltham, Senior Editor, and Sheila Collins OBE for their guidance, support and ideas which have been incorporated into the text.

I am deeply grateful to Professor Hildegard E. Peplau, not only for agreeing to write the foreword to this book but also for enabling me to develop a greater understanding of psychiatric nursing through her numerous publications. Thanks are also due to many colleagues and members of the multidisciplinary team who have offered comments and contributions: Dr Thomas Barnes, Dr Kate Tress, Maureen Ryan, Lyleanne Hopkins, Alison Cook, Jenny Harwood, Pauline Tanner, Niki Muir, Lynn Strickland, Fred Seechahid, Charlie Wood and the Reverend Geoffrey Johnson.

I should like to thank the library staff at the Royal College of Nursing, and Jacky Boothby and Margaret Paull of Horton Hospital, for their assistance.

The writing of this book has involved many discussions with learners and ward managers and I thank them for sharing their ideas and concerns.

I should like to thank two of my former colleagues for their support, John Scadden, Principal Nursing Officer (Research), and Stella Desai, Clinical Teacher, Horton Hospital, and finally Doris Crouch for typing the manuscript.

The author and publishers wish to thank the following who have kindly given permission for the use of copyright material:

Random House Inc. Alfred A Knopf Inc. for adaption of figure after Sabin, 1954, Role theory. In: *Handbook of Social Psychology*, Vol. 1, 1st edn (eds Lindzey and Aronson), Addison-Wesley, Reading, Massachusetts.

Rodale Press Inc. for figure from J. I. Rodale, *The Synonym Finder*, Copyright © 1978 by Rodale Press Inc.

Mayfield Publishing Company for 'The Johari window' from J. Luft, *Group Processes: An Introduction to Group Dynamics*, Copyright © 1984, 1970, 1963 by Joseph Luft.

John Wiley and Sons Ltd for material from *Senior Nurse*, **3**, No. 2, July 1985.

Every effort has been made to trace all the copyright holders but, if any has been inadvertently overlooked, the publishers will be pleased to make the necessary arrangement at the first opportunity.

Part 1: Concepts

Chapter 1

Introduction

Psychiatric nursing is a branch of nursing which uses interpersonal processes as a means of bringing about positive health changes in patients. The promotion of mental health is fundamental to the psychiatric nurses's role.

Health is an individually defined phenomenon with many variables and means much more than the absence of disease. A person who is mentally healthy is usually considered to have developed mature patterns of problem solving, is able to fulfil needs for love and work and is able to cope with crises within a network of family and social support systems (Crawford and Kilander, 1985). Health must therefore be viewed as an integration of the whole person. Watson (1979) suggests that health encompasses at least three of the following:

1. A high level of psychological, physical and social functioning.
2. An adaptive level of daily functioning.
3. The absence of illness or the presence of efforts that lead to its absence.

A person's state of wellness or illness moves along a continuum which is influenced by a great number of different factors. At times, there is a movement towards greater degrees of health and, at other times, movement towards ill health (Lancaster, 1980) (*Figure 1.1*). Definitions of mental ill health are

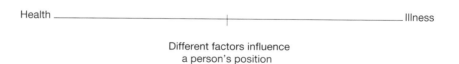

Figure 1.1   *The health–illness continuum*

closely related to the values and institutions within a society (Haber *et al.*, 1982). Ideas about mental health and mental ill health differ from one society to another and from time to time within the same society. For example, homosexuality was until recently considered to be an illness or a deviance from what was 'normal'; now, homosexuality has become more acceptable and is no longer regarded as an illness for which a person needs treatment. It is impossible to identify any one single cause of mental illness. People develop mental illness because of a variety of factors which interfere with their ability to adapt to the world they live in (Maddison and Kellehear, 1982). *Figure 1.2* shows some of the factors which influence the mental health–illness continuum.

In recent years, interest has been focused on life change events and their significance in contributing to a breakdown in health. Holmes and Rahe (1967) have attempted to express in qualitative terms the amount of stress associated

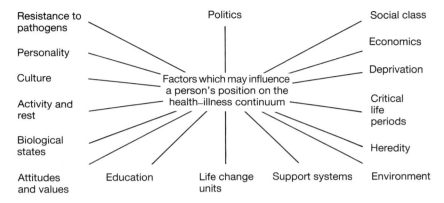

Figure 1.2   *Some of the factors which influence the mental health–illness continuum*

with a range of specific events (*Table 1.1*). Participants in their study were asked to comment on both pleasant and unpleasant events since both involved change. There was considerable agreement among the subjects as to which life event items required major adaptation and which were of less significance (Holmes and Rahe, 1967; Williams and Holmes, 1978).

Table 1.1   *Life change and stress*

Life events	Life change units
Death of spouse	100
Divorce	73
Marital separation	65
Jail term	63
Death of a close family member	63
Personal injury or illness	53
Marriage	50
Fired at work	47
Marital reconciliation	45
Retirement	45
Change in the health of a family member	44
Pregnancy	40
Sex difficulties	39
Gain of a new family member	39
Business readjustment	39
Change in financial state	38
Death of a close friend	37
Change to a different line of work	36
Change in the number of arguments with spouse	35

For the complete list, refer to Holmes and Rahe (1967).

The psychiatric nurse plays a vital role in the prevention of ill health and the promotion of health at three levels of intervention.

1. *Primary prevention* focuses on the maintenance and promotion of mental health, particularly among high risk groups.
2. *Secondary prevention* is concerned with the identification of maladaptive behaviours and strengthening a person's capacity to reduce stress.
3. *Tertiary prevention* is aimed at the rehabilitation of patients with mental illness, helping them to overcome difficulties and to return to useful lives in the community.

Today, psychiatric nursing is undergoing change and meeting new and exciting challenges. Nurses are finding greater opportunities to participate therapeutically with patients both in hospital and increasingly in the community. The nurse's prime tools in the promotion of health are the relationship that he or she has with the patient and the ability to communicate therapeutically. Therapeutic communication differs from every-day communication and involves a planned approach in which a conscious effort is made to influence the patient in directions that serve his interests and welfare (Hein, 1980). For the approach to be considered therapeutic, it must have a demonstrable and beneficial impact on the patient's maladaptive responses, so that the patient is able to mature and grow in the direction of mental health (Peplau, 1968). An important factor in the delivery of effective nursing care is the development of the nurse as a person. Peplau (1952) has long recognised that 'the extent to which each nurse understands her own functioning will determine the extent to which she can come to understand the situation confronting the patient and the way he sees it'.

The RMN Syllabus of The English and Welsh National Boards for Nursing, Midwifery and Health Visiting (1982) focuses on the development of major competencies necessary for the practice of professional nursing. Self-awareness skills are seen as an essential element of interactions with patients and determine the extent to which a nurse can effectively utilise the self in helping others.

The capacity to understand one's own feelings influences the effectiveness of communication and assists nurses to assess how their actions help or do not help patients (Gregg, 1963; Maloney, 1962). Developing an understanding of what happens when a nurse relates helpfully to a patient is an important step in defining the very nature of nursing itself.

REFERENCES AND FURTHER READING

References

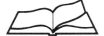

Crawford, A. L., and Kilander, V. C. (1985), *Psychiatric and Mental Health Nursing*, 6th edn, F. A. Davis, Philadelphia, Pennsylvania.

The English and Welsh National Boards for Nursing, Midwifery and Health Visiting (1982), *Syllabus of Training Professional Register*, Part 3.

Gregg, D. (1963), The therapeutic roles of the nurse, *Perspectives in Psychiatric Care*, **1**, No. 1, 18–24.

Haber, J., Leach, A. M., Schudy, S. M., and Sideleau, B. F. (1982), *Comprehensive Psychiatric Nursing*, 2nd edn, McGraw-Hill, New York.

Hein, E. C. (1980), *Communication in Nursing Practice*, 2nd edn, Little, Brown, Boston, Massachusetts.

Holmes, T. H., and Rahe, R. H. (1967), The social readjustment rating scale, *Journal of Psychosomatic Research*, **11**, 213–218.

Lancaster, J. (1980), *Adult Psychiatric Nursing*, Medical Examination Publishing, New York.

Maddison, D., and Kellehear, K. J. (1982), *Psychiatric Nursing*, 5th edn, Churchill Livingstone, Edinburgh.

Maloney, E. (1962), Does the psychiatric nurse have independent functions? In: *A Collection of Classics in Psychiatric Nursing Literature* (eds Smoyak, S. A., and Rouslin, S.), Charles B. Slack, New Jersey.

Peplau, H. E. (1952), *Interpersonal Relations in Nursing*, G. P. Putnam, New York.

Peplau, H. E. (1968), Psychotherapeutic strategies, *Perspectives in Psychiatric Care*, **6**, No. 6, 264–270.

Watson, J. (1979), *Nursing. The Philosophy and Science of Caring*, Little, Brown, Boston, Massachusetts.

Williams, C. C., and Holmes, T. H. (1978), Life change, human adaptation and onset of illness. In: *Clinical Practice in Psychosocial Nursing Assessment and Intervention* (eds Longo, D. C., and Williams, R. A.), Appleton Century Crofts, Norwalk, Connecticut.

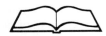

Further reading

Seedhouse, D. (1986), A universal concern, *Nursing Times*, **82**, No. 4, 36–38.

Chapter 2

The role of the psychiatric nurse

'The work of the nurse can be defined as that of a change agent who uses theory to guide nurse–patient interactions with the aim of promoting substantial change in patient behaviour.' (Peplau, 1978).

INTRODUCTION

A role can be defined as a patterned sequence of learned actions performed by a person in an interaction situation (Sinkler, 1970). Traditionally, a role is a part in a play about which the audience has a set of expectations (Downie, 1984).

THE NURSE STEREOTYPE

Everyone has expectations concerning the role of the nurse because the word nurse carries with it an expectation of certain skills and behaviours. The patient will have his own preconceived ideas about the nurse's role. His ideas about nurses may be influenced by romantic fiction, television and magazine articles rather than by personal experience. Traditionally, the role of the nurse has implied certain relationship skills, technical skills and symbols. The relationship skills have included caring and helping, while the technical skills have focused on concrete tasks such as giving medicines and carrying out procedures. The symbols which have been associated with the nurse are those relating to the female stereotype, e.g. frilly cap and black stockings (Jasmin and Trygstad, 1979). Cooper (1981) writes: 'Society only sees the nurse in terms of the actions she performs in carrying out her role. What they do not realize is that what they do not see is really what nursing is all about. The true practice of nursing lies in the nurse's ability to see, to listen and to feel beyond the ordinary person.'

THE NURSE AS AN INDIVIDUAL

The word nurse does not of course apply to a particular kind of person. Nurses come from all walks of life and represent a broad section of humanity. Like other people, they have their strengths and weaknesses and some have emotional problems of their own. Merely wearing a uniform and wanting to take on the role of the nurse does not mean that a person can be effective in that role. The ability to function effectively in the complex roles of the nurse depends very much on the kind of person that the nurse *is* and the personal qualities that he or she brings to the role.

NURSING AS A LEARNING PROCESS

Psychiatric nursing aims to enhance not only the personal growth of the patient but also the personal growth of the nurse. Peplau (1952) perceives nursing as a process which can promote constructive learning for both the patient and the nurse. Nursing functions are both educative and therapeutic when they lead people to develop the skills of problem solving. Peplau points out that problems relating to health are never completely solved because difficulties in living recur and, while solving a present difficulty is valuable, unless the individual learns how to meet the same or a similar difficulty in the future, the experience will not have taken the person towards greater maturity in living with others. In the therapeutic role the nurse consciously directs his or her own behaviour in the interaction with the patient and uses these interactive experiences towards therapeutic change. The patient is assisted to use his current living experiences towards greater self-understanding (Gregg, 1963).

The nurse's behaviour may influence not only the wellness behaviour of patients but also their illness behaviour as well (Peplau, 1978).

For this reason, nurses need to maximise their effectiveness by focusing on themselves and the presence that they bring to the health situation.

As Maloney (1962) points out, whatever label is given to the activities of daily living, it is clear that these activities must go on. It is the manner in which they go on that marks the difference between custodial care and creative psychotherapeutic nursing.

THE ROLES OF THE NURSE

The roles of the nurse can be illustrated as follows.

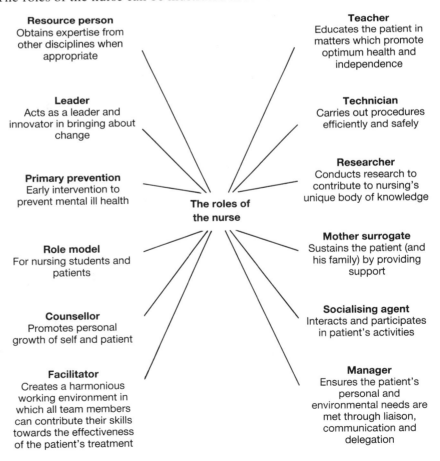

Resource person
Obtains expertise from other disciplines when appropriate

Leader
Acts as a leader and innovator in bringing about change

Primary prevention
Early intervention to prevent mental ill health

Role model
For nursing students and patients

Counsellor
Promotes personal growth of self and patient

Facilitator
Creates a harmonious working environment in which all team members can contribute their skills towards the effectiveness of the patient's treatment

Teacher
Educates the patient in matters which promote optimum health and independence

Technician
Carries out procedures efficiently and safely

Researcher
Conducts research to contribute to nursing's unique body of knowledge

The roles of the nurse

Mother surrogate
Sustains the patient (and his family) by providing support

Socialising agent
Interacts and participates in patient's activities

Manager
Ensures the patient's personal and environmental needs are met through liaison, communication and delegation

FACT SHEET

1. The nursing role is a caring role, different from but complementary to the medical role (McFarlane, 1983).
2. The nurse's concept of role can cause problems when it varies from what other team members expect. This can be observed when a nurse believes that she or he has a therapeutic role to play in purposely counselling patients, but the medical staff expect the nurse to behave in a soothing and reassuring 'have faith in the medication' fashion (Harries, 1976).
3. The 'role of the nurse' can be a barrier to human relatedness just as the role of the 'patient' may be a barrier (Travelbee, 1966).
4. Too often, nursing activities become an end in themselves and the reasons for the activities are overlooked. The nurse who focuses on what needs to be done, and not on the human being for whom the activities are planned, cannot perceive and respond to the human being who is the patient (Travelbee, 1966).
5. The therapeutic role of the psychiatric nurse cannot be described in terms of tasks or procedures. It must be discussed in terms of attitudes, feelings, understanding and relationships (Taylor, 1982).

REFERENCES AND FURTHER READING

References

Cooper, S. (1981), What is nursing?, *Nursing Times, Occasional Papers*, **77**, No. 34.

Downie, R. (1984), Nursing as a role job, *Nursing Mirror*, **158**, No. 4, 29.

Gregg, D. (1963). The therapeutic roles of the nurse, *Perspectives in Psychiatric Care*, **1**, No. 1, 18–24.

Harries, C. J. (1976), Modern developments in psychiatric nursing care. In: *Comprehensive Psychiatric Care* (ed. Baker, A. A.), Blackwell Scientific, Oxford.

Jasmin, S., and Trygstad, L. N. (1979) *Behavioural Concepts and the Nursing Process*, C. V. Mosby, St Louis, Missouri.

Maloney, E. (1962), Does the psychiatric nurse have independent functions? In: *A Collection of Classics in Psychiatric Nursing Literature* (eds Smoyak, S. A., and Rouslin, S.), Charles B. Slack, New Jersey.

McFarlane, J. (1983), Mirror, mirror on the wall, *Nursing Mirror*, **156**, No. 23, 17–20.

Peplau, H. E. (1952), *Interpersonal Relations in Nursing*, G. P. Putnam, New York.

Peplau, H. E. (1978), Psychiatric nursing: role of nurses and psychiatric nurses, *International Nursing Review*, **25**, No. 2, 41–47.

Sinkler, G. H. (1970), Identity and role, *Nursing Outlook*, **18**, No. 10, 22–24.

Taylor, C. M. (1982), *Mereness' Essentials of Psychiatric Nursing*, 11th edn, C. V. Mosby, St Louis, Missouri, 1982.

Travelbee, J. (1966), *Interpersonal Aspects of Nursing*, F. A. Davis, Philadelphia, Pennsylvania.

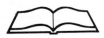

Further reading

Altschul, A. (1984), Does good practice need good principles 1?, *Nursing Times*, **80**, No. 27, 36–38.

Altschul A. (1984), Does good practice need good principles 2?, *Nursing Times*, **80**, No. 28, 49–51.

Anderson, E. R. (1973), *The Role of the Nurse*, Royal College of Nursing Research Project Series 2, No. 1.

Barber, P. (1986), The psychiatric nurse's failure therapeutically to nurture, *Nursing Practice*, **1**, No. 3, 138–141.

Campbell, W. (1979), The therapeutic community: problems encountered by nurses, *Nursing Times*, **75**, No. 47, 2038–2040.

Cormack, D. (1976), *Psychiatric Nursing Observed*, Royal College of Nursing, London.

Davis, B. D. (1984), What is the nurse's perception of the patient? In: *Understanding Nurses* (ed. Skevington, S.), John Wiley, Chichester, West Sussex.

Dietrich, G. (1976), Nurses in the therapeutic community, *Journal of Advanced Nursing*, **1**, 139–154.

Dotan, M., Krulik, T., Eckerling, S., and Shatzman, H. (1986), Role models in nursing, *Nursing Times, Occasional Papers*, **82**, No. 3, 55–57.

Duffy, D. (1984), Mental health nursing: a student's view, *Nursing Times*, **80**, No. 30, 67–68.

Hessler, I. (1980), Roles, status and relationships in psychiatric nursing, *Nursing Times*, **76**, No. 12, 508–509.

Hewitt, F. S. (1981), Role and the presentation of the self, *Nursing Times, Communication Skills*, **77**, No. 22, 17–20.

Kingey, J., and Kat, B. (1984), How can nurses use social psychology to study themselves and their roles? In: *Understanding Nurses* (ed. Skevington, S.), John Wiley, Chichester, West Sussex.

Peplau, H. E. (1978), Psychiatric nursing: role of nurses and psychiatric nurses, *International Nursing Review*, **25**, No. 2, 41–47.

RCN (1979), *Extended Clinical Role of the Nurse*, Royal College of Nursing, London.

Towell, D. (1975), *Understanding Psychiatric Nursing*, Royal College of Nursing, London.

Chapter 3

The nurse–patient relationship

'To understand another person the nurse must be able to realize not simply what he is thinking, but also what he is feeling. It is not enough to know what is in his mind; it is also essential to know what is in his heart.' (Jersild, 1962).

INTRODUCTION

The nurse–patient relationship is central to nursing and requires the active presence of the nurse. It is through this relationship that the goals of nursing are achieved. Through continuous contacts with the nurse the patient is able to learn more adaptive behaviours.

Whatever the setting in which the nurse–patient relationship is developed (whether it is in the patient's home or in hospital), it can have a major impact on his health care if the nurse has an understanding of how the nurse–patient relationship can be used as a definite therapeutic tool.

TRUST

During the initial phase of the relationship the nurse must work towards developing the patient's trust. Trust is an essential component of the relationship as it can provide the patient with a basis for learning and growth as a person. When a person learns to trust during the early stages of development, he is then able to transfer this feeling into later relationships. Many individuals

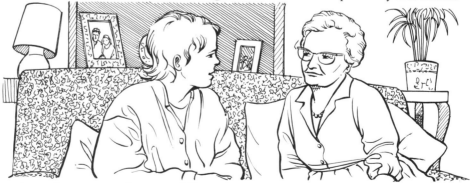

who seek treatment for mental illness have been denied the experience of trust. During childhood, they may have learned for a number of reasons that others cannot be trusted. Promises may have been made and then broken or confidences shared with significant people, who then betrayed these confidences to others. They will need time to build trust into their relationship with the nurse. When a patient is able to learn to trust the nurse, he is provided with the opportunity to transfer this learning to other life-enriching relationships.

For trust to be established in the nurse–patient relationship, the nurse must be a person who can be trusted. The nurse must be honest and genuine and show consistency towards the patient. Trust like respect cannot be demanded; it has to be earned. The trust of the patient is more likely to be gained when there is congruity between the nurse's words and actions. Unless the nurse is a person whom the patient feels he can trust, then the nurse–patient relationship is likely to be very superficial (Ruditis, 1979).

CONFIDENTIALITY

The very nature of the nurse–patient relationship implies confidentiality. The patient should be told that private information appertaining to himself is strictly limited to the health care setting. Sometimes the patient will tell the nurse something which he does not wish to share with others. This is understandable for each person chooses very carefully those he is willing to confide in; the patient may feel more at ease with some members of the multi-disciplinary team than with others.

If the patient gives the nurse information which is of particular significance, then the nurse can suggest that either he tells the doctor or, if he does not wish to do this, he may be willing for the nurse to share the information with the doctor. There are occasions when the nurse may have good reason to believe that the patient's actions or intended actions could bring harm to either himself or others. In these circumstances the nurse has a duty to go against the patient's wishes and to inform the medical staff.

THE NURSE–PATIENT RELATIONSHIP

The therapeutic value of the nurse–patient relationship very much depends on the kind of person that the nurse is and the competence with which therapeutic skills are employed. Travelbee (1971) believes that there is a direct correlation between the amount of expertise which a nurse possesses in interpersonal relationships and how well he or she is able to meet the needs of others. The nurse who is unable to face up to the reality of his or her own behaviour is unlikely to be able to help patients to do so. Each nurse must engage in a brave self-encounter; otherwise the nurse's own defence patterns may interfere with the development of the nurse–patient relationship. Nurses, like other human beings, have their strengths and weaknesses. While it is not possible to have a positive attitude towards every patient, self-awareness can assist the nurse to understand his or her own feelings and to plan an approach which is beneficial to the patient.

The nurse–patient relationship is a helping relationship in which the nurse facilitates the personal development and growth of the patient to grow and develop new insights. Talking to the patient is not the same as talking to a friend. A social relationship is reciprocal, while the nurse–patient relationship is goal directed and focuses on the patient. The patient should not be burdened with the nurse's problems or personal history; otherwise the focus on the patient's needs is lost (Peplau, 1960). Self-disclosure should only be used when it is an appropriate tool and assists the patient towards meeting his goals.

(a) Obstacles to the nurse–patient relationship

The obstacles which can occur in the establishment of a therapeutic nurse–patient relationship are as follows (Peplau, 1978):

1. Acting out one's own conflicts through a relationship with the patient.
2. Giving the patient personal information about oneself instead of focusing on him.
3. Feeling that he or she is the only person who can help the patient.
4. Spending a disproportionate amount of time with one patient.
5. Taking sides with the patient against his family.
6. Becoming so emotionally involved that the relationship is no longer beneficial to the patient.
7. Failing to fulfil promises made to the patient.
8. Labelling the patient, e.g. 'hysteric' or 'schizy'.
9. Avoiding the patient.
10. Denying the need for self-awareness, and therefore denying the need for change.
11. Prolonging a relationship when the therapeutic need for such a relationship no longer exists.
12. Entering the pseudochum relationship with a patient.
13. Having obvious favourites among patients.

(b) Stages of the nurse–patient relationship

1 Orientation phase

The first encounter with the patient is important. Not only does the nurse begin to assess the patient, but also the patient begins to assess the nurse; he may test the nurse with various questions and behaviours in order to learn about the kind of person that the nurse is.

The nurse needs to adopt a warm friendly manner, to smile appropriately and to be comfortable with the use of eye contact. The nurse should begin to establish trust by being honest and consistent in his or her own behaviours.

Finding a common interest or experience can help to establish rapport, as in the following example.

A newly admitted patient was reported as being uncommunicative. On entering the patient's room, one of the nurses noticed that the patient had pinned animal posters on the walls. Immediately the nurse who was also fond of animals was able to identify a common interest with the patient, which although established on a social level would later serve to facilitate more meaningful therapeutic communication.

2 Identification phase

As the nurse and patient become better acquainted and trust is established, the nurse is able to explore the patient's underlying needs and problems and to establish goals.

3 Working phase

During the working phase the nurse provides support as the patient works through his problems. This support may be provided by being physically and actively present, by listening or by showing understanding and empathy or setting limits. By being supportive the nurse helps the patient towards personal growth and independence.

4 Termination phase

Termination of the nurse–patient relationship occurs when the patient has accomplished his goals. Preparation for termination of the relationship should begin early on in the relationship, as both the nurse and the patient may experience feelings of loss or separation. Both will need to talk about the reality of termination.

The nurse must remember that the nurse–patient relationship is a professional relationship. It is not the same as two friends meeting and sharing confidences.

Personal feelings should never be allowed to impede the patient's progress towards independence and the nurse must always bear in mind that occasionally a patient may try to find a means of prolonging the relationship. His desire to be nursed may be greater than his desire to be cured.

BURN-OUT

The nurse–patient relationship can be very emotionally demanding and the nurse may be particularly vulnerable to 'burn-out'. Burn-out is physical and emotional exhaustion which leads to discernible negative responses and attitudes towards oneself and others (Lachman, 1983). It causes feelings of emotional fatigue, cynicism, depression, frustration, indifference, apathy, resignation and a sense of futility. Burn-out presents a troublesome barrier to human caring and separates the nurse from the original meaning and purpose of nursing. The nurse may find that the values taught in the nursing school are devalued in the work situation.

The nurse who is suffering from burn-out may withdraw from other people and use distancing manoeuvres to avoid patients. Sometimes a nurse will escape into a branch of nursing that requires less personal and emotional involvement (Beland, 1975).

Nursing is demanding; the nurse is faced with many life-and-death situations, each of which may leave its emotional toll. The nurse cannot be supportive to patients unless he or she feels supported by colleagues, and particularly by senior staff.

REFERENCES AND FURTHER READING

References

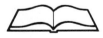

Beland, J. L. (1975), cited by Marriner, A. (1983), *The Nursing Process*, C.V. Mosby, St Louis, Missouri.

Jersild, A. T. (1962), Compassion, *Nursing Forum*, **1**, 61–72.

Lachman, V. D. (1983), *Stress Management: A Manual for Nurses*, Grune and Stratton.

Peplau, H. E. (1960), Talking with patients, *American Journal of Nursing*, **60**, No. 7, 964–966.

Peplau, H. E. (1978), Psychiatric nursing: role of nurses and psychiatric nurses, *International Nursing Review*, **25**, No. 2, 41–47.

Ruditis, S. E. (1979), Developing trust in nursing interpersonal relationships, *Journal of Psychiatric Nursing and Mental Health Services*, **17**, No. 4, 20–23 April, 18–20.

Travelbee, J. (1971), *Interpersonal Aspects of Nursing*, 2nd edn, F. A. Dans, Philadelphia, Pennsylvania.

Further reading

Altschul, A. (1970), Go and talk to the patients, *Nursing Mirror*, **130**, No. 15, 41–46.

Altschul, A. (1972), *Patient–Nurse Interaction, A Study of Interaction Patterns in Acute Psychiatric Wards*, Churchill Livingstone, Edinburgh.

Altschul, A. (1981), Issues in psychiatric nursing. In: *Current Issues in Nursing* (ed. Hockey, L.), Churchill Livingstone, Edinburgh.

Bailey, R. (1985), *Coping with Stress in Caring*, Blackwell Scientific, Oxford.

Bond, M. (1986), *Stress and Self-awareness: A Guide for Nurses*, Heinemann Nursing, London.

Brady, M. M. (1976), Nurse's attitudes towards patients who have a psychiatric history, *Journal of Advanced Nursing*, **1**, 11–25.

Burnard, P. (1985), How to reduce stress, *Nursing Mirror*, **161**, No. 19, 47–48.

Chilton, S. (1982), The nurse–patient relationship 1, *Nursing Times*, **78**, No. 10.

Chilton, S. (1982), The nurse–patient relationship 2, *Nursing Times*, **78**, No. 11.

Coltrane, F., and Pugh, C. D. (1978), Danger signals in staff/patient relationships in the therapeutic milieu, *Journal of Psychiatric Nursing and Mental Health Services*, **16**, No. 61, 34–36.

Cormack, D. (1982), Custodian or counsellor? *Nursing Mirror, Psychiatry/Mental Handicap Forum*, **154**, No. 4.

Cormack, D. (1983), *Psychiatric Nursing Described*, Churchill Livingstone, Edinburgh.

Cormack, D. (1985), The myth and reality of interpersonal skills used in nursing. In: *Interpersonal Skills in Nursing Research and Applications* (ed. Kagan, C. M.), Croom Helm, London.

Crews, N. E. (1979), Developing empathy for effective communication, *Association of Operating Room Nurses*, **30**, 536–545.

Davis, B. D. (1981), Trends in psychiatric nursing research, *Nursing Times, Occasional Papers*, **77**, No. 19, 73–76.

Dawkins, J. E., Depp, F. C., and Selzer, N. E. (1985), Stress and the psychiatric nurse, *Journal of Psychiatric Nursing and Mental Health Services*, **23**, No. 11, 9–15.

Dwyer, M. (1986), Why all this talk about communication? *Irish Nursing Forum*, **3**, No. 1, 32–34.

Firth, H., McIntee, J., McKeown, P., and Britton, P. (1986), Interpersonal support amongst nurses at work, *Journal of Advanced Nursing*, **11**, 273–282.

Gillespie, C., and Gillespie, V. (1986). Reading the danger signs, *Nursing Times*, **82**, No. 31, 24–27.

Hall, B. A. (1976), Mutual withdrawal: the non-participant in a therapeutic community, *Perspectives in Psychiatric Care*, **9**, No. 2, 75–79.

Hall, B. A. (1977), The effect of interpersonal attraction on the therapeutic relationship: a review and suggestions for further study, *Journal of Psychiatric Nursing and Mental Health Services*, **15**, No. 9, 18–23.

Hays, J. S., and Larson, K. (1963), *Interacting with Patients*, Macmillan, New York.

Heslop, A. (1985), Establishing therapeutic relationships, *Nursing Mirror*, **160**, 22, 28–29.

Heyman, B., and Shaw, M. (1984), Looking at relationships in nursing. In: *Understanding Nurses* (ed. Skevington, S.), John Wiley, Chichester, West Sussex.

Holderby, R. A., and McNulty, E. G. (1982), *Treating and Caring. A Human Approach to Patient Care*, Reston Publishing, Reston, Virginia.

Johnson, L. (1983), Burnout. In: *Handbook of Psychiatric Mental Health* (eds Adams, C. G., and Macione, A.), A Wiley Red Book, John Wiley, Chichester, West Sussex.

Kagan, C. M. (ed.) (1985), *Interpersonal Skills in Nursing Research and Applications*, Croom Helm, London.

Kasch, C. R. (1984), Interpersonal competence and communication in the delivery of nursing care, *Advances in Nursing Science*, **6**, No. 2, 71–88.

Kelly, H. S. (1969), The sense of an ending, *American Journal of Nursing*, **69**, 2378–2382.

Llewelyn, S. P. (1984), The cost of giving: emotional growth and emotional stress. In: *Understanding Nurses* (ed. Skevington, S.), John Wiley, Chichester, West Sussex.

Menzies, I. E. P. (1961), *The Functioning of Social Systems as a Defence against Anxiety*, Pamphlet No. 3, Tavistock, London.

Minshull, D. (1982), Counselling in psychiatric nursing 1, *Nursing Times*, **78**, No. 27, 1147–1148.

Minshull, D. (1982), Counselling in psychiatric nursing 2, *Nursing Times*, **78**, No. 28, 1201–1202.

Mooney, J. (1976), Attachment/separation in the nurse–patient relationship, *Nursing Forum*, **15**, No. 3, 259–264.

Murray, R. B., and Huelskoetter, M. M. W. (1983), *Psychiatric Mental Health Nursing: Giving Emotional Care*, Prentice-Hall, Englewood Cliffs, New Jersey.

Peplau, H. E. (1952), *Interpersonal Relations in Nursing*, G. P. Putnam, New York.

Peplau, H. E. (1957), Therapeutic concepts. In: *A Collection of Classics in Psychiatric Nursing Literature* (eds Smoyak, S. A., and Rouslin, S.), Charles B. Slack, New Jersey.

Peplau, H. E. (1962), Interpersonal techniques: the crux of psychiatric nursing. In: *A Collection of Classics in Psychiatric Nursing Literature* (eds Smoyak, S. A., and Rouslin, S.), Charles B. Slack, New Jersey.

Peplau, H. E. (1969), Professional closeness, *Nursing Forum*, **8**, No. 4.

RCN (1980), *Guidelines on Confidentiality in Nursing*, Royal College of Nursing, London.

Simmons, J. A. (1976), *The Nurse–Client Relationship in Mental Health Nursing*, W. B. Saunders, Philadelphia, Pennsylvania.

Simpson, R. (1980), Confidentiality in psychiatric nursing, *Nursing Times*, **76**, No. 19, 835–836.

Wilshaw, G. (1985), Are you trying to tell me something?, *Nursing Mirror*, **60**, No. 10, 33–35.

Yuen, F. K. H. (1986), The nurse–client relationship: a mutual learning experience, *Journal of Advanced Nursing*, **11**, 529–533.

Chapter 4

The nurse, the patient and the law
by *Bob Payne*

'Ignorance of the law excuses no man; not that all men know the law, but because 'tis an excuse every man will plead, and no man can tell how to refute him.' (John Selden, 1584–1654).

WHY BE CONCERNED WITH THE LAW?

Mention 'the law' to people and they think of police, courtrooms and very long words used by learned officials. You may also bring on feelings of unease as we try to remember what offence may have been unknowingly (or otherwise) committed. The language and ritual are formal, complex and hard at times to understand. When this is put together with a large volume of ever-changing legislation, it is not surprising that few nurses have a good enough understanding of their own legal position.

The position of nursing in law and society is changing very fast. Professional and government reports, stories in the media and research have all shown concern with current standards of nursing practice. The Nurses, Midwives and Health Visitors Act of 1979 requires nursing as a profession not just to maintain care standards but continuously to improve them. Since 1982 we have for the first time in this country a Code of Professional Conduct (revised, 1984). The Mental Health Act 1983 gives to the psychiatric nurse powers to restrict the freedom of patients. We are taking on increasing clinical responsibility and carrying out many tasks which before were performed by our medical colleagues. When this is taken together with a need to use limited resources more efficiently, the provision of which may be out of the hands of the nurse, we find ever-increasing accountability for care to patients, colleagues, the profession and society.

The nurse's understanding of the law should not solely be concerned with avoiding litigation. Such 'defensive nursing' as it might be called would lack imagination. The main wish should be to protect the rights of the patient. A clear definition of the role of the nurse, and a knowledge of the law, will ensure the nurse is not open to criminal or civil action over what he or she may not appreciate are his or her responsibilities.

WHAT IS THE LAW?

The legal system of the UK has developed over several centuries. A system organised to maintain order, with rules and scales of penalty, has existed since the seventh century. Most importantly the two parts, criminal and civil law, should be understood. A crime against the State, such as assault on a person or theft, is considered criminal and may be punished by removal of the offender's liberty. Breach of duty is a civil wrong, such as failure to complete a contract.

Civil action is taken by the person wronged, and the court is concerned to make sure that any loss or damage is made good through compensation, most often financial.

WHAT ABOUT THE DIFFERENT COURTS?

There are basically five types of court which the nurse may have to appear before. A criminal court can call a person by summons or warrant. In serious cases, warrants of arrest are issued by a magistrate, or justice of the peace; this allows the police to bring a person before the court. Witnesses can receive a subpoena requiring them to appear to give evidence.

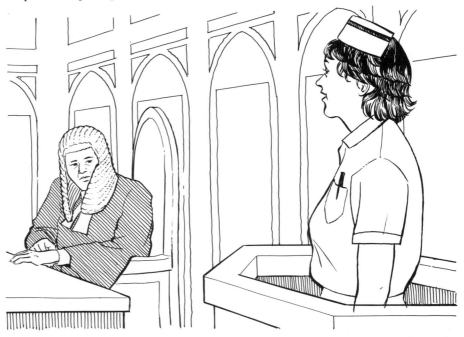

In ascending order of authority the criminal courts start with the magistrate's bench which has no jury. Intended for the trial of minor offences only, the defendant may choose whether he wishes to go before a crown court. Those accused of more serious offences will be seen first by the magistrates before being passed up to the crown court. Cases before a crown court are decided by a jury. (Nurses may be required to serve as jurors.) The defendant, if found guilty, may be given leave to appeal against judgement, or sentence, to a higher court. Appeals are mostly heard by the Criminal Division of the Court of Appeal. The highest level of appeal in the UK is to the House of Lords.

County courts deal with civil actions. Should claims for compensation be very high the action will be heard in the High Court, Queen's Bench Division.

A coroner's court examines evidence about the death of people in particular circumstances: if someone dies violently or unexpectedly, by notifiable disease, or where the cause or liability is unclear. The coroner must pass a verdict, which can be decided by a jury. If evidence of someone's behaviour suggests that they may be responsible, he will pass that evidence on to the Director of Public Prosecutions.

Concern with the effect of a court appearance on a young offender led to the establishment of the Juvenile Division. Headed by lay justices it is concerned with children under 14 and juveniles under 17 years of age. They have unique powers to deal with a young offender, designed to protect his best interest.

Difficulties that come from settling disputes between individuals and authority have led to the establishment of a number of tribunals. Different tribunals sort out rents, employment rights or entitlement to statutory benefits. The law profession has its own tribunal, as do doctors and midwives.

This chapter is only the briefest of introductions dealing with problem areas typical of those commonly met by the psychiatric nurse. Employment legislation is not covered. The case histories are intended only as examples of common situations; in reality, circumstances will vary considerably. Should a nurse be at all concerned with their specific legal position they should seek qualified help. This can be obtained privately or through their professional organisation or union. There is enough provision in the UK to make sure that those without enough money are not left without legal advice or representation.

POWERS OF RESTRAINT

The final right of the mental nurse is to detain a patient already in hospital.

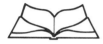

SUGGESTED READING

HM Government (1983), Mental Health Act 1983, HM Stationery Office, London.

Mental Health Division, DHSS (1983), Draft code of practice, Mental Health Act 1983, Department of Health and Social Security, London.

CASE STUDY

Gareth Henry, a 24-year-old local man, had been admitted to Larch Ward of the Bailey Hospital the previous weekend. His was a formal admission under the provision of the Mental Health Act 1983, Section 4. This section allows for compulsory admission to hospital for assessment in the case of emergency and lapses after 72 hours. Gareth had settled on the ward soon after admission and the holding section had been allowed to lapse. He was made fully aware of the change to informal status.

On arrival, Gareth had been very tired, dirty, hungry and cold, not having slept for 2 days. After these priorities had been dealt with, it left his major problems of bizarre thoughts and an obvious difficulty in separating reality from fantasy. The nursing staff had no reason to be concerned about his leaving the ward until during afternoon tea on Sunday. He approached Tom, the charge nurse, saying that he was off to see about a job. Tom talked with him to discover just what he intended to do. Gareth's thoughts were disjointed; he had no plan of action, no money and no specific place to go. It was February and very cold outside. He continually referred to a plan of preaching peace to the world from a boat that he would find at the local docks. Tom spent time with Gareth to persuade him that staying on the ward was in his best interests. Unfortunately, although remaining pleasant and cheerful, Gareth grew increasingly determined to leave. Tom tried to contact the duty doctor but discovered that he would be unavailable, except in the event of dire emergencies, for at least 3 hours.

(a) Discussion

Civil law requires every person to exercise common sense when presented with another person who may be considered to be in distress. This includes preventing a person from harming himself. Although there are circumstances where such action might be seen as a trespass, for a nurse not to take action for a patient in their care may be considered to be a breach of duty.

The Mental Health Act, 1983, Section 5, Subsection 4, allows for a person who is currently an in-patient receiving treatment for a mental disorder to be restrained from leaving by a nurse 'of the prescribed class'. The term prescribed means as defined by an order from the Secretary of State. Current interpretations of this definition vary. All state that the nurse must be a registered mental nurse. Most require the unit nursing officer or his deputy; some accept the charge nurse.

The Act states that the criteria to be met for the nurse to involve section five are that:

(a) The patient is at risk to himself or others.
(b) It is not practicable to obtain the immediate attendance of a medical officer.

In the case of Mr Gareth Henry these criteria are met.

Gareth would be at considerable risk of coming to harm. The circumstances which led to his admission have evidently not been resolved. The weather conditions and Gareth's lack of any coherent plan should lead Tom into considering the need to detain him. A medical officer is also not immediately available. Against this, Tom must be aware that to act against his patient's will would change the nature of their relationship, perhaps permanently. Tom must balance this against the immediate danger that Gareth would be in.

When invoking Section 5, the nurse must record the facts in writing, using the prescribed form. Form 13 of Schedule 1 to the Mental Health (Hospital Guardianship and Consent to Treatment) Regulations 1983. This report must be given to the hospital managers as soon as is practical. The period of detention is for up to 6 hours. The Act itself is not clear whether this period is renewable, but some are of the opinion that it is not. In any case the reason why a medical officer is still not available after the first period would be a cause for concern. The nurse must inform the hospital managers of when the period has lapsed, either after 6 hours or when a medical officer arrives.

In short, the nurse may be considered to be negligent in not exercising good judgement by detaining a patient, especially if the patient or another person comes to harm. However, the nurse may be concerned about actions leading to wrongful detention. The law does not ask for perfection, but only that all actions are taken in good faith and that decisions are reasonable for an average person with similar qualifications and experience (see Mental Health Act 1983, Section 139).

(b) Further information

The Mental Health Act 1983 is long and complicated and contains several other sections which allow a person to be compulsorily detained in hospital. The provisions of these other sections and how they work are best understood by referring directly to the document or to one of the many detailed guides now available. The nurse must be able to ensure that patients detained are fully aware of their restrictions and rights. For example, knowing when and how to apply to the Mental Health Review Tribunal, how the Court of Protection works and voting rights. The Royal College of Nursing suggests that all patients admitted to a psychiatric hospital are given a booklet outlining their rights.

Attention should also be paid to the Mental Health Act 1983, Part 9, which lays out the criminal offences shown in *Table 4.1.*

Table 4.1   Criminal offences in the Mental Health Act 1983, Part 9

Section	Offence
126	Forgery, false statements, etc., of documents concerned with the execution of the Act
127	Ill treatment or wilful neglect of a patient receiving treatment for a mental disorder
128	Helping patients to absent themselves without leave. This includes harbouring or acting with the intention of hindering his return to a place where he should be
129	Obstruction. Without reasonable cause, obstructing an authorised inspector from visiting any person or viewing any document required by him to do his job

The old Mental Health Act 1959, Section 128, has not been repealed. This section makes it an offence for a man to have sexual intercourse with a woman or to commit homosexual acts with a man if employed by the home in which the person is being cared for as a result of mental disorder.

Section 134 is about a patient's mail. No restriction can be placed on the mail of an informal patient. Mail from a detained patient may be stopped if the person to whom it is addressed requests this in writing. Mail for the patient or addressed by him to any of the following may not be obstructed:

(a) Government minister or member of parliament.
(b) Court of Protection.
(c) The Mental Health Review Tribunal.
(d) A health authority, including the Mental Health Act Commission.
(e) The managers of the hospital.
(f) Legal representative.
(g) European Commission on Human Rights.

The Public Health Act 1936, which was amended in 1961 and 1968, allows for a person suffering from any notifiable disease to be detained in hospital. The list is long and mostly consists of diseases which are very infectious or dangerous. Examples are acute meningitis, tetanus, rabies and yellow fever.

Subject to the powers conferred by the Mental Health Act 1983, if any other patient wishes to discharge himself, he may. A nurse will avoid problems if it can be shown that effort was made to persuade the patient to act in his best interest. The responsible medical officer must be told of a patient who intends to leave or has left hospital against advice. The nurse must record in writing what has happened. Other nurses involved should be prepared to sign as witnesses. Many units provide a standard form which the patient is asked to sign; this shows the patient that he is taking responsibility for his own behaviour and is in effect a release of the hospital authority from responsibility. However, because of the emotional condition of many of these patients, they often refuse to sign.

NEGLIGENCE AND LIABILITY

Nurses should be loyally answerable for a lack of proper care.

CASE STUDY

One Tuesday morning on a busy ward for the elderly mentally ill, Peter Bellwood, the charge nurse, discussed care with Malcolm Pears, staff nurse and second team leader. Mr Oscar, a large and heavy gentleman who was unsteady on his feet, required an increase in his daily exercise to help him to sleep and to reduce nightly wandering. The two learners working with Malcolm were not strong, and Peter was anxious that nobody should be put at risk. Following this, he discussed care with his own team; plans were reviewed and objectives for the day's care identified. Two learners were asked to assist a small, frail and confused lady with a bath before she had breakfast. Her husband was due to take her home for the day soon after. They readily agreed and left.

Peter was left alone for a short time to complete some paperwork. That done, he got up to leave the office and was startled to see the bath thermometer still on its shelf. Picking it up and moving quickly to the bathroom, he was met by one of the learners coming to get it. Relieved, he turned towards the dormitory and saw Malcolm, with a learner, carefully helping Mr Oscar to the breakfast table.

(a) Discussion

Because of the very varied and changing role of the nurse, many are left confused as to what they may be held accountable for and to whom. The individual nurse can define that role; with all people, you are expected to act with good intention and reasonable care. Professional skill must be of the standard of a nurse of similar age, qualification and experience. No nurse can be expected by themselves or others to assume any role for which they are not adequately prepared.

For negligence to be proven against a nurse in law, three requirements must exist: firstly, there must be a duty of care; secondly that duty must be breached in some way; lastly, damage must result. That damage may be physical, psychological, permanent or short term.

(b) Comment

If a supervising nurse requires a junior to perform a duty which is beyond what could reasonably be expected of them, and harm results, then the senior would be liable for negligence through an act of delegation. For example, in the case study, Malcolm could have been negligent if a small nurse had tried to assist Mr Oscar on her own, and either had been injured. The charge nurse, Peter Bellwood, could reasonably expect an 18-year-old learner to run a bath of the correct temperature. If the patient had been harmed by a too hot a bath, the learner would have been responsible in law. The ward was evidently managed with a team approach, using individualised and progressive care planning. Every effort was being made to ensure that the patients received nursing care to meet their specific needs. If a patient's unique strengths and weaknesses are identified, the care planned for them can be not only more efficient in the use of resources but safer as well. Potential hazards when identified can be avoided by good management.

(c) Negligence by omission

It is possible to be negligent by doing nothing. If a nurse failed to notice change or to notify any significant difference in a patient's condition to a medical officer, they could be guilty of negligence by omission.

(d) The employer's responsibility

All employers are responsible for the actions of those that they employ. This principle is known as vicarious liability. Increasingly, those who employ nurses, in both the public and the private sector, are seeking to recover costs from nurses whose actions have resulted in the employer's being sued. When nurses were even more poorly paid it was often not worth the cost of suing them. The greater use of professional indemnity insurance and the fact that society is becoming less resistant to legal action have resulted in a large increase in the number of nurses appearing in court.

(e) Safety at work

The Health and Safety at Work Act 1974 deals with safety at work.

Accidents at work are common causes of civil action. Wet floors, trailing electrical flex, smoking, and damaged furniture are hazards which cause injury to patients, visitors and staff. Particularly vulnerable patients must be observed and assisted in carrying out potentially dangerous tasks such as smoking or drinking hot liquids. No nurse can be expected to observe all patients throughout a span of duty. Careful assessment and individual care planning can do much to reduce hazards by identifying specific precautionary care.

Electrical flex must not trail across walkways. Appliances must have their serviceability checked regularly by qualified engineers, and this fact recorded. Hazards such as wet floors which cannot easily be removed must be clearly marked. Laboratory specimens should be kept in clean and clearly marked containers, and any specific danger known or suspected to be shown.

(f) Reporting

The details of any accident that occurs should be recorded in writing. The nurse involved must inform the care authority via the supervising nurse or manager. If the employer has produced a standard report, it should be used. Any report will include sufficient factual and descriptive material as the human memory is very unreliable, especially over what may become months or even years. The date, time, place and who was involved will be included. Witnesses should be named and they would be advised to make their own statements. The nurse should record who else was on duty and any action, such as first aid, taken. Note should be made of when any assistance was called and when it arrived.

(g) Further comments

No person can be held responsible for the actions of a rational man, unless he in some way incites them. However, if a nurse fails to supervise adequately a patient who is a known suicide risk, he or she is failing in his or her job. It is really very hard to structure a balance between safety for the patient, preserving his dignity and restoring self-esteem. The level and type of observation must be planned to meet the needs of the individual, and the effectiveness of such care clearly and regularly reviewed. It is impossible to remove all the possible methods that a person could use to harm themselves, but records should be kept of all prudent efforts that are made.

STANDARDS OF CARE

The delivery of the highest quality of nursing service to the individual patient is essential. Exactly what this is can only be decided with regard to unavoidable limitations.

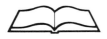

FURTHER READING

UKCC (1984), *Code of Professional Conduct for Nurses, Midwives and Health Visitors*, 2nd edn, UK Central Council for Nurses, Midwives and Health Visitors.

RCN, SPN (1985), *Standards of Care in Psychiatric Nursing Practice*, Royal College of Nursing, Society of Psychiatric Nursing, London.

CASE STUDY

Clive Craig, a qualified community psychiatric nurse, worked within a team of five nurses, managed by a community nursing officer. They were based at a day hospital and provided a service for the local people accepting referrals from general practitioners and consultants in both the hospital and the community. Clive's manager received a complaint from the husband of a patient. He stated that his wife had been suffering from what he decribed as agoraphobia and that Clive had been treating her for 1 month. He stated that, at the beginning of treatment, Clive had described a programme that would make his wife more independent. He was angry that, after a whole month, his wife was still not better and doing her full share of work around the house. He believed that Clive was not up to the job and wanted a more able and senior nurse to take over.

The nursing officer made Clive aware of the complaint and asked to discuss it with him. Examining the original referral from the general practitioner, he saw that the doctor had unwisely described the husband as 'interfering . . . overbearing . . . thoroughly unpleasant . . . and arrogant' and then went on to suggest that he was the sole cause of his wife's problems. The nursing notes contained a detailed assessment and included an objective description of the family dynamics. A plan which had been drawn up in discussion between nurse and patient showed their respective roles in treatment. Intended outcomes were specified, and objectives to be met on the road to success listed in order. The notes were factual, clearly written, dated and signed. Record was kept of every treatment session, and progress evaluated. Improvement was fast at first but slowed after a few sessions. The nursing officer noted an entry which quoted the patient as saying that her husband was very envious of the attention which she was receiving.

(a) Discussion

The Nurses, Midwives and Health Visitors Act 1979 requires that all care delivered by nurses should be progressive and planned to meet the individual needs of the specific patient. All nurses are required to deliver the best possible care, allowing for the situation which they find themselves in, the resources available and the experience which they have had. No one nurse can be held totally liable for failure to achieve the desired outcome, as no nurse is fully in control of all the influencing factors. The patient must keep some responsibility to make every effort in his own best interest. The nurse is accountable for efficient activities on her behalf towards a mutually agreed goal. Psychiatric patients are recognised as being particularly vulnerable and, with so many models of psychiatric nursing, the job of identifying success is very difficult. Research into psychiatric nursing is still very limited, although care should, whenever possible, be based on sound theory. All nurses are obliged to keep themselves up to date with the latest developments. As a profession, we have relied in the past on custom and practice, some of which has no basis other than that it has always been done that way. When having to justify actions before a court, a nurse will find such a defence little use.

The UK Central Council for Nurses, Midwives and Health Visitors has produced a code of professional conduct (2nd edition, 1984) evolved in part from the International Council of Nurses' Code. It is far reaching, and some of the sections should be read carefully to understand just what can be meant. For example it requires that anything that interferes with the delivery of proper care, from a lack of resources to conscientious objection, be made known to supervisors. Managers are charged with making certain that those under them have what they need to do a proper job. It is no longer enough to complain to colleagues about overwork or undermanning and then to carry on, always coping as nurses are inclined to do. The nurse must make these problems known and refuse to condone them by working on in situations where standards cannot be maintained. The code is relatively recent and, as yet, little tested in cases before the courts. Some difficulty has been experienced in its use as a defence before an industrial tribunal. Experience will doubtless clarify this.

(b) Action

If a complaint is received, the nurses affected must understand that a patient or relative under stress may be acting without their usual care and consideration. An opportunity for the complainant to discuss the problem and to be given an account of the nurse's action can serve to satisfy most people. If the complaint is justified, all action should be taken to rectify and reduce any adverse effects. When serious, the complaint must be put in writing as no action should be taken on the spoken word alone. The hospital authority should receive the complaint first and be given enough opportunity to put things right. If the person is not satisfied with the action taken, he can inform the Health Service Commissioner. The Commissioner cannot act if the complaint is currently being investigated by a court or if more than a year has passed since the incident. He is also prevented from investigating a person's clinical judgement or decisions to appoint staff. After investigation, he can submit a report to the person complaining and the authority concerned.

(c) Comment

The need to keep clear and factual records should be emphasised. However, defensive nursing to avoid complaints will restrict opportunity on the part of the nurse and patient, allowing neither to take calculated risks or to respond instinctively. It is therefore to be avoided but must be replaced by informed care. As the profession builds a body of knowledge based on carefully evaluated plans of care, this process will become easier.

CONSENT AND CONFIDENTIALITY

The patient's agreement should be obtained. The patient's right to privacy should be respected and maintained.

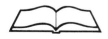

FURTHER READING

Mawson, D. (1986), Seeking informed consent, *Nursing Times*, **82**, No. 6, 52–53.

RCN (1981), *Guidelines on Confidentiality in Nursing*, Royal College of Nursing, London.

RCN (1977), *Ethics Related to Research in Nursing*, Royal College of Nursing, London.

CASE STUDY

The nursing team on an acute admissions ward were keen to start a programme of practical stress management skills for suitable patients. Trina, the deputy charge nurse, was also interested in investigating the effectiveness of the programme for research. She completed a literature search on the subject and was surprised to discover that none of the work previously published had been performed by nurses.

The team wrote a research protocol which was submitted and approved by the authority research ethics committee. They also approved the methodology and rating scales used.

The patients' questionnaire was improved following the pilot study. The survey lasted 6 months and was considered to be successful. Only two patients refused to participate. One felt hurt that he was being used; another thought that the whole idea was a waste of time.

(a) Discussion

Before involving a patient in any activity which will affect them, the nurse must first obtain their consent. All surgical procedures, except in life-saving emergencies when it may be unobtainable, require written consent. A nurse taking a consent form to a patient must understand that he or she can only sign it as a witness. Nurses are not sufficiently prepared by nurse education to inform the patient of all the implications of surgery and to ensure that the patient understands them. The task of explaining the details must remain the medical officer's. Even if given in writing, consent will only be valid if it can be shown later that the patient fully understood what was going to happen. If the patient was delirious or drowsy because of drugs, e.g. pre-medication, this would be very difficult. Employing authorities will have policies listing which procedures require written consent. It is important that they are followed; otherwise, actions could be regarded as negligent.

For small procedures such as intramuscular injections or participation in surveys or research, consent may be implied by the person's willingness to participate. Lying on a bed prior to removal of sutures or returning a completed questionnaire could be examples of implied consent. Any person collecting information for research must ensure that all involved know what is required, who will have access to the information and, provided that knowing will not interfere with results, to what use it will be put. All involved retain the right to withdraw their consent at any time and may request that their responses be withdrawn from results.

The issue of confidentiality must be raised. The right of an adult to demand that the nurse respects his privacy is close to sacrosanct. Even the presence of a person over 17 years of age in a nurse's care must not be made known to anybody outside the care team without his consent.

As will be discussed in the section on the nurse as a witness, a court can demand that professional confidences held by nurses be revealed. However, with all aspects of moral and social duty considered, an individual nurse may wish to choose to remain silent, perhaps by not revealing that she has information. Before deciding which course to take, the advantages or otherwise to all involved must be understood. This requires a high level of moral reasoning. Whether or not many nurses are well enough prepared for this during basic nurse training is open to doubt.

When using Department of Health and Social Security documents for surveys, it must be understood that they, and the information contained, remain the property of the Department of Health and Social Security. Permission should be obtained from the employing authority before use.

With increasing use of group techniques for patients, only those patients or staff who have agreed to maintain confidentiality should be included in groups where confidences are shared. This may be implied if the rule has been explained and a person stays in the group.

(b) Comment

To ensure that the nurse respects a patient's confidence, he or she must be aware of the patient's expectations of them. Conversely the nurse is a member of a team and must make clear to the patient the responsibility to them. If necessary, the nurse must not accept a patient's confidence if it prevents the proper care being given.

COMPLAINING AND DEFAMATION

To complain is to give a formal statement of grievance or dissatisfaction. Defamation is to make a statement which exposes a person to the hatred or contempt of other right-thinking persons.

SUGGESTED READING

Beardshaw, V. (1981), *Conscientious Objectors at Work*, Social Audit, London.
Committee on Hospital Complaints Procedure (1974), The Davies Report, HM Stationery Office, London.

CASE STUDY

Bob Irwin left nursing in his second year of RMN training. He had been unable to resolve the anxiety that he was left with as a result of being taught one standard in the school of nursing and being expected to perform at a different standard on the ward. The school talked of the need to deliver the best possible care to the individual, and this is what Bob had expected. The ward was concerned with surviving under the pressures of limited time, staff and resources. He recognised that both groups were caring concerned people, and he had a high regard for them. Unfortunately, he could not adapt to the social pressures that he felt.

(a) Discussion

Standards of care within mental hospitals have caused such concern within the profession and amongst the public. This is best illustrated by the allegations of, and investigation into, ill treatment during the last 16 years. Although it is hoped that improvements are always taking place, there may unfortunately still be occasions when an individual nurse must stand up and complain. This section is intended to ensure that a difficult situation will not be made worse through lack of preparation.

There are two legal forms of defamation, either of which if proved against a person would make them liable for damages.

The first, libel, is a statement made in permanent form which falsely or maliciously accuses a person. The second, slander, concerns the spoken word. Defamation will have occurred if the person complaining can produce evidence of actual harm as a result of either. This harm could be public hate, contempt or ridicule. The exception is where the defamation suggests criminal behaviour, social disease or a person's unfitness to fulfil their present professional position.

A nurse writing to the employing authority suggesting that another nurse was sleeping with a patient and was wrong would be committing a libel. A student telling patients that a charge nurse was incompetent would be slanderous. In these cases, actual damage does not need to be shown. If the comments are true or fair, there need be no fear of action. Privileges will allow a senior nurse to write fair and accurate reports on juniors.

(b) Action

If a nurse feels compelled to take action in an unacceptable situation, the first step must be to obtain the counsel of an experienced person who can be trusted. Professional representation should be obtained either privately, through such as the Royal College of Nursing, or a union. Make private notes as soon as practical of what was witnessed or reported. Only those facts which are certain should be noted, avoiding inference or conjecture. The concern should be reported to the nurse's immediate superior. Record must be maintained of all actions, noting the time, place and responses. If no action has been taken after a reasonable time, the process should be repeated. If no action is still forthcoming, the nurse must pass on to the next level of supervision.

The nurse should identify issues clearly, double checking facts. He or she must know and be able to refer to codes of professional conduct, hospital policies and relevant legislation. No statement, written or verbal, should be released to any person until the nurse is sure of its factual content, to whom it will be made available and what they intend to do with it. If at all possible, written statements are best checked first by the nurse's representatives. There will be considerable pressure from many sources when a complaint is made; no action that the nurse feels uncomfortable about should be taken. Time to consider can always be requested. The nurse must not allow himself or herself to be interviewed without an independent representative present.

Just occasionally the organisation may not take sufficient action to remedy the situation. Before going outside the organisation, inform the senior manager that this is intended, giving time for appropriate action to be taken. Any person who complains must be prepared to offer solutions. Most importantly, the person that will suffer most if the problem remains unresolved must be identified. To whom the information is then given is of course an individual decision. That decision must consider what the recipient is intended to achieve, their authority to do so and the resources available to them.

(c) Further information

The nursing profession has its own disciplinary process, designed not to punish but to protect the public. The Nurses, Midwives and Health Visitors Act 1979 allowed for significant changes in the disciplinary process. The committees will act on information received about the conduct of a nurse from other nurses or care workers, patients or relatives, and the courts are obliged to inform them of any conviction against a person known to be a nurse.

The four national boards have preliminary proceeding committees who investigate in the first instance. They may decide that no case exists or pass the findings directly to the Professional Conduct Committee of the UK Central Council for Nurses, Midwives and Health Visitors. In cases where there is a possibility of illness, the case may be passed to a Panel of screeners by either the appropriate preliminary proceedings committee or the Professional Conduct

Committee. The Panel consists of three members of the UK Central Council selected with regard to the professional field in which the person works. The Panel may ask for the opinion of medical officers. Where no evidence exists, the case may be closed. In other cases the evidence will be heard by the Health Committee of the UK Central Council. The Health Committee can dispose of the case in the same way as the Professional Conduct Committee except that it may also require specific conditions to be satisfied before a person may be reinstated to the register. For example a nurse may need to show that he or she has overcome an illness which led to the allegation in the first place. As previouly stated, the Professional Conduct Committee does not see its role as being to punish but to protect and where possible to rehabilitate. Depending on the findings, four different courses of action may be followed: no action at all; alternatively, no action but the person concerned is referred to the code of conduct; judgement may be postponed for a stated period to see whether this was an isolated incident; alternatively, the Committee may elect for removal of the person from the register or parts of it.

(d) Comment

The sensational stories that reach the media do not demonstrate the real cost to the nursing profession. Far more common are those who enter nurse education and who leave before or just after qualification because, what they hope is a caring profession, turns out not to be so, when it comes to its own members. All levels of nursing need peer support and ready access to supervisors. The maintenance of good standards of care depends largely on free communication and a positive attitude towards and between all levels of nurses and other members of the care team.

THE NURSE AS A WITNESS

The nurse sometimes has to act as a witness.

CASE STUDY

Jacqueline Palmer was still shaking. She had heard that such things happened, but never before to her. This was her first set of nights as a newly qualified staff nurse on a brand new acute admission ward. The fight had started so suddenly. First, George's brother had started shouting and then, before you could blink, he had been hit by an ashtray. She was surprised that the police had arrived so quickly. Another few minutes and she would phone the local casualty department to see how George was. The other patients were worried. Now the police wanted a statement; this could mean being in court as a witness. What would that involve?

(a) Action

The sensible nurse should always get legal advice before entering a court in any capacity. Confidential information obtained in the course of duty is not regarded by the court as privileged, and the nurse may be ordered by the court to reveal it. If asked, the nurse should inform the judge that the information was divulged as a professional confidence, and ask for specific direction.

As a witness, you may ask permission from the court to refer to your own notes. The court may well want to know how long after any incident they were made and under what circumstances. Notes must only record factual information, no assumptions or suppositions. Any record must be dated and signed, with no gaps between consecutive entries into which extra details may have been inserted. When making records or writing statements, care must be taken in the use of language. Technical terms, although carefully defined, are often applied loosely and occasionally wrongly. The punctuation of a sentence can change its whole meaning. As examples, consider the following:

1. 'Woman without her man is nothing'.
2. Bath in wheelchair in hall.

Each can be made to mean very different things depending on your standpoint. An opposition lawyer may easily reduce the credibility of a nurse by exploiting such common errors. If details or facts have genuinely been forgotten, then that fact must be admitted. As a professional witness a nurse is considered competent to give an opinion on issues which are covered by her professional duties, e.g. the amount and type of nursing care required by a particular patient.

During a hearing in the English courts, the plaintiff (or victim's) case is heard first; this will include expert evidence. The defence case is second. All witnesses are required to swear on oath, although this may soon be superceded by a promise to tell the truth. Answers to a barrister's questions should be addressed to the judge and should stick to what is asked. The temptation to elaborate or expand must be avoided as it may work against the witness and waste time. The purpose of the court is to establish the truth, and the right of just treatment applies equally to all involved. As stated previously in this chapter, the law only ever requires that the individual acts always in good faith and with reasonable care. To assume the rights of the nurse is inevitably to assume the responsibilities.

REFERENCES AND FURTHER READING

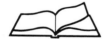

Reference

Selden, J. (1584–1654), *Table Talk*, LXXVII.

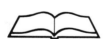

Further reading

Beardshaw, V. (1981), *Conscientious Objectors at Work*, Social Audit, London.
Carr, P. (1984), Legal and ethical perspectives in the nursing care of the mentally ill, *Community Psychiatric Nursing Journal*, **4**, No. 5, 14–18.
Carson, D. (1986), How the law affects nursing, *Professional Nurse*, **1**, No.10, 275–277.
Mental Health Division, DHSS (1983), Draft Code of Practice, Mental Health Act 1983, Section 118, Department of Health and Social Security, London.
HM Government (1975), The Employment Protection Act 1975, HM Stationery Office, London.
HM Government (1974), The Health and Safety at Work Act 1974, HM Stationery Office, London.
HM Government (1979), The Nurses, Midwives and Health Visitors Act 1979, HM Stationery Office, London.
HM Government (1983), The Mental Health Act 1983, HM Stationery Office, London.
Katz, F., *et al.* (1976), *Stepping Out. Nurses and Their New Roles*, New South Wales University Press.

Martin, J. P. (1984), *Hospitals in Trouble*, Basil Blackwell, Oxford.

Mawson, D. (1986), Seeking informed consent, *Nursing Times*, **82**, No. 6, 52–53.

McNulty, B. (1980), *Accountability Shared with Other Professions*, Royal College of Nursing, London.

RCN (1977), *Ethics Related to Research in Nursing*, Royal College of Nursing, London.

RCN (1981), *Guidelines on Confidentiality in Nursing*, Royal College of Nursing, London.

UKCC (1984), *Code of Professional Conduct for Nurses, Midwives and Health Visitors*, UK Central Council for Nurses, Midwives and Health Visitors.

Chapter 5

The multi-disciplinary team in mental health

'Teams are co-operative groups in that they are called into being to perform a task or tasks that cannot be attempted by the individual.' (Douglas, 1983).

INTRODUCTION

The mental health team is made up of a group of people each of whom possesses particular skills and expertise. As well as nurses, the team consists of a consultant psychiatrist, his registrar and housemen, clinical psychologists, social workers, occupational therapists, speech therapists, physiotherapists, dietician and hospital chaplain. Some members of the team may meet daily or weekly to discuss patient treatment and progress. Other members will provide their services as and when necessary.

TEAMWORK

Teamwork is an essential part of patient care and has a significant influence on treatment within the field of mental illness. Every person who comes into contact with the patient can in some way contribute to his welfare, provided that they fully understand the aims of treatment (Davies and Grove, 1976).

THE ROLES OF TEAM MEMBERS

Each member of the multi-disciplinary team needs to have an understanding of other members' roles in meeting the needs of patients. There is usually some blurring of roles in the therapeutic milieu and team members will not relate equally to every patient. Some team members may act as key workers with particular patients or groups of patients. The person who acts as the key worker for a particular patient may be selected from any member of the team, and therefore from a number of different disciplines. This person may be the nurse, the social worker, the psychologist or another professional with appropriate training.

A THERAPEUTIC ALLIANCE

The member may elect to work with a particular patient because he or she has been able to establish a meaningful relationship with him. It would be wasteful if all the team members did the same work and concentrated on the same patients (Altschul, 1980). As Ruch (1984) suggests: 'Imagine the patient who is receiving psychotherapy from several nurses, a psychologist and a minister of religion!' He suggests that, when various team members feel that it is their responsibility to encourage patients to talk about their problems, the team can become involved in a 'staff treasure hunt' with each person trying to link up with patients in moments of catharsis and 'get the goods' from them. This is a situation that is fraught with problems as some patients may encourage staff members to take on the role of being their psychotherapist, or staff may be manipulated by certain patients who claim that they are unable to talk to their assigned therapist. Some patients may migrate from one team member to another in an attempt to avoid being involved in a therapeutic relationship. Furthermore, the potency of psychotherapy can be considerably reduced if a patient talks about things that have already been discussed with other team members.

Psychotherapy is therefore best left to one person; when a patient has a close relationship with several members of the multi-disciplinary team, it diminishes the potential for the establishment of an effective therapeutic alliance (Ruch, 1984).

SUPPORTIVE ROLES OF TEAM MEMBERS

Because a patient may be assigned to a particular key worker for psychotherapy, this does not lessen the importance of other team members, who can provide interventions which are supportive and not disruptive to the therapeutic alliance (Ruch, 1984). Most importantly, team members can provide powerful models of normal behaviour. Despite the fact that the patient may have a therapeutic alliance with one particular member of the team, it is important for the patient to perceive the staff as a team who communicate well and work in harmony. The patient will have more confidence in the staff if he feels that each member of the team is fully aware of the goals of his overall care plan.

The nurse must be realistic about the limitations of the nursing role. One nurse cannot be all things to all patients. The nurse will not like every patient that he or she encounters and similarly the patient will not like all the nurses. Even a nurse who is disliked by a patient can fulfil a useful function if the patient learns to cope with his feelings of rejection or anger in a more appropriate way than he did before (Altschul, 1980).

MEMBERS OF THE MULTI-DISCIPLINARY TEAM

The nurse plays an important role in creating an environment for the patient which is both safe and therapeutic (Altschul, 1980). The community-based nurse plays an essential role in the primary prevention of mental illness by accepting referrals directly from general practitioners and also provides support and counselling for discharged patients. The nurse acts as a resource person and has access to a wide range of agencies and expertise.

The harmonious functioning of the multi-disciplinary team is dependent on the nurse's ability to be an effective communicator and to have an understanding of the roles and functions of other team members.

The hospital-based nurse is the member of the team who is actually present throughout the patient's stay in hospital. Equally the community-based nurse may be the professional who has most frequent contact with the patient. Other team members are particularly dependent on the nurse's observations of patients' behaviour. The nurse should remember that observation is of value only if the results are conveyed to other people concerned with the patient's care (Trick and Obcarskas, 1976).

(a) The consultant psychiatrist

The psychiatrist is usually acknowledged as the leader and organiser of the multi-disciplinary team. He carries a legal and social responsibility for making medical and psychiatric diagnoses and for prescribing treatment. As the team leader the psychiatrist is responsible for creating an atmosphere which allows other members of the team to feel confident in making their contribution to the patient's care plan. He helps team members to understand what information can be usefully fed back into the group.

The psychiatrist is particularly reliant on the information that he receives from nurses because of their 24-hour contact with patients. The knowledge that he seeks does not necessarily include psychiatric phenomena; he is especially interested in the nurse's observations of patients' behaviour. When nursing care is based on patient allocation, with each nurse taking responsibility for their own small group of patients, this can be advantageous for all concerned.

The nurse has a greater opportunity to get to know the patient well and this can enhance the quality of information given at ward rounds or team meetings.

Some psychiatrists are actively engaged in research and depend on the goodwill and cooperation of nurses in achieving the aims of their studies. Because of his specialised training the psychiatrist is ideally placed to make initial patient assessments.

The team can then discuss the patient's needs and problems and decide which member or members would be best able to make a positive contribution to the patient's treatment and management. One or more team members may act as key workers.

The role of the consultant psychiatrist as leader of the team is surrounded by controversy and there are numerous views concerning the leadership of the multi-disciplinary team, both in hospital and in the community.

(b) The psychologist

The psychologist, who has a scientific background, has a number of roles in the multi-disciplinary team. Having made a study of normal as well as abnormal behaviour, one of the psychologist skills lies within the field of psychological testing. Assessment of a patient's social skills, intelligence or neuropsychological functioning will enable information to be conveyed to other team members about what a patient can or cannot do. This information is vital in planning realistic goals for the patient. In a teaching capacity the psychologist is able to assist other professionals to apply their skills more effectively. For example, if the speech therapist is teaching a patient whose attention span and concentration are poor, to overcome a communication problem, the psychologist may suggest that a teaching input of more frequent but of shorter duration may be the most effective way to help the patient. Nurses may also find the psychologist's advice invaluable, particularly when faced with patients who have behavioural problems.

The psychologist is involved in the monitoring and evaluating of all aspects of psychiatric care (including cost-effectiveness) from service provision down to individual treatments.

A training in research design and statistics enables the psychologist to make a valuable contribution in this area.

(c) The social worker

The social worker has a wide role in the community but in the hospital works as part of the multi-disciplinary team. It is the responsibility of the social worker to assess the influence and impact of social factors in relation to the patients' presenting symptoms. The social worker also advises on and implements a plan of rehabilitation, helping the patient to maintain or establish links in the community to try to minimise the trauma of his or her illness. In order to effect this, the social worker may be involved in a wide range of tasks from solving basic practical problems to intensive case work with a patient and his or her family.

The social worker also has a statutory responsibility under some sections of the Mental Health Act 1983 to make an independent social assessment in relation to compulsory admission to, or detention in, hospital. Linked to this aspect is an important role for the social worker regarding civil rights.

(d) The hospital chaplain

With the inauguration of the National Health Service in 1948, important changes took place in the provision for the spiritual needs of a hospital community. As part of a national policy of setting standards and issuing 'guidance', the then Ministry of Health issued an important circular (RHB(48)76) advising hospital authorities that they 'should give special attention to provide for the spiritual needs of both staff and patients', 'should provide, where the size of the hospital justified it, a room for use as a chapel' and 'should appoint chaplains . . . consultations with the appropriate church authorities'.

A later circular HM(63)80 established further principles by which Anglican, Roman Catholic, Free Church and Jewish chaplains should be appointed to all hospitals.

Responsibilities of chaplains could include:

1. Providing for the spiritual needs of patients and staff by conducting regular services for those who could not attend their normal place of worship. Services may be in the chapel or on wards, as is appropriate.
2. Visiting wards and departments to talk with patients and staff and to listen to their anxieties, problems and fears. In visits, aiming to build up good relationships so that support and comfort may be offered in particular times of need, especially when a patient is dying.
3. Offering support to staff and families of those who have died, in order that grief may be expressed in a normal therapeutic way.

4. Being available to medical staff where particular knowledge of a patient may be of value—chaplains may at times be closer to patients because of time spent listening to them.
5. Being generally concerned for the rights of patients and staff; as he is involved in the life of the hospital and yet separate from the promotional structure, he can often view developments from a slightly more objective position.
6. Taking responsibility for baptism, marriages or burials as required and seeing that the chapel is always available and prepared for use.

(e) The occupational therapist

The aim of the occupational therapist is to use the interpersonal relationship between the therapist and the patient, and between patients themselves, within a framework of purposeful activities in such a way that patients are helped to gain an understanding of, and modify if necessary, their individual patterns of behaviour.

The occupational therapist working in conjunction with the multi-disciplinary team assesses the rehabilitative needs of patients and provides purposeful work and leisure activities which achieve short- and long-term goals for individual patients.

The relationship between the patient and the therapist is of vital importance. Through occupational therapy, patients are helped to reach their maximum functioning level.

The therapist looks at the whole life of the person, their work skills and their relationships. Emphasis is placed on independence and patients are encouraged to do things for themselves. The occupational therapist caters for specialist groups such as the elderly and provides reality orientation programmes and reminiscence groups.

Many activities such as role play and drama groups, domestic and social skills groups, and music therapy are used to help patients to lead fuller and more productive lives.

(f) The speech therapist

The speech therapist is an essential member of the multi-disciplinary team, as it is impossible to provide effective treatment for a patient whose ability to communicate is impaired, without fully understanding the extent and nature of his speech and language problems.

Many elderly patients suffer from high-frequency hearing loss and this difficulty can lead a person to appear to be withdrawn, depressed or confused. The speech therapist can assist by recognising and screening the hearing loss.

Early signs of impaired cognitive functioning often present in linguistic or memory difficulties, and language assessment is vital to assist the doctor in reaching a differential diagnosis or in the identification of neurological conditions such as Parkinson's disease. Once linguistic impairment has been identified, the speech therapist has an irreplaceable role in advising relatives and staff in the management of the patient. Intervention and advice in the early stages of confusion can help to prevent further deterioration. The speech therapist is often able to offer practical suggestions for improving and maintaining orientation, as many of the skills hopefully being maintained are language based. Some patients have swallowing and feeding difficulties. The speech therapist is able to assess their dysphagia and to set up treatment programmes to assist in the remediation of chewing, swallowing and other problems.

Patients who have very impaired linguistic function, severe dysarthria or dyspraxia may require alternative means of communicating. The speech therapist would be responsible for assessing which signal system or communication aid would be most suitable for the patient and would teach the use of the system or aid to the patient, his relatives and staff.

The speech therapist may also help patients with disorders of fluency, e.g. stammering, or with disorders of articulation in which case the patient will need skilled help in order to learn how to pronounce sounds correctly.

Speech therapy input is invaluable in social skills learning and the therapist plays a vital role in assessing and eliciting verbal and non-verbal communication.

(g) The physiotherapist

Physiotherapy is defined as a systematic method of assessing muscular–skeletal and neurological disorders of function including pain and those of psychosomatic origin and dealing with or preventing those problems by natural methods based essentially on movement, manual therapy and physical agencies. The physiotherapist working in the mental health unit deals with a whole range of physical problems similar to those found among patients in any general hospital. In addition to the patients' physical problems the physiotherapist must also be responsive to the patients' emotional needs. Physiotherapists specialising in psychiatry have to adapt their physical treatment programmes taking into account the patients' other difficulties and sometimes find that treatment may need to be carried out over a long period of time to achieve good results. Good working relationships with patients are essential for the promotion of health goals.

Another important role of the physiotherapist is that of a teacher who enables other professionals, and particularly nurses, to learn skills which enable patients to achieve a better quality of life through greater mobility, comfort and freedom from pain. The physiotherapist not only works with individual patients but also facilitates a wide range of group activities. Group exercises provide essential activities for elderly patients, helping to retain muscular integrity and mobility skills; vigorous physical activities provide a healthy outlet for aggressive energy and may be of particular value for groups of young emotionally disturbed patients; relaxation exercises may reduce stress and anxiety among many different patient groups as well as among nurses themselves who are particularly vulnerable to physical as well as emotional stress.

Teaching lifting skills and back care to nurses and other hospital workers plays an important part in the prevention of morbidity caused by back problems.

The physiotherapist plays an important role within the multi-disciplinary team and may advise on the suitability of equipment and furnishings to enable a safe environment to be maintained for patients.

Through working with physiotherapists, nurses will learn to minimise stress for themselves and for their patients.

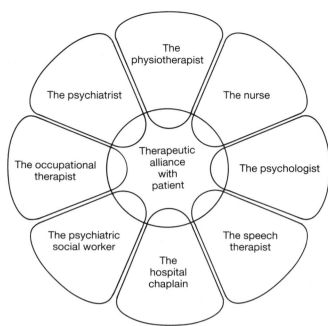

Any member of the multi-disciplinary team may have a therapeutic alliance with a particular patient or group of patients.

REFERENCES AND FURTHER READING

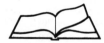

References

Altschul, A. (1980), The team approach to psychiatric care, *Nursing Times*, **76**, No. 18, 797–798.

Davies, M., and Grove, E. (1976), *Contribution of the Remedial Professions in Comprehensive Psychiatric Care*, Blackwell Scientific, Oxford.

Douglas, T. (1983), *Groups: Understanding People Gathered Together*, Tavistock, London.

Ruch, M. D. (1984), The multidisciplinary approach. When too many is too much, *Journal of Psychosocial Nursing*, **22**, No. 9, 18–23.

Trick, L., and Obcarskas, S. (1976), *Understanding Mental Illness and its Nursing*, 2nd edn, Pitman Medical, London.

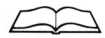

Further reading

Allison, M. (1984), Is the practice of community psychiatric nursing becoming too technical?, *Community Psychiatric Nursing Journal*, **4**, No. 6, 16–18.

Black, E., and John, W. G. (1985), Leadership of the multi-disciplinary team in psychiatry—a nursing perspective, *Nursing Practice*, **1**, No. 3, 177–182.

Bradshaw, P. (1986), Advocating change, *Senior Nurse*, **5**, No. 1, 34.

Brunning, H., and Huffington, C. (1985), Altered images, *Nursing Times*, **81**, No. 31, 24–27.

Clifford, C. (1985), Nurse–doctor relationships: is there cause for concern?, *Nursing Practice*, **1**, 102–108.

Fordwour, D. (1985), The counsellor, the doctor and the patient in general practice, *Community Psychiatric Nursing Journal*, **5**, No. 2, 22–27.

Haber, J., Leach, A. M., Schudy, S. M., and Sideleau, B. F. (1982), *Comprehensive Psychiatric Nursing*, 2nd edn, McGraw-Hill, New York.

Pasquali, E. A., Alesi, E. G., Arnold, H. M., and DeBasio, N. (1981), *Mental Health Nursing: A Bio-psycho-cultural Approach*, C. V. Mosby, St Louis, Missouri.

Peplau, H. E. (1966). Nurse–doctor relationships, *Nursing Forum*, **5**, No. 1 60–87.

Peplau, H. E. (1980), The psychiatric nurse: accountable to whom for what?, *Perspectives in Psychiatric Care*, **17**, No. 3, 128–134.

Rafferty, A. M. (1986), Teamwork or threat, *Senior Nurse*, **4**, No. 1, 22–23.

Ritter, S. (1984), Does the team work?, *Nursing Times*, **80**, No. 6, 53–55.

Stein, L. I. (1978), The doctor–nurse game. In: *Reading in the Sociology of Nursing* (eds Dingwall, R., and McIntosh), Churchill Livingstone, Edinburgh.

Sturt, J., and Waters, H. (1985), Role of the psychiatrist in community based mental health care, *Lancet*, **1**, 507–508.

Vaughan, B. (1985), Ward games, *Nursing Practice*, **1**, No. 2, 72–75.

Whitehouse, C. R. (1986), Conflict and co-operation between doctors and nurses in primary health care, *Nursing Practice*, **1**, 242–245.

Chapter 6

The therapeutic use of self

'Psychiatric nursing is a voyage into self-exploration and awareness.'
(Lancaster, 1980).

INTRODUCTION

The therapeutic use of self is the central focus of nursing and requires that the nurse is aware of his or her own thoughts, feelings and actions.

The therapeutic use of self is based on self-awareness, through which the nurse attempts to gain self-knowledge about the kind of person that he or she is. This is by no means an easy process since the self cannot be spontaneously discovered or dramatically unmasked (Stuart and Sundeen, 1983). Self-discovery is not necessarily a comfortable pursuit since each person may discover facets of himself that he would rather disown (Jourard, 1971). Nevertheless, time spent in the development of self-awareness is a worthwhile investment since the person without self-understanding can hardly be expected to understand others.

The nurse who lacks self-awareness may allow personal needs to act as a barrier to the formation of a meaningful relationship with patients, whereas the nurse who understands his or her own needs and motivations is in a better position to focus on the patient's needs as it is then possible to differentiate between each set of needs (Ludemann, 1968).

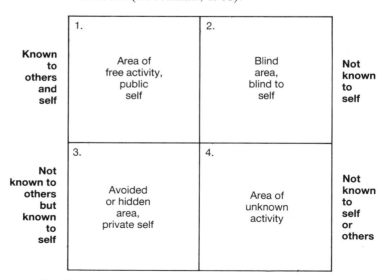

Figure 6.1   The Johari window

A MODEL OF SELF-AWARENESS

The Johari window (*Figure 6.1*) is one way of viewing relationships in terms of self-awareness (Luft, 1970). The model is composed of four quadrants. Quadrant 1 indicates an open area where behaviour and motivation is known to the self and others. Quadrant 2 illustrates the blind area in which other people can see things in a person of which he is unaware. Quadrant 3 is the hidden area representing the private self, things that the person knows about himself which are not revealed to others. Quadrant 4 is the area of unknown activity, in which neither the person nor others are aware of his behaviour and motives. A change in any one quadrant will affect the other quadrants. In *Figure 6.2* the Johari window is shown as it may appear at the beginning of a relationship, when people are usually less open with other people. *Figure 6.3* shows the Johari window after self-awareness has developed through learning about oneself and through feedback from others.

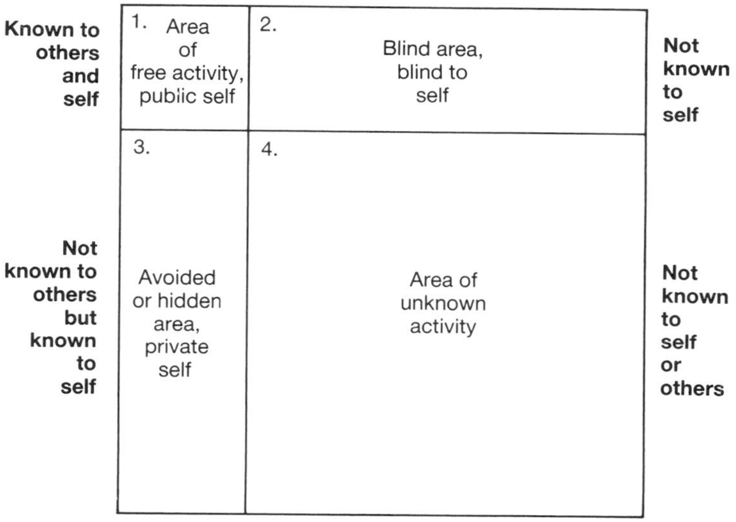

Figure 6.2   *The Johari window at the beginning of a relationship*

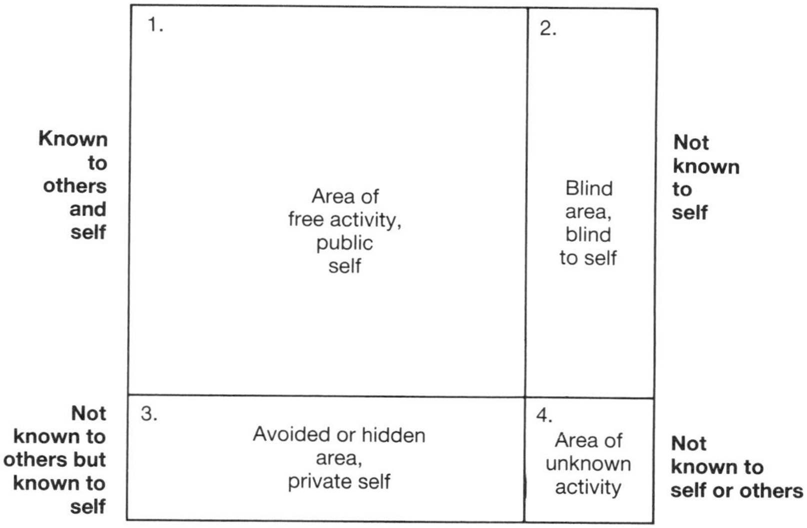

Figure 6.3   *The Johari window after a relationship has developed*

THE VALUE OF SELF-AWARENESS

In becoming more self-aware, the nurse is able to be more objective about a patient's behaviour and to understand the patient in the light of his or her own experience and from his or her own point of view (Stuart and Sunden, 1983). Self-awareness allows the nurse to identify weaknesses as well as strengths and to have more realistic self-expectations.

Jourard (1971) suggests that alienation from one's real self not only arrests one's growth as a person but also tends to make a mockery of one's relationships with other people.

The degree of self-awareness that the nurse brings to a patient relationship influences the entire nursing process. If the nurse is aware of his or her own beliefs and values in a situation, then it is easier to ascertain the degree of influence these beliefs and values have in judging the situation (Seeger, 1977). Furthermore, nurses who are self-aware have increased observation and assessment skills and are able to differentiate more easily between subjective and objective data (McGoran, 1978).

In the therapeutic relationship the nurse affects the patient's behaviour and is also affected by him. The nurse communicates through everything that he or she says and does and must be willing to assume responsibility for self-behaviour. For the nurse to use self-behaviours in a therapeutic manner, there must be an awareness of how this can be purposely useful to the patient.

THE MENTAL, PHYSICAL, PSYCHOSOCIAL AND SPIRITUAL ASPECTS OF SELF

Uys (1980) has attempted to categorise the therapeutic self into four operational definitions covering the mental, physical, psychosocial and spiritual aspects of self.

The mental aspects of self include the knowledge required in empathy, problem solving, developing nursing care plans, organising and interpreting information and using theoretical knowledge to make nursing care more effective.

The physical aspects of self are used to collect data through the senses. Psychomotor skills may be involved in the nurse's use of physical presence, while touch and body language may enhance communication.

The nurse's physical appearance and manner of dress may be used as an aspect of role modelling. Socialising skills can help to create an atmosphere for optimal mental health.

The nurse may express the spiritual self through his or her own experiences and spiritual values or seek help for the patient in this area.

Finally, Uys suggests that, the more fully functioning the nurse is in all these domains, the more he or she will be able to use the self therapeutically to help the patient.

THE DEVELOPMENT OF NURSE–PATIENT COMMUNICATION SKILLS FOR THERAPEUTIC PURPOSES

(a) Empathy

'In an empathic relationship I am with the other but I know I am not the other.' (Zderad, 1969).

Empathy means feeling into. It is a process through which the feelings and experiences of the other person are shared. It involves a movement towards another person for the purpose of knowing and understanding him and an ability to perceive accurately his current feelings. This mutual sharing of experiences is aptly summarised by an old Indian proverb which says 'You cannot know my experience unless you have walked in my moccasins.' (Hardin and Halaris, 1983). The ability to empathise is a fundamental element of the helping relationship since it allows the nurse to view the patient from his own perspective. The ability to empathise varies from person to person and within the same person from time to time. While it is possible to appreciate another person's feelings, it is not possible to empathise without a similar background of experiences. Spontaneity and flexibility within the empathiser's personality promote the process of empathy while a tendency to suppress feelings can impede the process. The conditions required for empathy include a kind of letting go in which the empathiser responds to the cues of the other person (Zderad, 1969). These cues are often non-verbal and form a particularly important element of the empathic process if the other person's feelings are to be accurately perceived.

Four phases of empathic understanding have been described by Ehmann (1971).

1. *Identification* in which the nurse loses consciousness of self and becomes totally engrossed in the personality and situation of the other person; for example the nurse may become engrossed in a patient's feelings of grief. The nurse than takes in the experience of the other person.
2. *Incorporation* which provides the reality of the other person's experience. If the nurse has also experienced grief, there will be an interplay between the two sets of experiences—the internalised feelings of the patient and the experiences of the nurse.
3. *Reverberation* which Ehmann describes as the interaction between the actual me and the me that has identified itself with the patient as the source of possibly the truest insight.
4. *Detachment* in which the nurse withdraws from subjective involvement and resumes his or her own identity. At this point, some sharing with colleagues may help to aid the nurse's detachment from empathic involvement. The ability to step back is very important.

During the process of empathic involvement the nurse must maintain a balance between objectivity and subjectivity. The nurse needs to be subjective enough to allow the creation of feelings but to retain the ability to offer helpful and objective responses to the patient in a language that he can comprehend.

Empathic understanding not only serves to increase the nurse's understanding of the patient's difficulties but also enables appropriate feedback to be given, since the nurse is in a better position to understand what the patient is experiencing.

(b) Touch

> '*Reaching out a hand can be the most important act of the nurse for the patient. It tells him "I am here, you are not alone. I understand. I want to give you comfort."* ' (Drummond, 1970).

Touch is an important aspect of the nurse's therapeutic use of self and can be used to facilitate more positive nurse–patient interactions. Touch can convey sensitivity towards and understanding of the patient (Mason and Pratt, 1980).

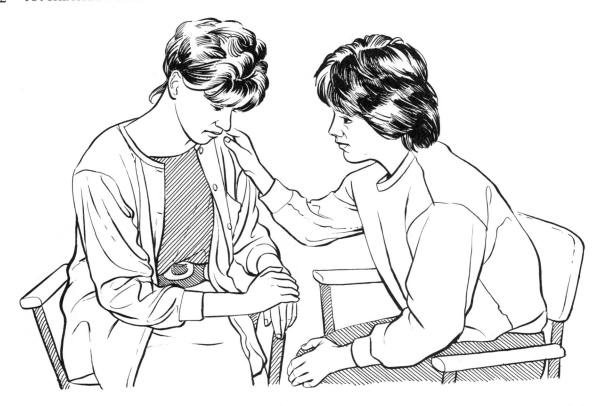

Touch can lower a patient's anxiety in a crisis situation and it may help to alleviate pain. While there are cultural differences in the use of touch, it is socially permissible for a nurse to touch a patient although he may be a total stranger (Mercer, 1966), as in the following example.

PATIENT PROFILE

Carl was in his seventies and had just been admitted to hospital. Carl was born in Poland and, although he had lived in the British Isles for many years, his grasp of the English language was very poor. Communication problems were further compounded by his failing eyesight and deafness. A nurse used touch as a means of reaching out to Carl. She sat by him and touched his hand, meeting his need for human contact. When the nurse told Carl that she must leave now, he responded by saying, 'You're very kind. Please come and see me again.' This illustrated how touch was used effectively with a total stranger.

Iveson-Iveson (1983) describes the nurse's hands as his or her most prized possession in carrying out the art and science of nursing. The nurse's hands may be used to gain information about the patient as well as to provide security, comfort and human warmth.

Touch has the power to enhance the transmission of verbal messages and in some instances may replace verbal messages completely. Touch is undoubtedly an important aspect of the nurse–patient relationship. However, when considering the use of touch as a communication tool in nursing, it is essential for the nurse's behaviour to be consistent with the particular rules and mores of the patient's culture (Johnson, 1965).

(c) Acceptance

'Acceptance is an active process, a series of positive behaviours designed to convey to the patient a respect for him as an individual human being who possesses worth and dignity.' (Topalis and Aguilera, 1978).

Acceptance means taking another person at face value without feeling the need to change him to fit into one's own frame of reference (Ujhely, 1968). To accept another person in a non-judgemental non-critical way is by no means easy since it is difficult to be free of the judgemental feelings that arise from a person's own values. The first step towards acceptance of another person is the ability to tolerate the pain of self-examination. Self-understanding is important because any inconsistency between feelings and actions towards the patient will only serve to lessen the effectiveness of the nurse–patient relationship. Intellectual acknowledgement of the patient must therefore be accompanied by an emotional state of acceptance that is conveyed through behaviour.

Acceptance conveys an attitude of positive recognition and respect for a person. While the nurse accepts the patient as he is, this does not mean that the nurse has necessarily to sanction or approve of his behaviour. What acceptance should convey to the patient is that he is a worthwhile human being.

(d) Listening

'Sounds full of meaning, yet often disguised by words, and motives hiding subjects too painful, too revealing or too difficult to share directly. Listen to them—they come from our patients.' (Hein, 1980).

Listening requires the investment of self.

Good listening habits are acquired by first learning to keep quiet. This means not interrupting when the other person pauses to clarify his feelings; it means refraining from 'putting words in his mouth' and it means not thinking about what one is going to say the moment that he stops talking.

Listening is an active process in which the nurse makes an effort to enter the other person's world of thought and feeling. By identifying and clarifying feelings when the meaning is not clear the nurse can convey to the patient a desire to understand his problems.

The quality of listening depends on involvement; to hear well, the nurse must be willing to listen. This willingness to be involved can make the difference between an effective and an ineffective nurse. The nurse needs to be familiar with the tools of communication and to use these tools appropriately. The nurse's body language will convey to the patient whether he is being listened to totally.

The factors that can enhance good listening are as follows (Hargie *et al.*, 1981):

1. Nods of the head indicate a readiness to listen.
2. Direct eye contact indicates an interest in what is being said.
3. Mirroring the facial expression of the speaker reflects and expresses sympathy with the emotional message being conveyed.
4. Adopting an attentive posture, such as leaning forward, arms at the side or placed in the lap.

5. Abstaining from the use of distracting mannerisms.
6. Smiling appropriately.
7. Responding with appropriate para language such as tone of voice and emphasis on certain words according to the patient's mood and circumstances.

The following factors may interfere with effective listening (Hargie *et al.*, 1981):

1. Slouched posture.
2. Lack of eye contact or staring.
3. Doodling.
4. Fidgeting.
5. Yawning.
6. Reading or writing while the speaker is talking.
7. Poor use of para language, e.g. flat tone of voice.
8. Turning one's back on the speaker.
9. Giving time grudgingly, e.g. clock watching.
10. Arms folded.

Acceptance is part of the listening process. The nurse must be able to accept what the patient says without making judgements. If the patient talks about something that is disturbing to himself or to the nurse, it is not helpful to change the subject. It may relieve the nurse's discomfort temporarily but it prevents the patient from working through his problem.

Not all nurses find the role of listener easy. Some nurses feel guilty because they are not actually '*doing*' for the patient.

(e) Silence

'*In the area of interpersonal relationships what is not said is just as important, if not more important, than the spoken word.*' (Smoyak, 1963).

Silence is a significant and powerful means of communication. It provides a time for reflective thinking; it allows a person to find the right words to express what he wants to say and it can convey meaning when words are inappropriate.

In nursing, periods of silence are important as they allow the patient to be observed unobtrusively when a patient is silent; the nurse should try to ascertain the type of silence being conveyed. The silence may be thoughtful, or it may be conveying anger or resistance. Silence can be linked to a stressful situation which can either impair the person's ability to think or provide him with a means of escape through non-involvement. Silence is one of the most difficult things for the nurse to come to terms with. Being comfortable with silence is something which has to be learned. If the nurse is uncomfortable with silence, then the cues as to what the patient is communicating may be missed.

When a patient's patterns of communication are unproductive or difficult, then it is very important that the nurse should not let self-anxiety enter the interaction. Many people are not good listeners because they are unable to use silence as a means of communication.

Silence is an important means of communication, and the nurse must avoid the urge to fill periods of silence with words or to leave the patient alone because he does not talk.

When the nurse is unsure as to the meaning of the silence being communicated by the patient, it may be as well to follow Hobart's (1964) advice. He suggests that when in doubt, sit it out. It is always the sounds underlying the silence that should be sought (Auvil, 1984). Unfortunately, some nurses have learned that 'good' nurses keep themselves busy. The busy nurse who has no time to listen to patients cannot claim to give total patient care.

Listening is an essential skill, if the nurse is to get to know the patient as a person, and an inherent part of the helping relationship.

(f) Caring

> 'Human caring is important because without it the spirit sickens and the body refuses to heal.' (Naugle, 1973).

When a patient approaches a nurse for help, he is essentially looking for two things: someone who is honest and someone who really cares about him (Irving, 1978). Mayeroff (1971) defines caring as helping the other person to grow, while Leininger (1980) describes caring as those human acts and processes which provide assistance for another individual. This assistance is basic.

Caring requires a commitment of one's self as well as an investment of one's time. Caring responses which promote health require the nurse to provide a facilitating environment, i.e. an environment in which the nurse responds with perception, thought and feeling. Reactions to another person that fail to initiate the process of caring set in motion a different set of behaviours which may be characterised by submission, dominance, anxiety or withdrawal (Winder, 1984).

(g) Self-disclosure

> 'Self-disclosure is a symptom of personality health and a means of ultimately achieving healthy personality . . . .' (Jourard, 1971).

In the nurse–patient relationship the patient discloses more about his personal circumstances and feelings than the nurse does, because he is the recipient of the helping relationship. Self-disclosure is the act of making oneself manifest, so that others can perceive you. To disclose means to unveil, to show and to divulge information about oneself. Auvil and Silver (1984) point out that it is neither desirable nor feasible to exclude the 'person' of the nurse in nurse–patient interactions: yet the question that many nurses will ask themselves is how much should they disclose. Weiner (1978) has established guidelines to enable nurses to evaluate the potential value of self-disclosure. The nurse needs to assess the usefulness of self-disclosure to determine whether it will facilitate the goals of nursing. For example, will the disclosure help the patient to learn more about himself or help him to deal more effectively with his problems or will the disclosure help the patient to discharge emotional feelings which have previously been withheld or suppressed?

The use of self-disclosure that is appropriate to a relationship or situation can provide a basis for trust, empathy and understanding.

Through the therapeutic use of self the nurse accepts his or her self as part of the learning experience. Essentially, it is the kind of person that the nurse *is* that will influence the effectiveness of nursing, and through this therapeutic use of self that the art and science of nursing finds its existence (Jasmin and Trygstad, 1979).

REFERENCES AND FURTHER READING

References

Auvil, C. A. (1984), The sounds of silence, *American Journal of Nursing*, **84**, No. 8, 1072.

Auvil, C. A., and Silver, B. W. (1984), Therapist self disclosure: when is it appropriate?, *Perspectives in Psychiatric Care*, **22**, No. 2, 57–61.

Drummond, E. E. (1970), Communications and comfort for the dying patient, *Nursing Clinics of North America*, **5**, No. 1, 55–63.

Ehmann, V. E. (1971), Empathy: its origin, characteristics and process, *Perspectives in Psychiatric Care*, **9**, No. 21, 72–80.

Hardin, S. B., and Halaris, A. L. (1983), Non-verbal communications of patients and high and low empathy nurses, *Journal of Psychiatric Nursing and Mental Health Services*, **121**, No. 1, 14–20.

Hargie, O., Saunders, C., and Dickson, D. (1981), *Social Skills in Interpersonal Communication*, Croom Helm, London.

Hein, E. C. (1980), *Communication in Nursing Practice*, 2nd edn, Little, Brown, Boston, Massachusetts.

Hobart, J. E. (1964), The problem of silences in a nurse–patient relationship, *Perspectives in Psychiatric Care*, **11**, No. 5, 29–34.

Irving, S. (1978), *Basic Psychiatric Nursing*, 2nd edn, W. B. Saunders, Philadelphia, Pennsylvania.

Iveson-Iveson, J. (1983), The art of touching, *Nursing Mirror*, **156**, No. 20, 48–49.

Jasmin, S., and Trygstad, L. N. (1979), *Behavioural Concepts and the Nursing Process*, C. V. Mosby, St. Louis, Missouri.

Johnson, B. S. (1965), The meaning of touch in nursing, *Nursing Outlook*, **13**, No. 2, 59–60.

Jourard, S. M. (1971), *The Transparent Self*, Van Nostrand Reinhold, New York.

Lancaster, J. (1980), *Adult Psychiatric Nursing*, Medical Examination Publishing, New York.

Leininger, M. (1980), Caring: a central focus of nursing and health care, *Nursing and Health Care*, **1**, No. 3.

Ludemann, R. S. (1968), Empathy: a component of therapeutic nursing, *Nursing Forum*, **7**, No. 3, 275–287.

Luft, J. (1970), *Group Processes, An Introduction to Group Dynamics*, 2nd edn, Mayfield Publishing, California.

Mason, A., and Pratt, J. W. (1980), Touch, *Nursing Times*, **76**, No. 23, 999–1001.

Mayeroff, M. (1971), cited by Winder, A. E. (1984), A mental health professional looks at nursing care, *Nursing Forum*, **21**, No. 4, 184–188.

McGoran, S. (1978), Teaching students self awareness, *American Journal of Nursing*, **78**, 859.

Mercer, L. S. (1966), Touch: comfort and threat, *Perspectives in Psychiatric Care*, **6**, No. 3, 20–25.

Naugle, E. H. (1973), The difference caring makes, *American Journal of Nursing*, **73**, 1890–1891.

Seeger, P. (1977), Self awareness and nursing, *Journal of Psychiatric Nursing and Mental Health Services*, **15**, No. 8, 24–26.

Smoyak, S. A. (1963), Non-verbal communication. In: *Some Clinical*

Approaches to Psychiatric Nursing (eds Burd, S. F., and Marshall, M. A.), Macmillan, New York.

Stuart, G. W., and Sundeen, S. J. (1983), *Principles and Practice of Psychiatric Nursing*, C. V. Mosby, St Louis, Missouri.

Topalis, M., and Aguilera, D. (1978), *Psychiatric Nursing*, 7th edn, C. V. Mosby, St Louis, Missouri.

Ujhely, G. (1968), *Determinants of the Nurse–Patient Relationship*, Springer, New York.

Uys, L. R. (1980), Towards the development of an operational definition of the concept 'therapeutic use of self', *International Journal of Nursing Studies*, **17**, 175–180.

Weiner, M. (1978), cited by Auvil, C. A., and Silver, B. W. (1984), Therapist self disclosure: when is it appropriate?, *Perspectives in Psychiatric Care*, **22**, No. 2, 57–61.

Winder, A. E. (1984), A mental health professional looks at nursing care, *Nursing Forum*, **21**, No. 4, 184–188.

Zderad, L. (1969), Empathic nursing. Realization of a human capacity, *Nursing Clinics of North America*, **4**, No. 4, 655–662.

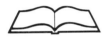

Further reading

Burnard, P. (1984), Developing self awareness, *Nursing Mirror*, **158**, No. 21, 30–31.

Burnard, P. (1985), Listening to people, *Nursing Mirror*, **161**, No. 3, 28–29.

Collins, M. (1983), *Communication in Health Care*, C. V. Mosby, St Louis, Missouri.

Forsyth, G. L. (1980), Analysis of the concepts of empathy: illustration of one approach, *Advances in Nursing Science*, **2**, No. 2, 33–42.

Gaut, D. A. (1986), Evaluating caring competencies in nursing practice, *Topics in Clinical Nursing*, **8**, No. 2, 77–82.

Goodykoontz, L. (1979), Touch: attitudes and practices, *Nursing Forum*, **18**, No. 1, 4–17.

Griffin, A. P. (1983), A philosophical analysis of caring in nursing, *Journal of Advanced Nursing*, **8**, 289–295.

Hambrick-Butter, S. K., and Sarasin, K. (1986), The 24 hour stay. Senior nursing students experience psychiatric hospitalisation from the patient's perspective, *Journal of Psychosocial Nursing*, **24**, No. 4, 23–25.

Hargie, O., Saunders, C., and Dickson, D. (1981), *Social Skills in Interpersonal Communication*, Croom Helm, London.

Iveson-Iveson, J. (1985), Developing self awareness, *Nursing Mirror*, **161**, No. 5, 25.

Klotkowski, D. (1980), Self disclosure: implications for mental health, *Perspectives in Psychiatric Care*, **18**, No. 3, 112–115.

Lawson, K. (1980), Listening to patients, *Nursing Times*, **76**, No. 41, 1784–1788.

Lenarz, D. M. (1971), Caring is the essence of practice, *American Journal of Nursing*, **71**, 704–707.

Leonard, R. (1984), Attending: letting the patient know you are listening, *Journal of Practical Nursing*, **23**, No. 8, 28–29.

Leung, J. K. C. (1981), A touching moment, *Nursing Mirror*, **153**, No. 12, 36–37.

O'Brien, M. (1978), *Communication and Relationships in Nursing*, C. V. Mosby, Missouri.

Stetler, C. B. (1977), Relationship of perceived empathy to nurses' communication, *Nursing Research*, **26**, 432–438.

Uys, L. R. (1980), Towards the development of an operational definition of the concept 'therapeutic use of self', *International Journal of Nursing Studies*, **17**, 175–180.

Wainwright, G. R. (1985), *Teach Yourself: Body Language*, Teach Yourself Books, Hodder and Stoughton, London.

Wolf, Z. R. (1986), The caring concept and nurse identified caring behaviours, *Topics in Clinical Nursing*, **8**, No. 2, 84–92.

Chapter 7

Conceptual models in nursing

'Basic to any professional discipline is the development of a body of knowledge that can be applied to its practice.' (Torres, 1980).

WHY USE A MODEL?

Nursing has been dominated in the past by theories borrowed from other disciplines, particularly medicine (Fitzpatrick, 1984). Consequently, nursing has been difficult to define in relation to other disciplines.

In the past, ideas about nursing have been centred around the labels of physical and mental disorder. Lectures about nursing in schools of nursing have usually followed and incorporated the medical model of care.

While the borrowing of concepts and theories from other disciplines has not necessarily been detrimental, effective nursing requires its own theoretical knowledge base, which is grounded in research and based on the reality of nursing practice.

As a relatively young profession, nursing is now beginning to develop a body of knowledge in terms of theories and concepts which are unique to nursing. These theories and concepts have been developed by nurses with a university education, e.g. Peplau, Orem, Roy, Roper, Logan and Tierney, and others.

WHAT IS A MODEL?

A conceptual model or framework is a way of looking at (conceptualising) a discipline (e.g. nursing) in a clear unambiguous way that can be communicated to others. It is a way of representing the reality of nursing practice, although the model is not, of course, the actual reality.

FUNCTION OF A MODEL

If nurses are to be considered as health professionals, then it is essential for them to communicate that what they do is unique and important within the multi-disciplinary team (Kozier and Erb, 1983). Conceptual models provide a means by which nurses can examine what they do. Before these are introduced, some clarification of terms is necessary. Concepts are abstract notions similar in definition to an idea. The term is adopted as a way of labelling and naming things: human beings, relationships communications and other realities that we perceive and think about (Kim, 1983). Concepts are the elements used to build theories. The word theory means vision—a theory can be viewed as an interrelationship of basic concepts that can be used systematically to explain approaches to nursing care and to predict outcomes (Torres, 1980).

June Clark (1985) compares a nursing model with the analogy of a shoe. A shoe, although recognisable by its shape, will not fit any foot. Each person's shoes are selected and moulded to the unique attributes of their feet. Similarly the nursing model must be moulded to fit the nursing needs of each individual patient, and not the patient moulded to fit the model.

Some models may be found to be more appropriate in certain situations than in others. Conceptual models provide frames of reference which give clear and explicit direction to nursing practice. They give nurses the opportunity to examine what they do and provide a framework for patient assessment. The first step in choosing a model for an individual patient's care is for the nurse to have a knowledge about models for nursing practice. Secondly, there must be agreement among the nursing team about the adoption of a particular model and a willingness to experiment and adapt models for patients within various nursing settings.

While some health authorities have selected a particular model for practice, Wright (1986) has strong reservations about the blanket application of one model of nursing to a variety of nursing settings. He argues that models should be varied and dynamic and should help nurses to explore and define their work. A model should never be allowed to become rigid and solid. It should be perceived as a growing and evolving structure with input from research, practice and education to keep it alive. He suggests that 'the ultimate test of the model is not the nurse's view but the patient's'.

A number of nursing models have been used in this book and an overview of these models is presented here. Readers are referred to the original texts for more comprehensive information.

A DEVELOPMENTAL MODEL

Hildegard Peplau has her roots in psychiatric nursing and was the first theorist to provide a conceptual model for psychiatric nursing. The publication of her book *Interpersonal Relations in Nursing* in 1952 is a landmark in the history of nursing and has played a part in advancing the role of the psychiatric nurse.

Peplau defines Man as an organism living in an unstable environment who strives to reduce tension generated by needs; health is perceived as a forward movement of personality and other ongoing human processes in the direction of creative, constructive, productive, personal and community living. Peplau considered nursing as a significant therapeutic interpersonal process in which the nurse and patient have equally important parts to play; she sees both the nurse and the patient learning and growing as a result of the interaction.

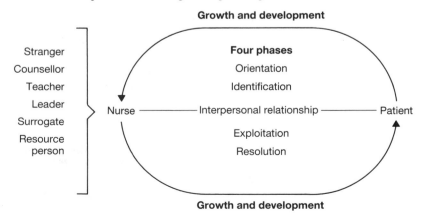

Peplau's developmental model

Nursing is defined as a 'human relationship between an individual who is sick or in need of health services and a nurse especially educated to recognise and to respond to the need for help'.

Peplau's writing has been greatly influenced by the theories of Harry Stack Sullivan. She observed that stress created energy which could be used either positively or negatively. Energy used negatively was wasteful, whereas energy used positively could be used as a productive force towards personal growth and maturation. The aim of the nurse is to use energy created by the person in stress in a positive manner.

Peplau's model consists of four phases in which the nurse and patient play an active role.

1. In the initial stage, *orientation*, the nurse and patient meet as two strangers (Peplau, 1952). The nurse gets to know the patient as a person and works towards a relationship in which concerns can be identified.
2. During the *identification* phase the patient begins to respond to the nurse, roles are clarified, and the patient's problems and needs are identified.
3. The third phase, *exploitation*, can be described as the working phase of the developmental model. The nurse intervenes therapeutically to help the patient and works towards the intended consequence for both, i.e. maturity. In this phase the patient derives full benefit from the nurse–patient relationship and any services necessary to meet the patients needs are utilised.
4. During the final phase, *resolution*, the nurse and patient work towards termination of the nurse–patient relationship. Dependence is relinquished and the patient resumes independence. The nurse evaluates the mutual maturation that has occurred through the educational, therapeutic and interpersonal processes of nursing (Chinn and Jacobs, 1983).

Peplau believes that the nurse–patient relationship is purposeful and goal centred. She suggests that the nurse's function is to help to reduce anxiety by channelling the patient's energy towards interpersonal growth. In order to facilitate this growth process the nurse adopts a number of roles in accordance with the level of maturity of interaction that the individual demands. The roles occur as a result of the patient's problems and includes the roles of stranger, teacher, leader, counsellor, resource person and surrogate as follows (Peplau, 1952, Chapter 3).

(a) Roles in nursing

1 The role of stranger
At first the nurse and patient are strangers to each other Peplau (1952) states that 'respect and positive interest accorded a stranger is at first non-personal and includes the same ordinary courtesies that are accorded to a new guest who has been brought into any situation'. She suggests that the patient is accepted as he is and that the patient should be treated as an emotionally able stranger. He should be related to on this basis until evidence shows him to be otherwise. Peplau emphasises that an appropriate approach 'arises out of the personality of the nurse and the way she sizes up the situation'. The greeting cannot be stereotyped if the nurse is to sound genuine.

2 The role of resource person
'A resource person provides specific answers to questions usually formulated with relation to a larger problem' (Peplau, 1952).

Giving a patient advice and answers to questions may shut out a patient's wish to work through his own problems; Peplau suggests that competent nurses will learn to identify opportunities to enable the patient to learn constructively.

3 The role of teacher

Teaching always proceeds from what the patient knows and develops around his interest in wanting and being able to use the information (Peplau, 1952). When the nurse promotes learning through experience, it may enable the patient to meet problems and difficulties that recur throughout life.

4 The role of leadership

Leadership functions are demanded of nurses in many different situations. The type of leadership that a nurse offers can create different kinds of group atmosphere.

'Democratic leadership encourages participation by everyone engaged in an endeavour.' Goals are determined by the group, and courses of action are discussed by group members. Peplau states that 'democratic leadership in nursing situations implies that the patient will be permitted to be an active participant in designing nursing plans for him'. She suggests that democratic nursing is a goal to aim for and requires attitudes of respect for the dignity and worth of each human being.

When autocratic leadership prevails, the patient may learn to 'overvalue the nurse and substitute the nurse's goals and successes for his own wish to struggle'.

5 The role of surrogate

Nurses are cast into surrogate roles more frequently than they realise. Outside his awareness the patient views the nurse as someone else. For example the nurse may symbolise a mother figure or some other person in his life. The patient then relates to the nurse in terms of the older relationship.

Substitute figures are brought to the mind of the patient when psychologically he finds himself in a situation that reactivates feelings generated in previous relationships. Permitting the patient to re-experience previous feelings in new situations with acceptance that promotes personality development requires a relationship in which the nurse recognises and responds in various surrogate roles.

6 The role of counsellor

As a counsellor the nurse uses certain skills and attitudes to help the patient to recognise, accept and resolve problems. Peplau suggests that all counselling functions in nursing are determined by the purpose of the nurse–patient relationship, i.e. the promotion of experiences leading to health. Peplau goes on to say that counselling has a great deal to do with the *way* in which nurses respond to the demands made of them, rather than to what those demands are. The counselling process is concerned with expanding experiences which are only dimly intelligible to the patient at first so that these experiences are better understood by both the patient and the nurse.

Pocock (1984) has compared Peplau's developmental model with the RMN Syllabus of The English and Welsh National Board for Nursing, Midwifery and Health Visiting (1982). He found compatibility between the writings of Peplau and the educational philosophy of the English and Welsh National Board for Nursing, Midwifery and Health Visiting; both place emphasis on the interpersonal aspects of nursing and the acquisition of these skills through experiential methods of learning.

Belcher and Fish (1980) suggest that the interpersonal process is an integral part of present-day nursing. While today the nurse may take the patient's total environment into account, Peplau's theory facilitates an increased understanding of the interactions which take place in the nurse–patient relationship; the nurse–patient relationship is after all the central focus of nursing.

AN ADAPTATION MODEL

Adaptation is the key concept in Roy's (1980) adaptation model. Man is viewed from a holistic perspective—a biopsychosocial being, with integrated functioning who is in constant interaction with his environment, striving to maintain equilibrium. This interaction is characterised by internal and external change. The process of adaptation occurs when the individual responds positively to internal and external change and moves along the health–illness continuum. A person's ability to respond to the stimuli that affect one or more of his modes depends on the cognitive and regulative mechanisms. The regulative mechanism operates through the autonomic nervous system and the cognitive mechanism operates through the central nervous system and is psychologically orientated. Roy believes that any change is one part or element within Man's integrated system will lead to a reaction that affects the whole rather than the parts separately.

Roy identifies four modes of adaptation which are activated when need deficits or excesses occur as a result of environmental change. These modes are as follows:

1. *The physiological mode* which relates to the need to maintain physiological integrity through fluid and electrolyte balance, exercise and rest, nutrition and elimination, and oxygen and temperature regulation.
2. *The self-concept mode* refers to the psychological integrity of the person as an inner need.
3. *The role mastery mode* which is the mode in which a person's self-concept is determined by his interaction with others. Interaction can help to establish a person's identity in relation to others. If elements of interpersonal behaviour are lacking, e.g. if a person is denied access to others for the purpose of interaction or if a person is receiving double messages and meanings, then a need deficit will occur.
4. *The interdependent mode* through which a person's life gains meaning and purpose. It involves relationships with others and ways of meeting needs for help, affection and attention.

At any point along the health–illness continuum, human beings are exposed to and acted on by a variety of stimuli. Roy describes three classes of stimuli that impinge on individuals:

1. Focal stimuli which immediately confront a person.
2. Contextual stimuli which include all other stimuli present.
3. Residual stimuli which are based on beliefs, values, attitudes and past experience which have an effect on the person's present situation.

When making an assessment, the nurse assesses the patient's needs in each mode and takes into consideration the classes of stimuli and how these influence needs.

The nurse's interventions are primarily aimed at assisting the patient's adaptation process.

AN ACTIVITIES-OF-LIVING MODEL

The activities of living are the focus of the Roper–Logan–Tierney model and central to their view of nursing. The model is composed of five components: the 12 activities of living, the lifespan, the dependence–independence continuum, the factors which influence the activities of living and the individuality in living. While their model is suitable for any nursing situation, in psychiatric nursing it seems probably more relevant for care of the elderly (see Chapter 17).

Roper, Logan and Tierney (1986) suggested that priorities among the activities of living will change according to circumstances. Although there are 12 activities of living, the nurse will need to collect information about only those activities which are relevant and not necessarily in the order depicted (Roper and Logan, 1985) (*Figure 7.1*).

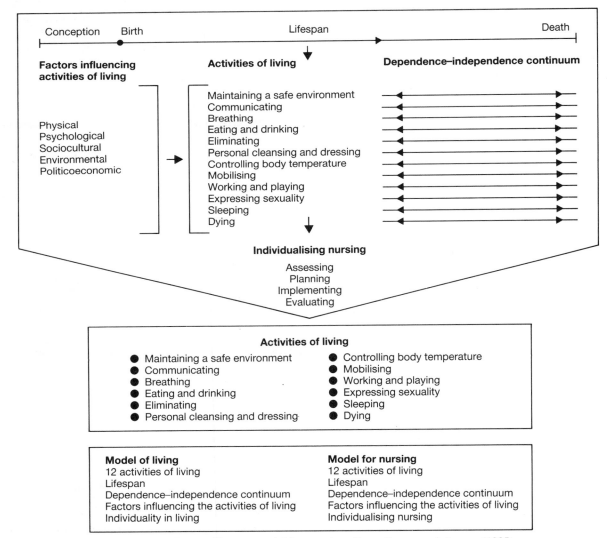

Figure 7.1   The revised Roper–Logan–Tierney model for nursing. From Roper and Logan (1985)

The lifespan begins at conception and ends in death and is the second component of the model. It serves as a reminder that nurses are concerned with people of all ages who are being constantly changed and shaped by their experiences.

The third component of the model is the dependence–independence continuum along which there can be movement in both directions. Roper and Logan (1985) stress the importance of assessing a person's level of independence in each of the activities of living and judging the direction and the amount that he should be assisted to move along the continuum. A nurse may sometimes assist a patient to move towards independence in the activities of living and other times to accept dependence.

Each activity has to be considered in the light of its complexities and influencing factors; each person carries out their activities of living differently because of physical, psychological, sociocultural, environmental and politico-economic factors. For example, control of body temperature will be influenced by a person's level of activity or inactivity, the type of clothing worn and its suitability for the external environment, knowledge attitudes and values, and their ability to purchase sufficient heat in winter.

The fifth component of the model is concerned with individuality. Individualised nursing care can be achieved through the process of nursing with the framework of a conceptual model, Roper and Logan (1985) suggest that 'a knowledge of a person's individuality in living is an essential prerequisite to individualising nursing'.

The data collected from the ongoing process of assessment is reviewed and the actual potential problems mutually identified and arranged in order of priority. Each are then set in relation to the activities of living and emphasis is placed on what the patient can as well as cannot do. If possible, the goals are stated in an observable and measurable way. Some nursing goals will be derived from medical or other prescriptions rather than the nursing assessment but also need to be included in the nursing plan.

A SELF-CARE MODEL

Orem's (1980) self-care model places the emphasis on the capacities of clients to manage their own self-care. She suggests that individuals have self-care needs for which they perform learned self-care behaviours.

Orem describes three categories of self-care requisites from which a person's total self-care demand can be assessed along a continuum of self-care activities.

1. *Universal self-care needs* are common to all human beings during the life cycle and include needs for sufficient air, food, water, elimination, activity, rest and solitude, the social interaction protection from hazards and the promotion of human functioning and development.
2. *Developmental self-care needs* are those for living conditions which support life. These vary according to the person's age and stage of development and are met either by a person's own abilities (in adulthood) or by others (in the case of a baby or young child).
3. *Health deviation self-care needs* relate to the adjustments that a person has to make when faced with an illness or disability.

If a person's self-care activities are therapeutic, then they support life processes and promote normal functioning, maintain normal growth, development and maturation, prevent, control or cure disease processes or injury and prevent or compensate for disability.

Orem describes three nursing systems.

1. *The partially compensatory system* is implemented when a person can carry out certain aspects of his care but needs assistance in some areas.
2. *The wholly compensatory system* is implemented when the nurse carries out all the activities that enable a person to meet his self-care needs.
3. *The educative developmental system* is applicable when a person is in control of his own self-care activities but the nurse necessarily acts in an educative role towards the individual and/or his family.

The role of the nurse is to give assistance to a person to meet his own self-care demands within the three categories of self-care requisites that Orem describes. The aim of nursing is to help the person to move along a self-care continuum so that he can progressively meet his own self-care demand. When a person has deficits in his health care ability and the nurse's abilities with regard to therapeutic self-care exceed those of the individual, then the nurse responds to the person's self-care deficits. The nurse seeks to prevent imbalances in self-care abilities between the client and the nurse so that a valid reason for nursing ceases to exist.

SUMMARY

Peplau, whose writings have been very influential, sees the nurse–patient relationship as a vehicle for promoting mutual growth and maturation, Roy views nursing as promoting man's adaptive abilities towards biopsychosocial homeostasis, Orem's self-care model seeks for man to achieve optimal self-care activities, and the Roper–Logan–Tierney model aims to assist a person with their activities of living.

According to McFarlane (1980), 'all theorists are concerned with nursing as a discipline that assists man to reach his optimal health state, but they differ in their descriptions as to how this is achieved'.

The development of these models as a tool for the nursing process is still at a relatively early stage and nursing models are not generally substantiated by research. This emphasises the need for the nurse:

1. To think critically about a model before using it.
2. To make sure that the model has been adapted to suit the patient and not vice versa.
3. To consider the advantages and limitations of using models for treatment (Green, 1985), and to keep up to date with current views on nursing models so that he or she can continually improve his or her treatment plans.

REFERENCES AND FURTHER READING

References

Belcher, J. R., Fish, L. J. B., and Peplau, H. E. (1980), *The Nursing Theories Conference Group. Nursing Theories: The Base for Professional Nursing Practice*, Prentice-Hall, Englewood Cliffs, New Jersey.

Chinn, P. L., and Jacobs, M. K. (1983), *Theory and Nursing: A Systematic Approach*, C. V. Mosby, St Louis, Missouri.

Clark, J. (1985), Paper presented at The Senior Nurse/Models for Nursing Conference, Manchester University, 1985.

The English and Welsh National Boards for Nursing, Midwifery and Health Visiting (1982), *Syllabus of Training Professional Register*, Part 3.

Fitzpatrick, J. J. (1984), Points of view, should nursing models be used in psychiatric nursing practice?, *Journal of Psychiatric Nursing and Mental Health Services*, **22**, No. 6.

Green, C. (1985), An overview of the value of nursing models in relation to education, *Nurse Education Today*, **5**, 267–271.

Kim, H. S. (1983), *The Nature of Theoretical Thinking in Nursing*, Appleton Century Crofts, Norwalk, Connecticut.

Kozier, B., and Erb, G. (1983), *Fundamentals of Nursing*, 2nd edn, Addison-Wesley, Reading, Massachusetts.

McFarlane, E. A. (1980), Nursing theory: the comparison of four theoretical proposals, *Journal of Advanced Nursing*, **5**, 3–19.

Orem, D. E. (1950), *Nursing: Concepts of Practice*, 2nd edn, McGraw-Hill, New York.

Peplau, H. (1952), *Interpersonal Relations in Nursing*, G. P. Putnam, New York.

Pocock, P. (1984), Models of nursing: Peplau and the 1982 syllabus for mental nursing, Unpublished seminar paper, for BEd(Hons), Nursing Education, Polytechnic of the South Bank.

Roper, N., and Logan, W. W. (1985), The Roper/Logan/Tierney model, *Senior Nurse*, **3**, No. 2, 20–26.

Roper, N., Logan, W., and Tierney, A. (1986), *Elements of Nursing*, revised edn, Churchill Livingstone, Edinburgh.

Roy, C. (1980), The Roy adaptation model. In: *Conceptual Models for Nursing Practice* (eds Riehl, J. P., and Roy, C.), Appleton Century Crofts, Norwalk, Connecticut.

Torres, G. (1980), The place of concepts and theories within nursing. In: *The Nursing Theories Conference Group. Nursing Theories: The Base for Professional Nursing Practice*, Prentice-Hall, Englewood Cliffs, New Jersey.

Wright, S. (1986), Developing and using a nursing model. In: *Models for Nursing* (eds Kershaw, B., and Salvage, J.), John Wiley, Chichester, West Sussex.

Further reading

Aggleton, P., and Chalmers, H. (1984), Models and theories: 2. The Roy adaptation model, *Nursing Times*, **80**, No. 40, 45–48.

Aggleton, P., and Chalmers, H. (1984), Models and theories: 3. The Riehl interaction model, *Nursing Times*, **80**, No. 45, 58–61.

Aggleton, P., and Chalmers, H. (1985), Models and theories: 5. Orem's self-care model, *Nursing Times*, **81**, No. 1, 36–39.

Aggleton, P., and Chalmers, H. (1985), Models and theories: 7. Henderson's model, *Nursing Times*, **81**, No. 10, 33–35.

Aggleton, P., and Chalmers, H. (1986), *Nursing Models and the Nursing Process*, Macmillan, London.

Akinsanya, J. A. (1984), The uses of theories in nursing, *Nursing Times, Occasional Papers*, **80**, No. 14.

Arumugan, U. (1985), Helping Harry to relate to others (using Riehl model), *Nursing Times*, **81**, No. 21, 43–45.

Barker, J. (1984), A plan for Arthur and Mary (using Orem model), *Nursing Times, Community Outlook*, 14 November.

Fitzpatrick, J., Whall, A., Johnson, R., and Floyd, J. (1982), *Nursing Models and their Psychiatric Mental Health Application*, Robert J. Brady, Maryland.

Hardy, L. K. (1982), Nursing models and research—a restricting view, *Journal of Advanced Nursing*, **7**, 447–451.

Hoeffner, B., and Murphy, S. (1982), The unfinished task: development of nursing theory for psychiatric and mental health nursing practice, *Journal of Psychiatric Nursing and Mental Health Services*, **20**, No. 12, 8–14.

Hoon, E. (1986), Game playing: a way to look at nursing models, *Journal of Advanced Nursing*, **11**, 421–427.

Iveson-Iveson, J. (1982), Putting ideas into action (Orem model), *Nursing Mirror*, **155**, No. 18, 52.

Iveson-Iveson, J. (1982), A two-way process (Peplau model), *Nursing Mirror*, **155**, No. 18, 52.

Johnson, M. (1985), Model of perfection?, *Nursing Times*, **82**, No. 6, 42–44.

Kershaw, B., and Salvage, J. (eds) (1985), *Models for Nursing*, John Wiley, Chichester, West Sussex.

Marriner, A. (1986), *Nursing Theorists and their Work*, C. V. Mosby, St Louis, Missouri.

McGlynn, J. (1984), The quest for nursing knowledge, *Nursing Education Today*, **4**, No. 2, 46–47.

Moscovitz, A. O. (1984), Orem's theory as applied to psychiatric nursing, *Perspectives in Psychiatric Care*, **22**, No. 1, 36–38.

O'Rawe, A. M. (1982), Self-neglect—a challenge for nursing (using Orem model), *Nursing Times*, **78**, No. 46, 1932–1936.

O'Toole, A. W. (1981), When the practical becomes theoretical, *Journal of Psychosocial Nursing and Mental Health Services*, **19**, No. 12, 11–19.

Pearson, A., and Vaughan, B. (1986), *Nursing Models for Practice*, Heinemann, London.

Runtz, S. E., and Urtel, J. G. (1983), Evaluating your practice via a nursing model (two case examples using Orem and Peplau), *Nursing Practitioner*, **8**, No. 3, 30, 32, 37–40.

Smith, S. (1981), Oremization, the curse of nursing, *RN (US)*, **44**, 83.

Somociuk, G. (1985), Concept meets reality (Neuman model), *Nursing Mirror*, **161**, No. 11, 29–33.

Stockwell, F. (1985), An enhancement model of psychiatric nursing, *The Nursing Process in Psychiatric Nursing*, Croom Helm, London, p. 14.

Webb, C. (1986), Nursing models: a personal view, *Nursing Practice*, **1**, 208–212.

Chapter 8

The nursing process

'Hopefully nurses will soon learn that nursing is a special case of loving.' (Jourard, 1971).

INTRODUCTION

The nursing process provides a problem-solving approach to nursing care based on the needs and problems of the individual patient. Whenever possible, the patient and his relatives are encouraged to participate in decisions relating to his care.

The nursing process consists of four stages: assessment, planning, implementation and evaluation. Although it is usual to discuss the different stages separately, it must be borne in mind that a dynamic interrelationship exists between the various phases (McGilloway, 1980).

In describing the stages of the nursing process some writers include the term nursing diagnosis. This is a summary statement which describes the patient's actual or potential health problems (Stanton *et al.*, 1980).

A nursing diagnosis is not synonymous with a medical diagnosis and is more likely to be determined by the entire needs of the patient (Smitherson, 1981).

The use of the term nursing process has been traced from the 1950s in the USA by Henderson (1982), although the term did not become part of the nursing vocabulary in the UK until the 1970s.

According to De La Cuesta (1983) the earliest evidence of the use of the term has been attributed to Lydia Hall when she gave a lecture entitled 'The quality of nursing care' in 1955. However, Peplau used the term even before this in her book *Interpersonal Relations in Nursing* which was published in 1952.

Many people are not happy with the term nursing process. Nurses use many processes in the course of their work—the helping process, the communication process and the leadership process to name but a few. Therefore, it seems inappropriate to refer to any one process used in nursing as *the* nursing process (Smitherson, 1981). Wainwright (1984) suggests that British nurses are using the term as if it were something unique, a particular way of nursing rather than as an aspect of the nursing situation. He feels that the term nursing process should be abolished and that we should talk about nursing instead. Henderson (1982) argues that the nursing process is often used as a substitute for nursing. She suggests that the nursing plan is often a plan of medical management and that the medical model is followed with some modification in language which enables nurses to justify their role in therapy.

The nursing process provides a useful methodology which helps nurses to arrive at decisions and to evaluate consequences; on its own, it does not *do* anything (Tierney, 1983). It is important to realise that the nursing process is not nursing, but a tool or methodology that helps nurses to arrive at decisions and to predict and evaluate consequences (Stanton *et al.*, 1980).

The nurse must never lose sight of the fact that the quality of nursing that the patient receives is primarily dependent on his or her humanistic capacity to meet the patient's needs. While the nursing process provides a systematic approach to care, it is the therapeutic use of self, and not a process or a methodology, which fulfils the purpose of nursing.

REFERENCES AND FURTHER READING

References

De La Cuesta, C. (1983), The nursing process: from development to implementation, *Journal of Advanced Nursing*, **8**, 365–371.

Henderson, V. (1982), The nursing process—is the title right?, *Journal of Advanced Nursing*, **7**, 103–109.

Jourard, S. M. (1971), *The Transparent Self*, Van Nostrand Reinhold, New York.

McGilloway, F. A. (1980), The nursing process: a problem solving approach to patient care, *International Journal of Nursing Studies*, **17**, 79–90.

Peplau, H. (1952), *Interpersonal Relations in Nursing*, G. P. Putnam, New York.

Smitherson, C. (1981), *Nursing Actions for Health Promotion*, F. A. Davis, Philadelphia, Pennsylvania.

Stanton, M., Paul, C., and Reeves, J. S. (1980), An overview of the nursing process. In: *The Nursing Theories Conference Group. Nursing Theories: The Base for Professional Nursing Practice*, Prentice-Hall, Englewood Cliffs, New Jersey.

Tierney, A. (1983), cited by Ross, T. (1983), Activities of living, *Nursing Mirror*, **156**, No. 6, 28–29.

Wainwright, P. (1984), Not the nursing process, *Nursing Mirror*, **158**, No. 21, 22–24.

Further reading

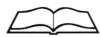

Aggleton, P., and Chalmers, H. (1986), Nursing research, nursing theory and the nursing process, *Journal of Advanced Nursing*, **11**, 197–202.

Glass, H. (1983), Interventions in nursing: goals or task orientated, *International Nursing Review*, **30**, No. 2, 52–56.

Johnson, J. (1984), The nursing process and psychiatry, *Nursing Mirror, Mental Health Forum*, **158**, No. 4, i–ii.

Keane, P. (1981), The nursing process in action 4. The nursing process in a psychiatric context, *Nursing Times*, **77**, No. 28, 1223–1224.

Martin, L., and Glasper, A. (1986), Core plans: nursing models and the nursing process in action, *Nursing Practice*, **1**, 268–273.

Miller, A. (1985), Are you using the nursing process?, *Nursing Times*, **81**, No. 50, 36–39.

Mitchell, J. R. A. (1984), Is nursing any business of doctors? A simple guide to the 'nursing process', *British Medical Journal*, **288**, 21 January, 216–219.

Roe, S., and Farrel, P. (1986), Shaping nursing process, *Nursing Practice*, **1**, 274–278.

Rowden, R. (1984), Doctors can work with the nursing process: a reply to Professor Mitchell, *British Medical Journal*, **288**, 21 January, 219–220.

Stockwell, F. (1985), *The Nursing Process in Psychiatric Nursing*, Croom Helm, London.

Syson Nibbs, L. (1980), Progress through a planned approach, *Nursing Mirror*, **150**, No. 7, 42–44.

Waters, K. (1985), The nursing process—methodology versus mythology, *Nursing Practice*, **1**, 92–97.

ASSESSMENT

> *'It seems difficult for professions to accept the fact that they cannot know any other person until they have taken steps to find out who and how he is. It is important to know the other person's self and how he is experiencing his world.'* (Jourard, 1971).

Assessment should lead to the richest possible view of the patient as a person: a person with successes and failures: a person with a culture that influences his values and beliefs and whose environment imposes conditions on the quality of his life; a person whose biological state affects his perception, thoughts and behaviour and who comes from a family that either prescribes or imposes roles on him (Banchik, 1983).

Assessment is an ongoing process and not a once-only event. It is unlikely that the patient will reveal matters which concern him deeply in an initial interview. Additional information will be gathered during daily interactions with the patient.

In psychiatric nursing, the establishment of trust is a primary goal. If the nurse–patient relationship is to develop within a framework of mutual trust and confidence, then the patient's first impressions of the nurse will be important. The relationship which begins between the nurse and the patient during assessment can form the basis for a better understanding of the patient during subsequent interactions. The amount of self-awareness that the nurse has will determine the extent to which the patient and the situation confronting him is understood (Peplau, 1952). The nurse should try to see the patient as an individual and not classify him into a certain type. To prejudge or label the patient may contribute to his stress and will therefore defeat the aims of nursing.

(a) Admission

> *'Too often admission documents form a barrier for the patient coming into hospital. If the nurse hides behind standard questions the whole greeting can be depersonalised.'* (Price, 1983).

When the patient is admitted, the nurse should go forward to meet him as he enters the ward. Price (1983) emphasises the importance of admitting the patient as a *process* rather than as a *procedure* with the focus being placed on the social skills of the admitting nurse.

Going into hospital is usually a major event in a person's life which may well mark the climax of weeks of tension and anxiety (Burr and Andrews, 1981). When a patient is admitted to hospital, his personal belongings and territorial space are left at home. The day before admission he may have a clear sense of identity reinforced by his own possessions and space, but suddenly he is faced with all the anxiety and insecurity of being placed in an unfamiliar environment without his personal space and with few possessions. Showing the patient around the ward and introducing him to other patients and staff can help to familiarise him with his new territory. He will need to have some space to call his own, even if it is only a

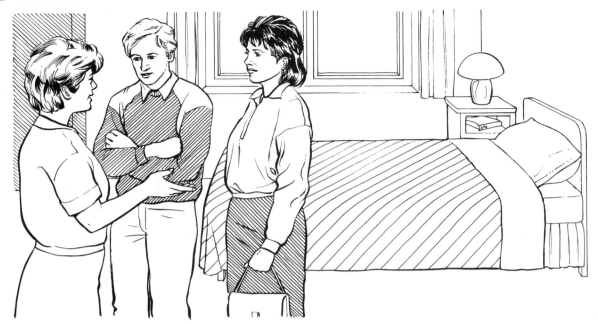

bed, a chair and a bedside locker. Once the patient is established in his territory, the space should be treated with respect as if it were his own home. Nothing should be moved or changed without asking his permission (Hayter, 1981).

The nurse should try to alleviate the patient's concerns about hospitalisation by telling him the things that he will need to know. However, when relating to the patient and his family, the nurse needs to bear in mind that something said once may not be picked up immediately. High anxiety levels may make connections between what is said and its relevance to a particular situation difficult (Ujhely, 1966). The nurse may need to repeat information over and over again.

(b) Interviewing

'Each person is unique and has something of his own that marks him off from other persons. This individuality is seen in both his person and his personality.' (Gillis, 1980).

An interview can be defined as a conversation conducted to achieve some preplanned objective of one or more persons usually through face to face communication (Edwards and Brilhart, 1981). The goal of the interview is to obtain as full a picture of the patient as possible. In nursing, interviewing is a specific kind of communication in which the nurse focuses attention on the patient and helps him to gain a better understanding of what is happening or what has happened to him in a particular situation. The climate which the nurse creates within the nurse–patient interaction will influence the substance of the interview; if the taking of a nursing history is viewed as a procedure rather than as a means of getting to know the patient, the purpose of the interview will be defeated. It is not always wise to interview the newly admitted patient immediately. He will need time to familiarise himself with his new environment (Kron, 1981). In some instances, the patient's mental state may not make an interview feasible and a history may have to be taken from the patient's family or friends, e.g. if the patient is very confused, disorientated or out of touch with reality. Furthermore, the patient may only be able to recognise and discuss his problems when the nurse has gained his trust and confidence, through ongoing interactions (Altschul, 1977).

1 Manner of interview
To interview the patient, the nurse needs to prepare a comfortable setting, free from distractions. The interview should be carried out in a flexible relaxed friendly way. The assessment interview provides the patient with an opportunity to define himself as a unique individual. He can be helped to share in his own words how he views himself and his problems (Eisenman and Dubbert, 1977). At the beginning of the interview the necessary introductions should be made and the purpose of the interview explained. Under no circumstances should questions just be read from a form and the answers filled in or just ticked off (Kron, 1981). Such a presentation would be counter-productive and prohibitive in enabling the patient to share his concerns. Ideally, the nurse should enable the patient to see what is being written about him on the assessment form, so that statements can be clarified; however, the nurse may feel that it is inappropriate to introduce 'a form' into the interaction and may prefer to write up the information immediately after the interview. The patient should never feel pressurised into discussing something which he does not yet feel ready to discuss and should never be asked questions which are unnecessary, irrelevant or asked merely out of curiosity.

2 Importance of interview in the nursing process
Understanding where the interview fits into the nursing process can enhance the nurse's effectiveness as an interviewer. If the patient can see that the information is necessary in order to plan his care, then he may be more willing to participate. At this point, it is as well to bear in mind that a nursing assessment is not a copy of the medical history; it is a tool with a different focus—that of uncovering the information necessary to *nurse* the patient (Kron, 1981). The assessment determines the baseline information which is used to evaluate the patient's achievement of goals and the effectiveness of nursing. Baseline observations are those which establish the condition of the patient at a particular time and provide a basis for future comparison.

3 Interview technique
Interviews are not made up entirely of questions and answers; together with silence, they set into motion patterns of thought that continue throughout the course of the interview (Hein, 1980). The nurse's skill as an interviewer will make all the difference between a productive interview and a non-productive one. Active listening and acceptance will encourage the patient to express himself. Words, of course, convey only part of the meaning of conversation. Non-verbal messages can convey meanings which are often more trustworthy than words.

4 Non-verbal communication
Some people try to control their facial expressions when they feel embarrassed or frightened by their feelings; few do so effectively. The patient's attempts to control his facial expressions may give the first indication that something is wrong. The observant nurse will notice a fake smile, a poker face or an attempt to camouflage a facial expression by rubbing the eyes or nose. These may be clues to the fact that the patient is trying to conceal his true feelings (Cooper, 1979). Non-verbal behaviours such as facial expressions, tone of voice, eye contact or lack of it, gestures, body posture and movements are much harder to

mask than verbal behaviour and can therefore serve to reinforce or contradict verbal communication (Snyder and Wilson, 1977).

All the patient's behaviour has meaning if only the nurse is willing to learn the language (Kron, 1981). The biting of nails, clenching of hands, stroking of fingers or restlessness can indicate distress signals to the discerning nurse.

5 Types of question
Questions that stimulate explanations are more effective than questions which may only require a 'yes' or a 'no' answer. 'Why?' questions, especially concerning the patient's behaviour, can create defensive attitudes. Stating an observation can allow him to respond without feeling threatened. He can be given the opportunity to confirm or correct the impression which the nurse has of him.

6 Reflection
Restatement of something that the patient expresses, using words similar to those that he uses, helps him to know that he has communicated successfully (Bootay, 1978). Reflecting the patient's previous statement or repeating what he has just said can encourage him to volunteer more information but this technique should not be overused (Kron, 1981).

7 Listening
Listening adds another dimension in learning about the patient; in listening to the patient's words the nurse attempts to identify those areas in which he experiences most conflict and disturbance (Bermosk, 1966).

8 Consideration of patient's disabilities
The value of the interview is clearly related to the skill of the person who conducts it. Interviewing is not just a skill of eliciting responses, but the ability to minimise the effects of one's own point of view on the response is important (Calnan, 1983). If the patient is elderly, sensory losses are more likely to be present, and the interviewer's placement of self is important. The patient is usually able to respond more readily if he can look directly at the interviewer. However, if he has better hearing in one ear than the other, then the nurse should sit nearest the good ear rather than in the face to face position (Metz, 1978).

9 Ending an interview
At the end of the interview the patient should be given the opportunity to ask questions or to add additional information. It is always important to close an interview properly. The way in which this is done matters a great deal to the patient. A successful interview will enable the patient to feel that he has played an effective part in planning his own care. Perceiving the patient's needs and problems through the process of assessment will involve a harmonising of the nurse's impressions.

10 Inferences
Cues observed from the patient's verbal and non-verbal behaviour and the inferences drawn from these cues must be recorded. An inference is a conclusion drawn from a chain of events, which may or may not be related, seen or experienced. Inferences are not necessarily untrue but indicate a higher or lower degree of probability to the truth. However, the more an inference is shared by other carers, the greater the likelihood that it is valid (Hein, 1980).

For an inference to be accurate it must be based on a number of cues; to rely on one cue only may lead to inaccurate information. For example, because a patient does not know what day it is does not mean that the nurse can infer from this information that the patient is confused. However, if other cues are evident such as constantly asking where he is, not knowing where he lives and trying to get out of bed on the wrong side, the nurse may infer that he is confused (Crow, 1979).

11 Patient's needs

The whole purpose of assessment is to identify the needs and problems of the patient. A need can be described as a lack of some necessary factor or condition which maintains adequate biological, psychological or social functioning (French, 1983). Biologists and physiologists define needs as those things in the environment that are essential to life and without which an organism could not survive.

Needs are concerned with the maintenance of self. They are specific areas related to the patient's health which are identified for intervention. If the needs are not met, their absence leads to illness in the mind, the body or the spirit (Rines and Montag, 1976). It is the nurse's responsibility to see that the patient's needs are met, either directly through nursing activities or indirectly by calling in the expertise of others.

12 Problems

A problem occurs when an unmet need exists. Actual problems are those problems experienced by the patient during assessment. They are readily identifiable through observation or because the patient indicates them to the nurse. Potential problems are not experienced by the patient during assessment, but problems could arise if no action is taken (Duberley, 1979). For example a patient who is depressed must be considered a potential suicide risk; a patient with a history of violent behaviour shows a potential for upsetting a safe ward environment. Duberley questions the wisdom of categorising problems into 'nursing problems', 'patient problems' and 'medical problems'. She suggests that it may be preferable to act in terms of problems experienced by patients which may be amenable to care by one or more health care disciplines. It is unlikely that one discipline acting alone would bring about the desired goals; through working together, the desired goals may be achieved. A patient's problems are dynamic and not static in nature; therefore, nursing care plans and interventions must be updated to meet the patient's changing needs. Just as the patient's problems and needs will change in the course of time, so will the priorities for his care.

(c) Recording

> 'I do not believe that we can formulate patient needs without consulting the patient.' (Haggerty, 1971).

Every hospital- or community-based service will have its own format for documentation of the nursing records. The most important thing to bear in mind is that the nursing record should be a written account of the process of nursing and not an additional doctor's record (French, 1983).

Descriptions should be accurate and concise. The use of psychiatric terminology and abbreviations is to be discouraged in objective recording. Abbreviations may be open to many different interpretations and can lead to a breakdown in communication. The notes should be written in every-day descriptive language, as it is important to describe exactly what the patient did or said.

The information collected can only be valid if it truly reflects what the patient did or said. If the data are filtered through the nurse's perception and depiction of events, then it is the nurse's story and not the patient's (Eisenman and Dubbert, 1977).

The nursing record should provide a means of communication not only for nurses providing care at different times of the day but also for other members of the multi-disciplinary team. It allows nurses and others to define the particular contribution of nursing towards the patient's achievement of goals.

FACT SHEET: INFORMATION-GATHERING TECHNIQUES

(a) Open-ended questions

Give the patient a wide range of options as to how he will respond. They allow him to describe his personal experiences in his own words giving as much or as little information as he wishes, e.g. 'How are you feeling today?'

(b) Focused questions

Limit the area to which the patient can respond but at the same time encourage more than a 'yes' or 'no' answer, e.g. 'You said that you felt anxious last time that I saw you. How have you been since then?'

(c) Probing questions

Probing questions are used to seek out further detail about a particular area, e.g. 'Can you tell me anything else about it?'

(d) Paraphrasing

Using simple and culturally relevant terms the nurse may immediately confirm the patient's previous message. In other words, paraphrasing is to give back the patient's meaning of what he has said in one's own words. The meaning is verified with the patient, e.g. for a patient's statement 'The doctor put me on some different tablets, but I stopped taking them because I felt so much better.' We have the nurse's statement 'You were taking some different tablets, but you discontinued them because you felt better.'

(e) Clarifying

Sometimes the patient may say or do something that the nurse does not understand and clarification will be necessary (however, if the patient is distressed, it may be better to leave this until a more appropriate time). If a request for clarification is presented with warmth and interest, it is likely to be perceived by the patient as a genuine attempt to understand, e.g. 'I'm not quite sure that I understand what you are saying.'

(f) Dealing with sensitive areas

An area of interviewing which can be difficult concerns asking the patient about very personal things. These topics may include sexual habits, drug usage and alcohol consumption. When information concerning such topics is essential to data collection, these subjects may be approached more easily once an atmosphere of trust has been established. The patient needs to be reassured that the information is both necessary and confidential. The nurse's approach to the patient is important, and he or she must have sufficient self-awareness to feel comfortable in exploring these areas with the patient. The nurse must be unhurried in his or her approach, because the patient may struggle to find words to describe very private experiences. Not to explore personal areas may be doing the patient a disservice, because it may be in these areas that the patient needs most help.

(g) Testing discrepancies

The patient may express feelings, explanations and body language which are inconsistent. When the nurse notes a discrepancy, he or she must decide on what action to take: he or she can ignore it, explore it or make a note of it and explore it at a later time, e.g. a patient looks sad but says that he feels great.

(h) Summarising

At the end of the interview, it is useful to summarise what the patient has said. Mutual understanding can be prompted when the nurse feeds back to the patient the general essence of the interview from the patient's viewpoint. This technique decreases assumptions and prevents the formation of inaccurate concepts.

(i) Closing

The nurse should give the patient a sense that the time has come to end the interview. Closure should be carried out smoothly so that the patient does not feel cut off. Remember that it is not possible to learn everything about the patient from one interview. Assessment is ongoing and other opportunities can be planned to get to know the patient.

FURTHER READING

Bradley, J. C., and Edinberg, M. A. (1982), *Communication in the Nursing Context*, Appleton Century Crofts, Norwalk, Connecticut.

Collins, M. (1983), *Communication in Health Care*, C. V. Mosby, St Louis, Missouri.

Spradley, B. W. (1981), *Community Health Nursing Concepts and Practice*, Little, Brown, Boston, Massachusetts.

REFERENCES AND FURTHER READING

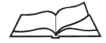

References

Altschul, A. T. (1977), Use of the nursing process in psychiatric care, *Nursing Times*, **73**, 1412–1413.

Banchik, D. (1983), Psychiatric assessment and case formulation. In: *Handbook of Psychiatric Mental Health Nursing* (eds Adams, C. G., and Macione, A.), John Wiley, Chichester, West Sussex.

Bermosk, L. S. (1966), Interviewing: a key to therapeutic communication in nursing practice, *Nursing Clinics of North America*, **1**, No. 2, 205–214.

Bootay, L. S. (1978), Interviewing your patient. In: *Nursing Skillbook. Documenting Patient Care Responsibility*, Nursing 78 Books, Horsham, Pennsylvania.

Burr, J., and Andrews, J. (1981), *Nursing the Psychiatric Patient*, 4th edn, Baillière Tindall, London.

Calnan, J. (1983), *Talking with Patients*, Heinemann Medical, London.

Cooper, J. (1979), Actions really do speak louder than words, *American Journal of Nursing*, **79**, No. 4, 29–32.

Crow, J. (1979), Assessment. In: *The Nursing Process* (ed. Kratz, C.), Baillière Tindall, London.

Duberley, J. (1979), Giving nursing care. In: *The Nursing Process* (ed. Kratz, C.), Baillière Tindall, London.

Edwards, B. J., and Brilhart, J. K. (1981), *Communication in Nursing Practice*, C. V. Mosby, St Louis, Missouri.

Eisenman, E. J. P., and Dubbert, P. M. (1977), The mental health assessment interview. In: *Psychiatric Mental Health Nursing Contemporary Readings* (eds Backer, B. A., Dubbert, P. M., and Eisenman, E. J. P.), Van Nostrand Reinhold, New York.

French, P. (1983), *Social Skills for Nursing Practice*, Croom Helm, London.

Gillis, L. (1980), *Human Behaviour in Illness*, 3rd edn, Faber and Faber, London.

Haggerty, V. C. (1971), Listening, *Nursing Forum*, **10**, No. 4, 382–387.

Hayter, J. (1981), Territoriality as a universal need, *Journal of Advanced Nursing*, **6**, 79–85.

Hein, E. C. (1980), *Communication in Nursing Practice*, 2nd edn, Little, Brown, Boston, Massachusetts.

Jourard, S. M. (1971), *The Transparent Self*, Van Nostrand Reinhold, New York.

Kron, T. (1981), *The Management of Patient Care*, W. B. Saunders, Philadelphia, Pennsylvania.

Metz, E. L. (1978), Assessing the older psychiatric patient. In: *Mental Health Concepts Applied to Nursing* (ed. Dunlap, L. C.), John Wiley, Chichester, West Sussex.

Peplau, H. E. (1952), *Interpersonal Relations in Nursing*, G. P. Putnam, New York.

Price, B. (1983), Just a few forms to fill in, *Nursing Times*, **79**, No. 44, 26–29.

Rines, A. R., and Montag, M. L. (1976), *Nursing Concepts and Nursing Care*, John Wiley, New York.

Snyder, J. C., and Wilson, M. F. (1977), Elements of a psychological assessment, *American Journal of Nursing*, **77**, No. 2, 235–239.

Ujhely, G. B. (1966), Basic considerations for nurse–patient interaction in the prevention and treatment of emotional disorders, *Nursing Clinics of North America*, **1**, No. 2, 179–186.

Further reading

Campbell, C. (1978), *Nursing Diagnosis and Intervention in Nursing Practice*, John Wiley, New York.

Frijda, N. H. (1982), The meanings of emotional expression. In: *Non-verbal Communication Today* (ed. Key, M. R.), Mouton, Berlin.

Hill, L. (1981), Don't stereotype your patient, *Journal of Practical Nursing*, **31**, No. 8, 34–35.

Joel, L., and Davis, S. (1973), A proposal for baseline data collection for psychiatric care, *Perspectives in Psychiatric Care*, **11**, No. 2, 48–58.

Maguire, P. (1985), Deficiencies in key interpersonal skills. In: *Interpersonal Skills in Nursing Research and Applications* (ed. Kagan, C. M.), Croom Helm, London.

O'Brien, M. (1978), *Communications and Relationships on Nursing*, C. V. Mosby, St Louis, Missouri.

Prange, A. J., and Martin, H. W. (1962), Aids to understanding patients, *American Journal of Nursing*, **62**, 98–100.

Smitherman, C. (1981), *Nursing Actions for Health Promotion*, F. A. Davis, Philadelphia, Pennsylvania.

Tissier, J. (1986), The development of a psychiatric nursing assessment form.

In: *Psychiatric Nursing Research* (ed. Brooking, J.), John Wiley, Chichester, West Sussex.

Tremlett, R. (1977), A dangerous practice, *Nursing Mirror*, **144**, No. 24, 33.

Whyte, L., and Youhill, G. (1984), The nursing process in the care of the mentally ill, *Nursing Times*, **80**, No. 5, 49–51.

Wilkinson, S. (1981), Factors influencing the relationship between the nurse and the client/patient. In: *Process in Clinical Nursing* (eds Leonard, B. J., and Redland, A. R.), Prentice-Hall, Englewood Cliffs, New Jersey.

Wilkinson, T. (1979), The problems and the values of objective nursing observations in psychiatric nursing care, *Journal of Advanced Nursing*, **4**, 151–159.

PLANNING

> '*Some nurses argue that they have always planned nursing care, but their care has been largely based on information gained from the doctor's notes. When using the nursing process nurses collect their own information.*' (Keane, 1981).

A nursing plan provides a guide for individual patient care, the focus being placed on the patient as a person rather than on his illness. Whenever possible, the patient should be actively engaged in the planning process. It is important for the patient to identify what he feels is important for him.

The nursing care plan serves as a basis for communicating information about the nursing needs of a particular patient to other nurses and to other professional members of the team.

In a multi-disciplinary setting, nurses cannot and should not work in isolation. The nursing plan helps nurses to identify their particular contribution to care within the overall treatment plan agreed by the team.

The nursing care plan consists of three main components.

1. Firstly, the patient's needs and problems are stated. Actual and/or potential problems are identified from the assessment data. Some of the problems identified will fall outside the realms of nursing and will need to be referred to the multi-disciplinary team. The nurse is not expected to meet every need or to solve every problem that a patient may have. A great deal of expertise is available within the team. Once identified, needs and problems must be placed in order of priority, with problems relating to survival and safety placed first. The more life threatening that a problem is, the higher its priority must be.

2. Secondly, a goal is written for each of the needs or problems of the patient in terms of the desired outcome. The goal is stated in such a way that the patient's goal achievement can be evaluated in terms of changed behaviour. The goal statement is written in terms of what the patient will do, e.g. Mr Marshall will sit at the table for his meals; Mr Marshall will develop a positive self-image. Goals must be realistic and achievable. In some instances a patient may take considerable time to meet the stated goals. In psychiatric nursing, the achievement of goals will depend on the development of the nurse–patient relationship. It will be essential for the nurse to observe small changes in the patient's goal-seeking behaviour. Reinforcement of adaptive behaviours will let the patient know that he *is* making progress and help to maintain motivation.

Figure 8.1   Nurse building interventions into a plan of care

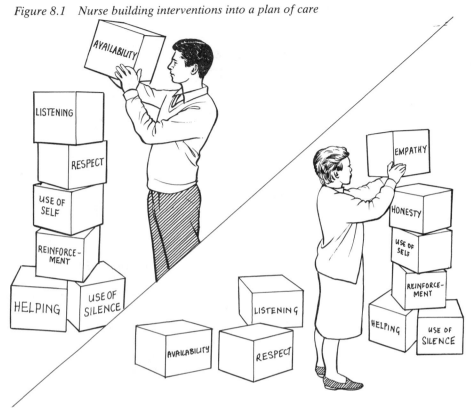

Figure 8.2   Replanning different interventions

3. Thirdly, the nursing orders are written into the care plan. These are statements which describe the prescribed nursing interventions which will be used to help the patient to achieve his goals (*Figure 8.1*). The nursing interventions will incorporate many of the low-visibility functions described in the next section on implementation. The choice of nursing interventions may be decided through discussion with others who can facilitate creative thinking.

In some instances the prescribed nursing interventions may not have the desired effect on the patient's goal achievement. When replanning nursing care, a different set of interventions may be built into the care plan (*Figure 8.2*).

When nursing care is planned, goals are essential for both the patient and the nurse. If nursing interventions are planned, it is easier to assess the achievement of goals so that care may be evaluated.

Without written goal statements, nursing is haphazard and may therefore be less effective. The planning of nursing helps nurses to seek more efficient ways to provide quality care in different health care settings (Bower, 1982).

REFERENCES AND FURTHER READING

References

Bower, F. L. (1982), *The Process of Planning Nursing Care*, 3rd edn, C. V. Mosby, St Louis, Missouri.

Keane, P. (1981), The nursing process in action 4. The nursing process in a psychiatric context, *Nursing Times*, **77**, No. 28, 1223–1224.

Further reading

Barnett, D. (1985), Making your plans work, *Nursing Times*, **81**, No. 2, 24–27.

Castledine, G. (1982), A poor record in writing, *Nursing Mirror*, **154**, No. 22, 31.

Duberley, J. (1979), Giving nursing care. In: *The Nursing Process* (ed. Kratz, C.), Baillière Tindall, London.

Hampshire, G. (1984), Defining goals, *Nursing Times*, **80**, No. 11, 45–46.

Hunt, J. M., and Marks-Maran, D. J. (1980), *Nursing Care Plans. The Nursing Process at Work*, H. M. and M. Publishers, Aylesbury, Buckinghamshire.

Matthews, A. (1986), Patient-centred handovers, *Nursing Times*, **82**, No. 24, 47–48.

Schrock, R. A. (1980), Planning nursing care for the mentally ill, *Nursing Times*, **76**, No. 16, 704–707.

Spradley, B. W. (1981), *Community Health Nursing Concepts and Practice*, Little, Brown, Boston, Massachusetts.

Vitale, B. A., and Schultz, N. V. (1974), *A Problem Solving Approach to Nursing Care Plans: A Program*, C. V. Mosby, St Louis, Missouri.

Wright, S. (1985), Real plans for real patients, *Nursing Times*, **81**, No. 34, 36–38.

IMPLEMENTATION

> '*Nursing is an experience lived between human beings.*' (Paterson and Zderad, 1976).

Implementation is the actual giving of nursing care. The nursing interventions relate to the goals in the nursing care plan and are based on the patient and the problem that he is experiencing.

While nursing interventions refer to the process of acting or doing, many of the skills practised by psychiatric nurses are not readily seen by others. Brown and Fowler (1966) describe nursing functions in terms of visibility and clearly distinguish between high- and low-visibility functions (*Table 8.1*).

Table 8.1   *High- and low-visibility functions*

High-visibility functions	Low-visibility functions
Bed making	Empathising
Aseptic technique	Accepting
Giving an enema	Establishing rapport
Oral hygiene	Being with
Bathing patients	Caring
Feeding patients	Reassurance
Recording blood pressure	Use of self
Giving medication	Love of humanity

Source: Brown and Fowler (1966).

(a) High-visibility functions

High-visibility functions are easily seen by others because they involve the use of manual skills and the manipulation of material objects. High-visibility functions are used in meeting a patient's physiological needs and may easily 'become routinised in a mass production and assembly line fashion'. Brown and Fowler suggest that, because high-visibility actions are readily identifiable and easily broken down into steps, they find their way into the host of procedure books which are to be found in hospitals. Furthermore, high-visibility functions have traditionally been the basis for reward, promotion and evaluation since they are easily controlled by high-status personnel.

(b) Low-visibility functions

Low-visibility functions do not require the employment of material goods and are therefore not easily seen by others.

Low-visibility functions relate to the psychological needs of the patient and require a high degree of cognitive and affective skill. Brown and Fowler suggest that low-visibility functions tend to make a lasting impression on others but that they are difficult to routinise, are less easy to control by high-status personnel as they cannot be broken down into steps and procedurised and traditionally they are not highly rewarded.

Many of the interventions used in psychiatric nursing can be described as low-visibility functions, particularly as psychiatric nursing is not merely a matter of *doing* but more importantly a matter of *being*.

(c) Reporting nursing interventions

In an article on nursing interventions, Anderson (1983) asks, 'What did you do that helped?' She suggests that the nurse who can actually state what he or she did with themselves when with a patient can actually help other members of the multi-disciplinary team to understand what a psychiatric nurse does.

Furthermore, if the nurse is able to specify clearly in the patient's nursing notes what nursing was carried out with the patient, not only does it increase the nurse's accountability but it also reduces the trial-and-error approach to nursing by specifically labelling interventions. Anderson gives an example of how the nurse may meet the goal of 'providing support' for two different patients. The nurse may provide support for Eddie, a withdrawn patient who seems comfortable with silence and having someone physically present, by sitting with him at planned intervals. Support for Robert, another withdrawn patient, may be provided through helping him to interact with others in order to reduce his feelings of isolation. When recording nursing interventions in the nursing notes, if the nurse only writes in general terms 'provided support', this will give little indication of what the nurse actually did to help the patient move towards his desired goals. If the nurse writes for Eddie 'Provided support for Eddie by using physical presence and sitting with him at hourly intervals' and for Robert 'Taught Robert the importance of interacting with others. Sat with him and encouraged him to participate in the small group activities programme', when the nursing notes are read by other nurses, it is then possible to see what the nurse actually did with the patient. If the responses of each patient are also recorded, it is then possible to see the change brought about in the patient's behaviour because of nursing intervention.

Anderson shows that the goal of providing support is met for both patients, but in each instance the nurse uses himself or herself differently. Although both patients are withdrawn, each is a unique individual with different needs and different ways of responding. More skill is required on the part of the nurse in giving a patient support than in performing complicated physical or technical tasks (Travelbee, 1971). Anderson suggests that, if each nurse writes in the nursing notes what she or he actually did with each patient, it will mean not only that a more effective approach can be adopted towards the patient but also that other nurses will be saved from learning by trial and error.

Another example of nursing intervention is providing reassurance for two different patients. The nurse may use touch to provide reassurance for one patient. By placing a hand on his arm or shoulder he may visibly appear to relax. Another patient may be in equal need of reassurance but may prefer not to be touched. Just sitting with this patient, leaning towards him and displaying an open posture may provide reassurances. Again, the most appropriate way of reassuring each patient should be entered in the nursing notes otherwise such statements as 'The patient was reassured' remain vague terms which give no indication as to how reassurance was achieved.

The recording of nursing interventions is important. The nursing notes should indicate the nursing interventions which have taken place for each patient and the effects of the interventions on patients' movements towards goals.

The more that nurses begin to verbalise and write about *nursing*, the nearer they will move towards developing a body of knowledge that is unique to their discipline and based on the reality of nursing practice.

FACT SHEET: SOME NURSING INTERVENTIONS

Examples of some nursing interventions are as follows:

1. *Accepting* another person and welcoming him as a living outcome of all his past experiences, attitudes and feelings and accepting that he is a product of life not always positive or endearing but a life that is ultimately his own (Hein, 1980).
2. *Allowing silence* can give a patient time to find the words that he wants to express (Bradley and Edinberg, 1982).
3. *Attending*, i.e. paying close attention to a patient through eye contact, proximity, posture and other non-verbal behaviours (Bradley and Edinberg, 1982).
4. *Being aware of self*, i.e. understanding the behaviour of others in the light of self-understanding (Burton, 1977).
5. *Being genuine*, i.e. being oneself, the person that you are; using one's total experience as a human being to blend naturally into interactions with patients (Adams, 1980).
6. *Being with* a patient in order to help him (Murray, 1975).
7. *Caring*, i.e. taking time and making an effort for the other person (Robinson, 1983).
8. *Communicating therapeutically*, i.e. communicating purposefully in order to contribute to a patient's recovery and to encourage the patient's participation in the problem-solving process (Marriner, 1983).
9. *Empathising*, i.e. appreciating fully how another person experiences his world (Bradley and Edinberg, 1982).
10. *Establishing rapport*, i.e. creating a sense of harmony between individuals (Murray and Huelskoetter, 1983).
11. *Giving time*, i.e. spending time with a patient when no procedure is being carried out communicates interest and caring to the patient (Blondis and Jackson, 1982).

12. *Health teaching*, i.e. helping a patient to learn what he needs to know in order to maintain or regain health (Ellis and Nowlis, 1981).
13. *Informing*, i.e. allowing a patient's repeated exposure to new information so that he can absorb it thoroughly (Ellis and Nowlis, 1981).
14. *Leading*, i.e. adopting a leadership style that is compatible with the purpose of a group and the feeling of its individual members (Ellis and Nowlis, 1981).
15. *Listening*, i.e. making a voluntary effort to understand what is being said (Burgess and Lazare, 1976).
16. *Modelling*, i.e. showing a patient a particular sequence of behaviour and using reinforcement if he successfully copies the behaviour (Butler and Rosenthall, 1978).
17. *Observing* what is evident about a patient from his mannerisms and style of communicating in order to have a better understanding of him as a person (Burgess and Lazare, 1976).
18. *Using body language*, i.e. placing actions into meaningful patterns to convey understandings (Collins, 1983).
19. *Reassuring* and ensuring that reassurance is based on fact (Burgess and Lazare, 1976).
20. *Problem solving*, i.e. using a step-by-step process of enquiry to facilitate the solution of a problem (Blondis and Jackson, 1982).
21. *Using self-reflection*, i.e. auditing and editing one's own behaviour during nurse–patient relationships (Peplau, 1986).
22. *Shaping*, i.e. allowing desirable behaviour to be built up in small steps by reinforcing only the behaviour which is a little better each time (Butler and Rosenthal, 1978).
23. *Supporting*, i.e. encouraging and promoting a persons's current assets (Grace and Camelleri, 1981).
24. *Talking* and encouraging a patient to talk; talking things over makes people feel better (Burgess and Lazare, 1976).
25. *Applying theory* as an observational framework to explain observed phenomena and to choose interventions (Peplau, 1986).
26. *Touching*; how the nurse touches her patient says a great deal about how she feels about him (Blondis and Jackson, 1982).
27. *Validating*, i.e. verifying inferences with other nurses; consensual validating of inferences of patients (Peplau, 1986).

REFERENCES AND FURTHER READING

References

Adams, D. M. (1980), Establishing therapeutic relationships. In: *Psychiatric Nursing, A Basic Text* (ed. Pothier, P. C.), Little, Brown, Boston, Massachusetts.

Anderson, M. L. (1983), Nursing interventions. What did you do that helped? *Perspectives in Psychiatric Care*, **21**, No. 1, 4–8.

Blondis, M. N., and Jackson, B. E. (1982), *Non-verbal Communication with Patients*, John Wiley, Chichester, West Sussex.

Bradley, J. C., and Edinberg, M. A. (1982), *Communication in the Nursing Context*, Appleton Century Crofts, Norwalk, Connecticut.

Brown, M. M., and Fowler, G. R. (1966), *Psychodynamic Nursing*, W. B. Saunders, Philadelphia, Pennsylvania.

Burgess, A. W., and Lazare, A. (1976), *Psychiatric Nursing in the Hospital and the Community*, Prentice-Hall, Englewood Cliffs, New Jersey.

Burton, G. (1977), *Interpersonal Relations*, 4th edn, Tavistock, London.

Butler, R. J., and Rosenthal, G. (1978), *Behaviour and Rehabilitation*, John Wright, Bristol.

Collins, M. (1983), *Communication in Health Care*, C. V. Mosby, St Louis, Missouri.

Ellis, J. R., and Nowliss, E. A. (1981), *Nursing, A Human Needs Approach*, Houghton Mifflin, Boston, Massachusetts.

Grace, H. K., and Camelleri, D. (1981), *Mental Health Nursing, A Socio-Psychological Approach*, Wm. C. Brown, Dubuque, Iowa.

Hein, E. C. (1980), *Communication in Nursing Practice*, 2nd edn, Little, Brown, Boston, Massachusetts.

Marriner, A. (1983), *The Nursing Process*, C. V. Mosby, St Louis, Missouri.

Murray, R. (1975), *Nursing Concepts for Health Promotion*, Prentice-Hall, Englewood Cliffs, New Jersey.

Murray, R. B., and Huelskoetter, M. M. W. (1983), *Psychiatric Mental Health Nursing: Giving Emotional Care*, Prentice-Hall, Englewood Cliffs, New Jersey.

Paterson, J. G., and Zderad, L. T. (1976), *Humanistic Nursing*, John Wiley, Chichester, West Sussex.

Peplau, H. E. (1986), A celebration of skills, Paper presented at the Third International Congress of Psychiatric Nursing, Imperial College, London.

Robinson, L. (1983), *Psychiatric Nursing as a Human Experience*, W. B. Saunders, Philadelphia, Pennsylvania.

Travelbee, J. (1971), *Interpersonal Aspects of Nursing*, 2nd edn, F. A. Davis, Philadelphia, Pennsylvania.

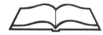

Further reading

Cooper, S. (1981), What is nursing?, *Nursing Times, Occasional Papers*, **77**, No. 34, 136.

Dirterle, J. A. (1983), Clinical validation of psychiatric nursing skills, *Journal of Nursing Education*, **22**, No. 9, 392–394.

Glass, H. (1983), Intervention in nursing: goals or task orientated, *International Nursing Review*, **30**, No. 2, 52–56.

Henderson, V. (1978), The concept of nursing, *Journal of Advanced Nursing*, **3**, 75–84.

McMahon, R. A. (1986), Nursing as a therapy, *Professional Nurse*, **1**, No. 10, 270–272.

Perry, J. (1985), Has the discipline of nursing developed to the stage where nurses do 'think nursing'?, *Journal of Advanced Nursing*, **10**, 31–37.

Schoenhofer, S. O. (1984), Support as legitimate nursing action, *Nursing Outlook*, **32**, No. 4, 218–219.

EVALUATION

> '*When looking at the effectiveness of nursing care we cannot omit the appraisal of the patient himself.*' (Dye, 1963).

Evaluation is the phase of the nursing process in which the nurse determines the effectiveness of nursing care in helping the patient to achieve the stated goals. In order to evaluate the quality of nursing care, it is necessary to be very clear about what nursing *is*, and to distinguish nursing from interventions by other members of the multi-disciplinary team. Bergman (1982) sees nursing care as 'the sum of interventions by nursing personnel, for the purpose of achieving (i.e. attaining, maintaining or recovering) the optimal health status of individuals, groups or communities'.

By differentiating nursing from the contributions of other health care workers within the multi-disciplinary setting, nurses are able to examine their own particular discipline more closely.

Like other phases of the nursing process, evaluation is a dynamic ongoing activity. It is not something that happens just because the patient is being discharged. Evaluation must occur periodically, so that the nursing care plan and interventions can be altered or modified to meet the patient's changing needs.

If each goal is accompanied by a date which it is expected that the goal will be achieved, the patient's progress can be monitored. Goals will need to be examined on predetermined dates.

To evaluate the effectiveness of care, the nurse must return to the goal statements of the nursing care plan and compare these statements with the patient's changed behaviour. The data baseline behaviours from the initial assessment are compared with present behavioural patterns to determine the patient's progress. The nursing notes can also be used for making comparisons, particularly if the nursing actions have been recorded accurately in relation to the set objectives.

Whenever possible, the patient and his family or those people of significance to him should be encouraged to participate in the evaluation as well as other members of the multi-disciplinary team who may be able to give additional information.

Lowe (1984) suggests that there are three elements which can be studied in evaluation.

1. *Structure evaluation* involves examination of the setting in which care is given. This includes factors such as numbers and grades of staff, patient dependency and management style.
2. *Process evaluation* focuses on nurses and what they do. A patient may be observed while he is receiving care or a nurse may be observed while giving care (concurrent process evaluation). Evidence that nursing care was given to a satisfactory standard may be obtained by examining nursing records after a patient has been discharged (retrospective evaluation).
3. *Outcome evaluation* focuses on the patient and patient's outcomes. The actual outcome of care is compared with the patient's goals. Lowe (1984) states that outcome evaluation can be carried out concurrently or retrospectively. Concurrent outcome evaluation takes place while the patient is receiving care, while retrospective outcome evaluation takes place after discharge.

Evaluation should be as objective as possible. Facts need to be considered, rather than opinions. Weaknesses, as well as strengths, should be revealed and acted on.

If a patient has failed to meet the set objectives or has only partially met them, it may be necessary to change or modify the nursing care plan, to examine the use of different nursing strategies or to reassess his needs and problems.

It cannot be suggested that evaluation is an easy process. Concrete activities are much more easily appraised than the less tangible low-visibility functions involved in developing and maintaining nurse–patient relationships in a psychiatric setting.

Nursing models may of course influence the kind of information which is sought in evaluation (Lowe, 1984). For example Orem's model focuses on the patient's ability to manage his own self-care, while Peplau's developmental model focuses on the personal growth which has occurred for both patient and nurse (see Chapter 7).

Nevertheless, a willingness to examine nursing care critically, together with a willingness to learn and implement change where necessary, can only serve to enhance future nursing practice.

REFERENCES AND FURTHER READING

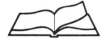

References

Bergman, R. (1982), Evaluation of nursing care—could it make a difference?, *International Journal of Nursing Studies*, **19**, No. 2, 53–60.

Dye, M. C. (1963), Clarifying patient's communication, *American Journal of Nursing*, **63**, 56–59.

Lowe, K. (1984), The fourth step of the nursing process evaluation. In: *A Systematic Approach to Nursing Care*, Open University, Milton Keynes, Buckinghamshire.

Further reading

Ceccio, J. F., and Ceccio, C. M. (1982), *Effective Communication in Nursing: Theory and Practice*, John Wiley, New York.

Hargreaves, I. (1975), The nursing process. The key to individualised care, *Nursing Times, Occasional Papers*, **71**, No. 35, 89–92.

Kron, T. (1981), *The Management of Patient Care*, W. B. Standard.

Luker, K. (1979), Evaluating nursing care. In: *The Nursing Process* (ed. Kratz, C.), Baillière Tindall, London.

Open University (1984), *A Systematic Approach to Nursing Care*, Open University, Milton Keynes, Buckinghamshire.

Waters, K. (1986), Cause and effect, *Nursing Times*, **82**, No. 5, 28–30.

Chapter 9

The nurse's role in group therapy

'No man can come to know himself except as an outcome of disclosing himself to another person.' (Jourard, 1971).

INTRODUCTION

Note that the terms nurse, therapist and leader are used interchangeably in this chapter.

The treatment of patients with psychiatric or emotional problems usually involves a number of different methods. Group therapy is one such method employed in both in-patient and out-patient settings which enables valuable insight to be given to one patient by another.

Group therapy is a controlled interactive interventive process which is conducted in small groups. The focus is placed on group interactions, and the emotional energy generated is directed towards change in the behaviour of individual group members (McManama, 1983).

People experience many emotional difficulties in every-day life—feelings of loneliness, isolation, rejection, unworthiness and problems of relating to others to form meaningful relationships.

Group therapy enables patients to work through their problems in the presence of others, to observe how group members react to their behaviour and to try out new and more adaptive ways of behaving.

Group involvement can provide a patient with valuable learning experiences which encourage him to develop greater self-understanding and help him to gain a different perspective of his problems. He is able to learn that his problems are similar to the problems experienced by others; through contact with other group members, he is able to learn new ways of approaching and solving these problems. The problem-solving skills learned within the group enable the patient to function more independently outside the group by enhancing his individual worth, relieving distress and increasing insight. Not only is he able to receive help but also he is able to give help as well.

While individual therapy can help a person to overcome some of his problems, group therapy offers wider experience for application to every-day life and the therapist has the advantage of being able to help several patients at one time.

SELECTION OF GROUP MEMBERS

The selection of group members should reflect the purpose for which a group has been designed. There needs to be some degree of homogeneity in the group so that objectives will reflect the patients' capacities and needs; personalities and problems should match sufficiently that group members can learn from one another without feeling isolated or estranged (Marram, 1978). At the same

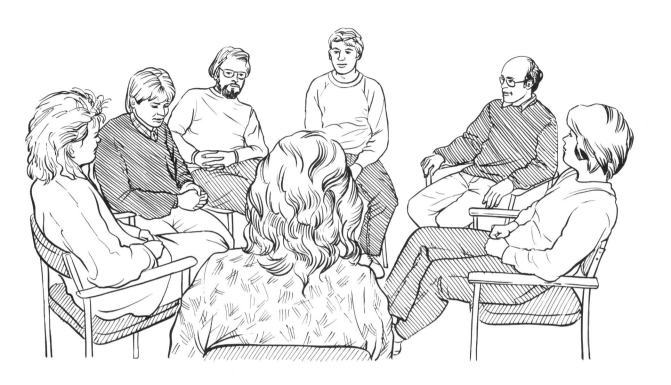

time the assembled personalities should reflect a variety of the problems found in every-day life situations so that members can locate a basis for identification and similarity.

The patient who is selected for group membership should be prepared for the experience by being given an explanation of what to expect. He will be inadequately prepared if he is just told that he is going to join a group without knowing what to expect or what is expected of him.

Grace and Camilleri (1981) propose the following explanations. 'Through talking to others, you will learn how to manage difficulties similar to yours' or 'Through participating in the group, you should be able to gain new understandings of how your behaviour affects others'. The patient must be told that the group, rather than the therapist, is the potential source of help, that he will be expected to communicate his feelings and problems and that a change in behaviour is the expected outcome for all group members.

If the patient is expected to take the risk of joining a group, the potential value of the experience must outweigh the cost of revealing himself in the group setting. The appropriateness of the group as a form of therapy for the individual must be assessed as well as the suitability of the individual for the group. Not all patients benefit therapeutically from groups, although this does not mean that they should be precluded from groups at a future date. In determining the suitability of members for a group, the nurse needs to assess a patient's thinking patterns; if he is deluded or hallucinated, others may not understand what he is saying. If he has a poor self-concept and low self-esteem, he may be easily hurt by critical feedback, however well meant. The withdrawn patient may feel threatened and block others attempts to know him or the suspicous patient may take offence easily and react with hostility and aloofness (Marram, 1978).

(a) Group size

The number of members selected depends on the purpose of the group. Groups which are too large or too small should be avoided. The optimum size for a group may be between six and ten members although the therapist may include one or two extra members in case someone drops out. Enough members must be present for free and spontaneous interaction to occur but, if numbers are too large, then the therapist will not be able to observe the relationships and reaction between members.

(b) Length and frequency of sessions

The length of sessions should be determined from the very beginning. If the sessions are too short, members may feel frustrated and lack a sense of achievement; if the sessions are too long, members may lose interest and find the groups exhausting. 1–2 hours is the usual length of time devoted to group therapy sessions. It must also be decided how frequently the group will meet, and the number of sessions to be held during the lifetime of the group.

(c) Type of group

The therapist needs to decide whether the groups are going to be open or closed. In a closed group, no new members are accepted once the group starts and, if a member leaves, he is not replaced. In an open group, new members are admitted and, over a period of time, there may be a complete turn-over of membership.

(d) Physical setting

The room chosen for group sessions should be free from noise and distractions. Such things as room temperature, acoustics and lighting need to be taken into consideration when arranging a suitable setting for the group. Chairs should be placed in a circle, so that each group member is in full view of the others. In this way, there is no obvious staff position.

While the physical setting is important, it does not make up for the therapist's ability to create an atmosphere and interpersonal exchange that facilitates self-disclosure (Marram, 1978).

STARTING A GROUP

Like other health professionals, the nurse may work with many different kinds of group. The nurse may function as the group therapist or act as a cotherapist working closely with another member of the health care team, such as the psychiatrist, psychologist or social worker.

Working in groups requires special preparation and training. While group therapy is largely based on the same theoretical principles as individual therapy, it has different dimensions and addresses itself to problems not always met in individual therapy. The nurse needs not only to learn through first-hand experience what it is like to be a member of a group but also to develop the skills to facilitate effective group change and to meet the demands and responsibilities of group work by working under the direction of an experienced supervisor.

Every new group goes through the process of developing as a group. Members are likely to experience increased tension and feelings of apprehension at the beginning but, after a period of orientation, these feelings generally diminish.

A period of orientation is important as it enables members to get to know each other and to learn each other's names. It also allows the therapist to work towards establishing a sense of rapport with group members. Groups usually progress from discussion of safe superficial subjects to matters of more emotional concern. The nurse must not consider that the superficial matters raised are a waste of time, simply because the group is not yet addressing itself to its real work (Ellis and Nowlis, 1981). Although trust and acceptance take time to establish, they are essential if members are to engage in self-disclosure during the working phase of the group. Members must be allowed to proceed at their own pace and should not be expected to deal with emotionally important areas prematurely (Yalom and Terrazas, 1968).

Group norms develop early in the course of a group and, once established, are difficult to change. A group norm is an expectancy regarding what is considered to be appropriate standard of behaviour for members (Hollander, 1981). Examples of norm that develop in groups are related to punctuality, mode of dress and topics which may or may not be discussed, safety and confidentiality in the group.

WORKING PHASE

As each person becomes more comfortable in the group situation, an atmosphere of mutual trust develops and members show a willingness to become involved with each other. As the group evolves, members experience a sense of belonging and cohesiveness and the amount of influence that members have over each other increases.

Group pressure is an effective way of bringing about behavioural change as the patient is far more likely to learn to modify his behaviour in response to the demands of the group than he is to respond to the demands of the individual nurse (Eisenberg and Abbot, 1967).

The goals of the therapist are different from those of group members. The therapist is interested in facilitating interaction between members to enable the group to engage in the problem-solving process. The therapist must not assume a superior position or adopt an authoritarian leadership role (see the boxed section entitled 'Leadership in groups' at the end of this chapter) in which responsibility is taken on for making decisions on behalf of members. Instead the therapist much reflect each patient's questions and comments back to the patient himself and to the group, asking for their reaction. The therapist needs to have a positive attitude to members' contributions even when some members' contributions may seem irrelevant. It is essential to create an atmosphere in which members feel that they can contribute.

There are some patients who do not want to have the responsibility and freedom to make their own decisions, as it is far easier for them to look to someone else to solve their problems. When they find that the therapist is not providing solutions, they will be forced to look for a different authority, that of the group itself (Smith, 1970).

Table 9.1   Roles adopted by group members

Role	Characteristics
The silent one	Does not talk or contribute
The monopoliser	Does all the talking and takes up a greater proportion of group time than other members
The conformist	Always agrees with others. Never expresses conflicting ideas
The scapegoat	Gets blamed by the others
The blocker	Does anything to keep the group from achieving its goals
The non-conformist	Will do anything to be different and to stand out in the group
The bored one	Is bored by the whole thing
The bore	Labours on a topic and bores everybody else
The opposition leader	Opposes the leader and works towards acquiring influence and power
The playmate	Sees the group as a social event. Refuses to focus on the goals of the group
The insignificant one	Ideas are disregarded by others
The expert	Knowledgeable. Opinions sought by others
The help seeker	Uses group to gain sympathy
The fool	Is not taken seriously
The debunker	Puts down other people's ideas but does not offer any contributions
The important person	Highly regarded. Respected
The aggressor	Acts negatively and denigrates others contributions

Adapted from Pffeifer and Jones (1977), Sampson and Marthas (1981) and Smith (1965).

During the working phase of the group, members may assume many different roles (*Table 9.1*). These roles may be assigned to individuals by members of the group. Interpretation of these various roles by group members may help an individual member to learn how he is perceived by others and may provide a valuable learning experience towards behavioural change. Because of the use of various defence mechanisms, not all members will behave appropriately or admit the need for the group experience. A member may resist participating verbally or make excuses to avoid meetings; the nurse will have to weigh up the advantages of keeping this member in the group, because the member may gain little growth within the group, and his behaviour may be detrimental to the group at large (Marram, 1978).

Throughout the working phase the type of attitude that the nurse needs to adopt is one which expresses to the group realistic, hopeful and therapeutic expectations for success and change (Kreigh and Perko, 1983). It is important to keep the group focused on these goals and to bear in mind that the nurse's own behaviour provides a powerful modelling force for group members.

TERMINATION

Eventually all groups must come to an end. Participants in an open and loosely structured short-term group may feel less a sense of loss than a closed and closely knit cohesive group. Members will come to terms with any sense of loss more easily if termination is planned from the beginning. Some members may feel a profound sense of loss when the group comes to an end, and there may be episodes of regression in some members. The therapist should provide members with the opportunity to express their feelings and to gain some perspective about their separation from the group. While it may seem logical for the therapist to equate members' sense of loss with other losses in the past the therapist must be aware of the risk in raising post-issues, particularly if there is no time to work through painful memories that arise. It may be better to focus on the present feelings that members have about the termination of the group, and the progress made (Marram, 1978).

DEALING WITH PARTICULAR PROBLEMS WITHIN THE GROUP

One of the nurse's important responsibilities is to allow the group freedom of expression, and this will mean dealing with anger. There may be occasions when the nurse will be the focus of a member's anger. While it is very threatening to be the object of another person's anger, it is unwise to retaliate. The nurse needs to feel secure enough to accept the patient's anger, to recognise its meaning and to understand that everybody feels anger at times, particularly when a goal is blocked or interfered with in some way.

As a first step towards helping the member to deal with his anger the nurse must come to terms with his or her own feelings towards the anger and to recognise that the angry individual needs to do something to expend the energy generated by the anger by expressing the emotion behind it (Rosenfeld, 1969). The group milieu is beneficial to the patient as he is able to ventilate a wide range of pent-up emotions in a safe protected environment, whereas this would not be acceptable in more usual social settings.

The monopolising patient often presents a problem in the group setting as he tends to dominate the discussion and to meet his own needs through excessive verbal output. His incessant talk may either cause other members to withdraw with a subsequent build-up of anger for which they have no release or give some members an excuse for not participating (Eisenberg and Abbot, 1967). The nurse must stop the monopolist from consuming all the group time; otherwise, members cannot benefit from the group. He must not be ridiculed or threatened in any way or other members may be afraid to speak for fear of similar treatment (Yalom and Terrazas, 1968). The person should be given the opportunity to become aware of himself in relation to others and to explore more appropriate forms of behaviour. Adams (1983) suggests four interventions which may be appropriate when a member monopolises the group.

1. *Supportive interruption*. 'You've made an important point—perhaps we could get some views about your ideas from other members.'
2. *Reflection*. 'Are you aware that no one else is talking?'
3. *Interpretation*. 'I don't know what you mean; perhaps you're anxious about something.'
4. *Confrontation*. 'Could you be quiet for a while? I wonder why the group is allowing itself to be monopolised?'

When confrontation is used, it must be timed appropriately; the patient must be emotionally ready to acknowledge the nurse's observations. Premature confrontation can inhibit rather than facilitate a therapeutic reaction because it disrupts the nurse–patient relationship. When confrontation is used appropriately, it can provide a valuable learning experience for the patient (Bromley, 1981).

Silence can present another problem. Silence requires skilled intervention in the group setting. Silence may describe the behaviour of the whole group or a single member. The nurse should bear in mind that communication occurs all the time in a group, even when members are silent (McManama, 1983). Therefore the nurse must try to assess the kind of silence being presented in order to decide on the most appropriate intervention. The silence may be reflective and relaxed or tense and awkward. If the silence is reflective, the best intervention is usually none at all; however, if the silence is awkward and uncomfortable, the nurses may feel that, by using words to manage the silence, discomfort will be relieved and group participation restored.

If a quiet patient is placed in a group, he may perceive himself as inferior because he feels unable to compete with others. If he is singled out and asked to speak, he may feel threatened and guilty because his silent behaviour is exposed before others. The quiet patient usually needs more time to build up the confidence to communicate verbally within the group.

If appropriate, the nurse may offer the patient the opportunity to contribute to the group in a non-threatening way by asking for his thoughts about what is happening in the group. This will show the patient that he is recognised as an individual, that his thoughts or opinions are important to the group and that the nurse is aware of the patient's silence.

When the patient feels accepted and understood by the nurse, he may find it easier to participate more actively in the group.

Finally, transference is a concept which occurs not only in groups, but also in one-to-one relationships. Transference in groups describes members unconscious tendencies to relate to the therapist in terms of some qualities they require people in authority to possess, although these are not usually the qualities the therapist actually possesses (Sampson and Marthas, 1981). By using transference, feelings and thoughts from former experiences in life may be conveyed to members of the group. If the therapist is able to provide a touch of reality to members' perceptions, then greater self-awareness may lead to an understanding of how present situations can be distorted in terms of past events.

LEADERSHIP IN GROUPS

Leadership styles vary, and each has its strengths and weaknesses. A leadership style can be said to be most effective when it is compatible with the purpose of a group and the feelings of its individual members (Ellis and Nowlis, 1981).

The leader's function is to help members to explore, validate and clarify thoughts and feelings so that seemingly insurmountable problems are reduced to realistic and manageable proportions and verifiable solutions (Dye and Pothier, 1980). The leader must have infinite patience and a willingness to emphathise with others, as well as the qualities of self-understanding and inner strength and a genuine desire to help members who respond with anger, sarcasm and disruptive behaviour.

During the orientation period of the group, Pasquali et al. (1981) suggest that the leader needs to adopt a moderately authoritative role, to enable group members to receive some direction. As members begin to feel a sense of trust and confidence in the leader, the leader relinquishes this role in order to facilitate interaction between group members. It is important for the leader to be sensitive to the feelings and meanings expressed by the group and to accept the group where it is now. The leader must also accept each member's degree of participation, confront members in a caring way and provide constructive feedback without attacking members' defences.

The leader must work to maintain a viable atmosphere so that all group members feel comfortable enough to work constructively (Dye and Pothier, 1980).

REFERENCES AND FURTHER READING

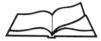

References

Adams, C. G. (1983), Group approaches. In: *Handbook of Psychiatric Mental Health Nursing* (eds Adams, C. G., and Macione, A.), A Wiley Red Book, John Wiley, Chichester, West Sussex.

Bromley, G. E. (1981), Confrontation in individual psychotherapy, *Journal of Psychiatric Nursing and Mental Health Services*, **19**, No. 5, 15–18.

Dye, C. A., and Pothier, P. C. (1980), Establishing therapeutic groups. In: *Psychiatric Nursing. A Basic Text*, Little, Brown, Boston, Massachusetts.

Eisenberg, J., and Abbot, R. (1967). The monopolising patient in group psychotherapy, *Perspectives in Psychiatric Care*, **6**, No. 2, 66–69.

Ellis, J. R., and Nowlis, E. A. (1981), *Nursing, A Human Needs Approach*, Houghton Mifflin, Boston, Massachusetts.

Grace, H. K., and Camilleri, D. (1981), *Mental Health Nursing, A Socio-Psychological Approach*, Wm. C. Brown, Dubuque, Iowa.

Hollander, E. P. (1981), *Principles and Methods of Social Psychology*, 4th edn, Oxford University Press, Oxford.

Jourard, S. M. (1971), *The Transparent Self*, Van Nostrand Reinhold, New York.

Kreigh, H. Z., and Perko, J. E. (1983), *Psychiatric and Mental Health Nursing*, 2nd edn, Reston Publishing, Reston, Virginia.

Marram, G. D. (1978), *The Group Approach in Nursing Practice*, 2nd edn, C. V. Mosby, St Louis, Missouri.

McManama, D. (1983), Working with groups. In: *Psychiatric Nursing as a Human Experience* (ed. Robinson, L.), W. B. Saunders, Philadelphia, Pennsylvania,

Pasquali, E. A., Alesi, E. G., Arnold, H. M., and DeBasio, N. (1981), *Mental Health Nursing: A Bio-psycho-cultural Approach*, C. V. Mosby, St Louis, Missouri.

Pffeifer, J. W., and Jones, J. E. (1977), *A Handbook of Structured Experiences for Human Relations Training*, Vol. VI, University Associates, California.

Rosenfeld, E. M. (1969), Intervening in hostile behaviour through dyadic and/or group intervention, *Journal of Psychiatric Nursing and Mental Health Services*, **7**, No. 6, 251–254.

Sampson, E. E., and Marthas, M. (1981), *Group Process for the Health Professions*, 2nd edn, John Wiley, Chichester, West Sussex.

Smith, A. J. (1970), A manual for the training of psychiatric nursing personnel in group psychotherapy, *Perspectives in Psychiatric Care*, **8**, No. 3, 107.

Smith, W. S. (1965), *Group Problem Solving through Discussion*, Bobbs–Merrill, Indianapolis, Indiana.

Malom, I. E., and Terrazas, F. (1968), Group therapy for psychotic elderly patients. In: *Psychiatric/Mental Health Nursing: Contemporary Readings* (eds Backer, B. A., Dubbert, P. M., and Eisenman, E. J. P.), Van Nostrand, New York, pp. 257–265.

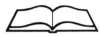

Further reading

Affonso, D. D. (1985), Therapeutic support during in-patient group therapy, *Journal of Psychiatric Nursing and Mental Health Services*, **23**, No. 11, 21–25.

Bloch, S., and Crouch, E. (1985), *Therapeutic Factors in Group Psychotherapy*, Oxford University Press, Oxford, 1985.

Brown, M. M., and Fowler, G. R. (1966), *Psychodynamic Nursing*, W. B. Saunders, Philadelphia, Pennsylvania.

Burrows, R. (1985), Group therapy, *Nursing Mirror*, **160**, No. 14, 41–43.

Cohen, R. G., and Lipkin, G. B. (1979), *Therapeutic Group Work for Health Professions*, Springer, New York.

Hargreaves, A. G., and Robinson, A. M. (1950), The nurse leader in group psychotherapy. In: *A Collection of Classics in Psychiatric Nursing Literature* (eds Smoyak, S. A., and Rouslin, S.), Charles B. Slack, New Jersey.

Platt-Koch, L. M. (1986), Clinical supervision for psychiatric nurses, *Journal of Psychiatric Nursing and Mental Health Services*, **24**, No. 1, 6–15.

Rogers, C. (1971), Carl Rogers describes his way of facilitating encounter groups, *American Journal of Nursing*, **71**, No. 2, 275–279.

Thomson, S., and Khan, J. H. (1976), *The Group Process as a Helping Technique*, Pergamon, Oxford.

Ward, J. T. (1974), The sounds of silence: group psychotherapy with non-verbal patients, *Perspectives in Psychiatric Care*, **12**, No. 1, 13–19.

Chapter 10

The nurse's therapeutic role in physical treatments and procedures

'The procedures nurses carry out must never be allowed to take precedence over the very human beings for whom these activities are performed. There is no nursing procedure that is not accompanied by a word or an unspoken message. It is the patient's understanding of that message that influences the outcome of the procedure.' (Blondis and Jackson, 1982).

INTRODUCTION

The nurse may be involved in a number of physical treatments and procedures. These may range from administering medicines, assisting with electroconvulsive therapy (ECT) to carrying out basic care techniques or preparing a patient for investigative procedures.

   The role of the nurse in physical treatments cannot be underestimated. The nurse has the opportunity to make any treatment or procedure less anxiety provoking and therefore more acceptable to the patient. The nursing procedure has been likened to a script for a play (*Figure 10.1*). If the nurse and patient are viewed as the main performers in a shared situation, then it is essentially the nurse's role that can enhance the well-being of the patient. The nurse is able to direct the play, to manage the setting and to influence the cast of characters (Paterson and Zderad, 1976).

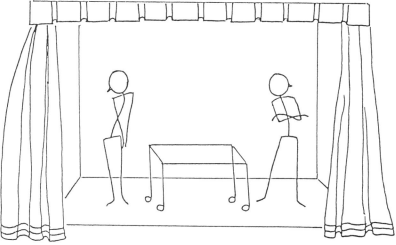

Figure 10.1   Enacting the nursing procedure. After Sarbin and Hardyck (1953)

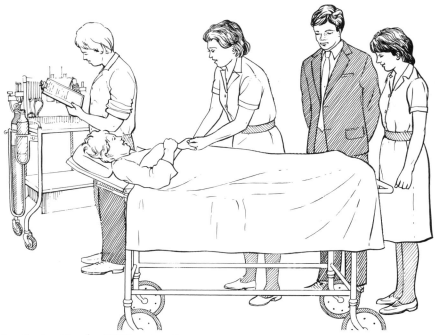

A patient waiting for ECT treatment

REASSURANCE OF PATIENT

The humanistic qualities of the nurse can promote the patient's well-being although, as well as demonstrating such qualities as kindness and compassion, the nurse must demonstrate technical competence. The patient cannot be reassured unless he observes that the nurse is an efficient and safe practitioner.

To reassure a patient prior to treatment, the nurse must try to ascertain his areas of concern. This is best achieved by listening rather than talking (Smith, 1972). Sometimes a patient will have misconceptions about a treatment which he is to receive. If he is able to discuss these misconceptions with a nurse whom he trusts, he may feel reassured by being given the correct information. Sincerity, honesty and warmth of feeling towards the patient are essential and he should never be told that a procedure such as an intramuscular injection 'won't hurt a bit'. Not only does this show a disregard for his feelings but also it is unlikely to gain his trust. Reassurance can only be experienced by the patient when he feels respected and understood by the nurse, who then assists him to recognise and develop his own resources in order to restore his self-confidence.

ELECTROCONVULSIVE THERAPY

One of the more controversial treatments used in psychiatry is ECT. It is essential for nurses to come to terms with their own feelings about ECT; otherwise the nurse's anxiety may be transmitted to the patient. ECT is most frequently given for severe depression and in some instances may be preferred to treatment with anti-depressants. Severe depression has a toll not only on the patient but also on his family and in some instances the doctor may consider the quicker results obtained with ECT desirable.

ECT involves giving a general anaesthetic and, although legally it is the doctor's responsibility to explain the treatment and to obtain consent, the patient will often require further information from the nurse. The way in which the nurse gives this information must be reflected by the patient's current problems, his intellectual capacity and his social background. It is easy to under-explain a procedure to a patient who conveys an air of sophistication or who dismisses the event as not being a cause of worry (Aasterud, 1973).

Some patients worry about having a general anaesthetic. If a patient who is about to have ECT asks the nurse, 'How many patients die from this treatment?', it is doubtful that he is seeking factual or statistical information; he may possibly have underlying fears about dying which he desperately needs to talk about (Gregg, 1955). If the nurse responds with a factual answer, this will convey to the patient that his underlying fears have not been understood. He may refrain from pursuing the matter any further, because the nurse's blocking mechanisms have denied him the opportunity to express his feelings. It is therefore essential for the nurse to be alert to both the verbal and the non-verbal cues that the patient presents and to respond appropriately.

The patient may also be concerned about the temporary confusion and memory loss that occurs after ECT. If the patient is told that this is usually of brief duration, he may not necessarily feel reassured. He may feel more comforted if he knows that he can rely on a nurse whom he trusts for clarification and maintenance of his safety. For any treatment or procedure to be acceptable to the patient, it may well depend on how something is done rather than on what is done (*Figure 10.2*). The effective nurse will recognise that particular interventions are called for at a given moment. The need for human touch is often heightened when a patient is anxious, and it is often the unspoken activities that are of prime importance at times of stress.

Procedural interventions		**Humanistic interventions**	
Technique	Treadmill	Amiable	Courteous
Routine	Second nature	Warm	Understanding
Method	Bureaucratic rigmarole	Kindly	Clement
Practice	Wont	Compassionate	Well meaning
System	Convention	Helpful	Attentive
Mode	Protocol	Good natured	Respectful
Rote	Formality	Gentle	Empathic
Style	Red tape	Benevolent	Forbearing
Ways and means	Regulation	Tender	Tolerant
Habitude	Consuetude	Lenient	Accepting
Regulation	Line of action	Generous	Condolent
Custom	Measure	Beneficient	Patient
Rut	Process	Gracious	Magnanimous
Rule	Policy	Sympathetic	Forgiving
Order	Plan of action	Charitable	Kind hearted
Pattern	Ritual	Considerate	Obliging
		Thoughtful	Accommodating

Figure 10.2   Procedural and humanistic interventions. After Rodale (1979)

GIVING MEDICINE

Giving medicines is a nursing activity that occurs not only daily but several times a day. Whatever the chemical formula of a drug, its placebo effects also need to be considered. The overall effectiveness of treatment depends just as much on creating the right conditions as it does on the doctor's choice of drug (Crammer *et al.*, 1978). Not only will the nurse as a person influence the beneficial properties of a drug but also the size, colour and shape of tablets may have some bearing on the desired effects. The nurse who has positive attitudes can influence the outcome of a drug favourably; however, negative attitudes on the part of the nurse may prevent a drug from achieving its full potential.

Undoubtedly, drug therapy plays an important part in the treatment of many mentally ill patients, and the nurse is able to teach patients about matters concerning their medication. Problems of non-compliance are frequently reported in the nursing literature. There are two main reasons why patients fail to take their medication, once discharged from hospital: firstly, the importance of continuing to take medication even when symptoms are no longer experienced may not have been sufficiently emphasised; secondly, the patient may not know what side effects to expect and may discontinue his medication as soon as side effects occur (Smith, 1981).

SIDE EFFECTS OF DRUGS

The patient should be educated about the side effects of the drug that he is taking and he must understand the importance of continuing with his medication to prevent the recurrence of symptoms. Teaching the patient about his medication is not something that should be left until the moment of discharge; it is far better if such education is incorporated into daily interactions with the patient. The nurse also has the opportunity to point out the possible dangers of self-medication, the inadvisability of taking alcohol with drugs, and the need to omit certain foods from the diet in conjunction with monoamine-oxidase inhibitor drugs.

REFERENCES AND FURTHER READING

References

Aasterud, M. (1963), Explanation to the patient, *Nursing Forum*, **2**, No. 4, 36–34.

Blondis, M. N., and Jackson, B. E. (1982), *Non-verbal Communication with Patients*, John Wiley, Chichester, West Sussex.

Cranmer, J., Barraclough, B., and Heine, B. (1978), *The Use of Drugs in Psychiatry*, Gaskell, London.

Gregg, D. (1955), Reassurance, *American Journal of Nursing*, **55**, 171–174.

Paterson, J. G., and Zderad, L. T. (1976), *Humanistic Nursing*, John Wiley, Chichester, West Sussex.

Sarbin, T. R., and Hardyck, C. D. (1953), cited by Argyle, M. (1972), *The Psychology of Interpersonal Behaviour*, Penguin, Harmondsworth, Middlesex.

Smith, E. (1972), Reassure the patient, *Nursing Times*, **68**, No. 42, 1334–1335.

Smith, J. (1981), Improving drug knowledge in psychiatric patients, *Journal of Psychiatric Nursing and Mental Health Services*, **19**, No. 4, 16–18.

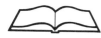

Further reading

Coohran, C. C. (1984), A change of mind about ECT, *American Journal of Nursing*, **84**, 1004–1005.

Hein, E., and Leavitt, M. (1977), Providing emotional support to patients, *Nursing (US)*, **7**, No. 5, 38–41.

Jourard, S. M. (1971), *The Transparent Self*, Van Nostrand Reinhold, New York.

Kyes, J. J., and Hofling, C. K. (1980), *Basic Psychiatric Concepts in Nursing*, J. B. Lippincott, Philadelphia, Pennsylvania.

Lindsay, M. (1981), The fantasy and reality of ECT, *Nursing (UK)*, **30**, 1337–1340.

Mawson, D. (1985), Shock waves, *Nursing Times*, **81**, No. 46, 42, 44.

Northcott, N. (1985), A day in bed, *Nursing Mirror*, **160**, No. 1, 24–25.

Paterson, J. G. (1976), The placebo effect, nursing implications, *Nursing Digest*, **4**, No. 4, 15–16.

RCN (1982), *Nursing Guidelines for ECT*, Royal College of Nursing, London.

Silverstone, T., and Turner, P. (1978), *Drug Treatment in Psychiatry*, Routledge and Kegan Paul, London.

Trekas, J. (1984), It takes two to achieve compliance, *Nursing (US)*, **14**, No. 9, 58–59.

Ujhely, G. B. (1979), Touch: reflections and perceptions, *Nursing Forum*, **18**, No. 1, 18–32.

Vissenga, C., and Whitfield, W. (1983), ECT: a balanced perspective?, *Nursing Times*, **79**, No. 29, 43–44.

Youssef, F. A. (1984), Adherence to therapy in psychiatric patients: an empirical investigation, *International Journal of Nursing Studies*, **21**, No. 1, 51–57.

Chapter 11

Relating to the physically ill patient

'The patient is affected by everything which is done for him (or not done for him) from the moment of admission to the time of discharge.'
(Bojar, 1958).

THE INFLUENCE OF THE HOSPITAL ENVIRONMENT ON THE PATIENT

Illness is a threatening event and the emotional stresses that a person experiences can be intensified if admission to hospital is necessary. The person not only loses the safety and security of his own home but also, while he is feeling very vulnerable, has to place himself in the care of strangers. He is required to adopt the role of a patient and to comply with the rules and regulations of the hospital. Furthermore, he is required to answer questions of a very personal nature addressed to him by people he does not know, and even his body may be viewed by complete strangers. To add to his sense of insecurity, his clothes may be sent home because of lack of space. His life patterns are completely changed in the uncustomary world of the hospital, and even his visitors may feel a sense of unease when they detect the peculiar hospital smell (Bojar, 1958).

When the patient is dependent on others for his needs, it may make it very difficult for him to be the kind of person that he really is. He may feel that he has to behave in the ways in which other people expect of him because, if he opposes them, he may feel threatened in case they should withdraw their care (Luckmann and Sorensen, 1975).

THE FEAR OF DEATH

The anxieties and fears aroused by the hospital situation are compounded on those already aroused by the patient's illness and he may ask himself profound questions regarding the meaning of life and death (Meiner, 1981).

Hospitalisation may make him realise that he is no longer invulnerable to suffering and even death.

THERAPEUTIC ROLE OF THE NURSE

The nurse who is accustomed to the world of the hospital should try to recognise how alien the environment must seem to the patient. The nurse who recognises the patient's fears can do a great deal to make the experience of hospitalisation less stressful to him. The nurse is after all with the patient more than the doctor is and, in this position of constant attendance, the nurse's function assumes increasingly greater importance as a psychotherapist. The pervasive factor in this function is the nurse's personal relationship with the patient (Bojar, 1958).

THE INFLUENCE OF THE PATIENT'S ILLNESS ON THE NURSE'S ATTITUDE

In the first instance the patient must be accepted as a person and not merely categorised as a disease entity. Nevertheless the nurse will have attitudes towards the patient's illness which may influence the patient's own feelings and self-image. The patient will quickly detect the attitudes of his carers through their non-verbal behaviour, particularly when such behaviours are incongruous with verbal statements.

Some illnesses are more socially acceptable and prestigious for the doctors treating the patient (*Table 11.1*). Other conditions may leave the patient feeling less worthy or even rejected and he may experience a lowering of self-esteem. Mutilating or disfiguring disorders such as burns or conditions where there is an offensive smell may evoke strong feelings of disgust and revulsion in others (Luckmann and Sorensen, 1975).

Table 11.1   Some socially acceptable and unacceptable diseases

Status conditions	Stigmatised conditions
Heart transplants	Skin diseases
Rare conditions	Epilepsy
Peptic ulcer	Venereal diseases
	Mental illness

THE PATIENT'S REACTION TO HIS ILLNESS

How a patient reacts to his illness may depend not only on the nature of the illness but also on his cultural background and his personality. The same illness will hold different meanings for different patients. Emotional responses may include anxiety, anger, withdrawal and depression. What is important is that the nurse accepts that emotional responses are normal in illness.

THE NURSE–PATIENT RELATIONSHIP

If the nurse is to help the patient to express his emotional responses to illness, then first and foremost it is necessary to develop a relationship with the patient. The nurse cannot know the patient without getting to know and understand him as a person (Jourard, 1971).

While the nurse will interact with the patient while carrying out the necessary procedures for his care, it is also essential to spend time with the patient when he has no practical nursing needs. There is some evidence to suggest that most conversations between nurses and their patients are task orientated and relate to technical rather than emotional matters (Faulkner, 1979; Macleod Clark, 1981).

While physical activities contribute to a patient's comfort and well-being, they should also be used as a vehicle for deepening the nurse–patient relationship. After all, when a patient has something on his mind, it may have direct pertinence to his overall health (Jourard, 1971).

If the nurse makes herself or himself available to the patient, he can be provided with the opportunity to discuss his feelings. Sometimes a patient will feel unable to discuss the matters which concern him among the daytime activities of a busy ward; for this reason the night nurse plays a particularly significant role in meeting the emotional needs of patients. When a patient is unable to sleep or wakes up in discomfort or pain, he may feel alone and uncertain. The night may seem endless and the patient's mind may be filled with fears concerning his predicament.

NURSING INTERVENTIONS

The nurse can minimise the patient's stress by providing appropriate interventions. The nurse may provide comfort and support by sitting and listening to the patient while he expresses his fears. His fears may relate to areas of the unknown and in some instances the nurse may be able to help to reduce these fears by increasing his understanding of what to expect.

(a) Touch

Touch is particularly helpful to the patient who is anxious or in pain. If the use of touch can facilitate the patient's comfort, then the nurse should not ignore its importance. When touch is used appropriately, it can provide an expression of care and compassion unmatched by words.

It is necessary for the nurse to know when and how and under what circumstances touch is therapeutically relevant. Not all patients like being touched; so the nurse must make judgements concerning the use of touch as a nursing intervention. Tactile contact is particularly important for the patient who is dependent on others or on machines for maintenance of his vital functions. Touch can tell the patient who is hanging on to life by a thread that he still *is* (Lewis, 1976).

(b) Empathy

Effective nursing calls for a high degree of interpersonal competence. Just sitting quietly with a patient who is distressed can convey empathy; sitting quietly with a patient who does not communicate can convey to him that he is worthwhile whether he speaks or not; the depressed patient may find comfort in knowing that the nurse is willing to spend time with him. However, he may ask to be left alone and the nurse may hesitate to approach him again for fear of being rejected. Nevertheless, the nurse should not reject the patient, and he should be encouraged to express his feelings rather than to repress or deny them (Auvil, 1984). The depressed patient is often helped if the nurse communicates directly by saying 'Mr Jones, you seem depressed. Would you like to tell me how you feel?' This communicates to the patient that his emotional state is perceived by the nurse and that the nurse is willing to listen. If the patient begins to cry, then the nurse should remain sitting nearby but should not move to touch or comfort the patient at the time, because immediate touching or speaking may stop the patient from revealing what is really bothering him (Barry, 1984).

THE DIFFERENT BEHAVIOURS OF PATIENTS

The anxiety of the hospitalised patient may manifest itself in many different

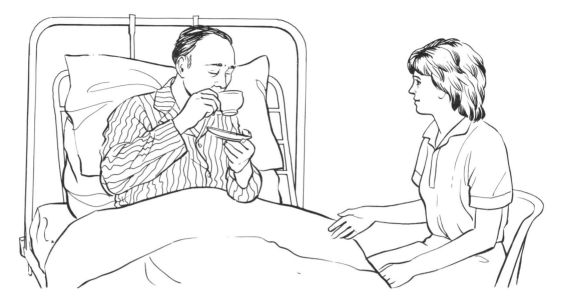

ways and through many different behaviours. Patients do not always express their anxiety overtly.

(a) The self-controlled patient

The nurse may find a particular patient difficult to talk to; he may seem to be so well in control of his emotions that it is difficult to know what he is really feeling. He may actually need to feel in control of himself at all times because any event that threatens his self-control will provoke an arousal of his anxiety. The controlled patient is often very questioning. He wants to know every detail concerning his illness and treatment. However wearing this may be, the nurse should bear in mind that the patient really does need honest answers to his questions to enable him to deal with his anxiety by maintaining self-control (Barry, 1984). The patient will usually feel more secure if he is given an explanation regarding his treatment, medication and diagnostic tests.

(b) The demanding patient

The nurse will find that other patients have exaggerated and dramatic emotional responses to illness. Such patients may challenge the tolerance of the nurse, but again it is helpful to remember that the basic dynamic which is operating is that of anxiety. The demanding patient often has an underlying fear of abandonment and being alone. His basic need is one of being cared for and the nurse who is able to recognise this need will sit and talk to him rather than react with anger or annoyance (Barry, 1984).

(c) The patient who does not seem to want to recover

Sometimes the nurse may encounter a patient who seems poorly motivated and whose rate of recovery is slow. The patient may have fears about coping independently and returning to work. His self-image may have changed as a result of illness and surgery and he may lack the confidence to resume former roles. The nurse can help the patient by encouraging him to talk about his fears and by ensuring that his care plan contains short-term goals that can be readily achieved, thereby giving him a sense of accomplishment.

THE NEEDS OF VISITORS

Finally, it is not only the needs of the patient that the nurse must consider but also the needs of the patient's visitors. Visitors often perceive the hospital as the doctors' and nurses' territory. The nurse's actions can make the patient's visitors feel comfortable and welcome. Simple courtesies such as providing chairs or directing visitors to the cafeteria, chapel or waiting room outlines the permissible space which they can feel free to occupy (Meisenhelder, 1985).

One of the greatest needs of relatives is information concerning the patient; by giving careful explanations the nurse can help to allay any worries that they may have. By meeting the needs of relatives the nurse indirectly aids the recovery of the patient, since a dissatisfied relative might well have an adverse effect on the patient's progress. Information should be given with the same consideration whether in a face-to-face encounter or over the telephone. It can be frustrating for relatives to be told in a parrot-like fashion that there is 'no change' or that the patient is 'as well as can be expected' (Roberts, 1971). Such well-rehearsed cliches do nursing a disservice. The nurse should remember that, when relatives cannot obtain the information which they seek from nursing personnel, then they will be forced to find other sources for providing the answers to their questions. They may ask other patients or approach the domestic staff (Little, 1963). Certain information may only be given with consideration for the doctor's wishes. He may wish to discuss certain aspects of the patient's illness and treatment with the relatives himself. The nurse needs to be absolutely clear as to what information the doctor will give and what information giving will fall within the nurse's area of responsibility. The nurse must bear in mind that the presence of anxiety will alter the way in which the patient hears, and it may be necessary to give the patient the same information on many occasions.

The nurse can provide support for the patient's visitors by anticipating their feelings. It is often the little things that visitors value, such as a welcoming smile, remembering their names and showing a willingness to listen to their concerns. Visitors often feel apprehensive in the unfamiliar hospital environment with its strange sights and sounds. They may be shocked by the effects of illness on the patient or they may feel intimidated by the tubes and equipment surrounding a loved one. The patient's visitors can be helped by being prepared as to what to expect and the offer of a friendly arm to lean on can provide the much needed support to approach the patient's bed (Meisenhelder, 1985).

THE PROVISION OF A LINK WITH OTHER PROFESSIONAL SERVICES

Undoubtedly, the nurse is in a unique position and can alleviate much of the patient's anxiety during hospitalisation by accepting the patient as a person and by providing the conditions for the patient in which problems may be discussed. The nurse will encounter patients with problems which may benefit from the services of other professionals. An anxious patient may benefit from relaxation exercises taught by the physiotherapist or the patient's problems may warrant the skills and expertise of a specialist nurse. The patient may wish to discuss matters relating to spiritual needs and the hospital chaplain may be the most appropriate person to help the patient. The nurse has an important role in acting as a resource person in meeting the patient's needs indirectly as well as directly through the development of a nurse–patient relationship. While the nurse sometimes uses tangible tools in the helping relationship, it is the nurse's use of self, warmth of personality and manifest interest in the patient that makes him or her a therapeutic person (Lewis, 1976).

HELPING THE PATIENT TO EXPRESS HIS EMOTIONS

Emotional responses to illness are quite normal and should be expected. In times of high stress, threatened loss or actual loss, it is quite usual for people to react with strong emotion (Nichols, 1984).

The nurse's function then is to provide the patient with the opportunity to express these responses. Nichols (1984) states that the prime commodity in emotional care is the response which the nurse makes towards the patient, for this he suggests will determine whether the nurse has a facilitating or a blocking effect.

The nurse's role is to provide a relationship and a setting which helps the emotional processes along. The nurse needs to communicate permission, acceptance and safety so that the patient will not feel ashamed nor the need to suppress emotion.

Eliminating emotional processes is not the primary target of emotional care. The nurse's objective must be to create the opportunity for the expression of emotion (Nichols, 1984).

REFERENCES AND FURTHER READING

References

Auvil, C. A. (1984), The sounds of silence, *American Journal of Nursing*, **84**, No. 8, 1072.

Barry, P. D. (1984), *Psychosocial Nursing, Assessment and Intervention*, J. B. Lippincott, Philadelphia, Pennsylvania.

Bojar, S. (1958), The psychotherapeutic function of the general hospital nurse, *Nursing Outlook*, **6**, 151–153.

Faulkner, A. (1979), Monitoring nurse–patient conversation in a ward, *Nursing Times, Occasional Papers*, **75**, No. 23, 95–96.

Jourard, S. M. (1971), *The Transparent Self*, Van Nostrand Reinhold, New York.

Lewis, L. (1976), *Planning Patient Care*, Wm. C. Brown, Dubuque, Iowa.

Little, D. E. (1963), The say something tell nothing concept of nursing, *Nursing Forum*, **2**, No. 1, 38–45.

Luckmann, J., and Sorensen, K. C. (1975), What patient's actions tell you about their feelings, fears and needs, *American Journal of Nursing*, **75**, 54–61.

MacLeod Clark, J. (1981), Communicating in nursing, *Nursing Times*, **77**, No. 1, 12–18.

Meiner, S. (1981), The patient in the middle, *Journal of Practical Nursing*, **31**, No. 8, 25–26.

Meisenhelder, J. B. (1985), Self esteem: a closer look at clinical interventions, *International Journal of Nursing Studies*, **22**, No. 2, 127–135.

Nichols, K. A. (1984), *Psychological Care in Physical Illness*, Croom Helm, London, Charles Press, Philadelphia, Pennsylvania.

Roberts, H. (1971), Talking to relatives, *Nursing Times*, **67**, No. 28, 860–861.

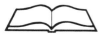

Further reading

Anon. (1981), Who am I? Where am I? Why do I hurt so much?, *Nursing Times*, **77**, No. 15, 633–634.

Anon. (1981), The great conspiracy, *Nursing Times*, **77**, No. 15, 635–639.

Anon. (1983), Emotional rescue, *Nursing Mirror*, **156**, No. 27, 24–25.

Boguslawski, M. (1979), The use of therapeutic touch, *Journal of Continuing Education in Nursing*, **10**, No. 4, 9–15.

Brown, L. (1986), The experience of care: patient perspectives, *Topics in Clinical Nursing*, **8**, No. 2, 56–62.

Clark, M. (1983), Diary of a stroke victim, *Nursing Times*, **79**, No. 34, 27–30.

Cohen, A. (1978), Reassurance unobtainable, *Nursing Mirror*, **147**, No. 6, 26.

Durr, C. (1971), Hands that help—but how?, *Nursing Forum*, **10**, No. 4, 392–400.

Fazey, N. (1985), Nurse as patient, ministering angels?, *Nursing Times*, **81**, No. 21, 26–27.

Field, W. E. (1985), Physical causes of depression, *Journal of Psychosocial Nursing and Mental Health Services*, **23**, No. 10, 31–35.

Frances, M. (1983), Shipwrecked in my body, *Nursing Mirror*, **156**, No. 25, 45–46.

Garant, C. (1980), Stalls in the therapeutic process, *American Journal of Nursing*, **80**, 2166–2169.

Hardy, J. (1975), The importance of touch for patient and nurse, *Journal of Practical Nursing*, **25**, No. 6, 26–27.

Hayward, J. (1975), *Information—A Prescription against Pain*, Royal College of Nursing, London.

Hein, E., and Leavitt, M. (1977), Providing emotional support to patients, *American Journal of Nursing*, **77**, No. 5, 38–41.

Hill, A. (1981), Care is relatives, *Nursing Times*, **77**, No. 45, 1945.

Hodgson, S. (1983), Enhancing patient–nurse communication, *Nursing Times, Occasional Papers*, **79**, No. 18.

Knight, F. (1985), Nurse as relative out in the cold, *Nursing Times*, **81**, No. 21, 28–29.

Lambert, J. (1983), A lousy rotten deal, *Nursing Mirror*, **157**, No. 21, 32–34.

Mallows, D. (1985), Communication—a patient's view, *Nursing (UK)*, **2**, No. 38, 1112, 1114.

Marshall, J. (1979), Altered image, *Nursing Mirror*, **160**, No. 23, 46–47.

Marshall, J. (1979), Reassurance, *Nursing Times*, **75**, No. 40, 1723–1724.

Orr, J. (1985), Nurse as patient: when the tables are turned, *Nursing Times*, **81**, No. 21, 24–26.

Peplau, H. (1964), Psychiatric nursing skills and the general hospital patient, *Nursing Forum*, **3**, No. 2, 28–37.

Pritchard, P. (1981), Stress and anxiety in physical illness—the role of the general nurse, *Nursing Times*, **77**, No. 4, 162–164.

Rieman, D. J. (1986), Non-caring and caring in the clinical setting: patient's descriptions, *Topics in Clinical Nursing*, **8**, No. 2, 30–35.

Robinson, J. (1983), Like a foreign country, *Nursing Mirror*, **157**, No. 2, 31–33.

Smith, E. (1972), Reassure the patient, *Nursing Times*, **68**, No. 42, 1334–1335.

Webster, R. A., and Thompson, D. R. (1986), Sleep in hospital, *Journal of Advanced Nursing*, **11**, 447–457.

Wilson Barnett, J. (1976), Patient's emotional reactions to hospitalizations: an exploratory study, *Journal of Advanced Nursing*, **1**, 351–358.

Wilson Barnett, J. (1979), *Stress in Hospital*, Churchill Livingstone, Edinburgh.

Part 2: Care

Chapter 12

Nursing care of the person who is depressed

'All of life's experiences—every thought and action, every human relationship—is registered in the brain's emotional centre as pleasurable or painful, life supporting or life negating. The brain keeps a tally.' (Collins, 1983).

INTRODUCTION

It is normal to experience feelings of sadness after an unhappy event or failure. It is also normal to feel sadness and grief following the death of a significant person. After any normal period of sadness, time eventually heals, and the person adjusts and carries on with his daily living activities.

A state of sadness becomes an illness when it occurs as a mood of such persistence and severity that it interferes with the person's daily routine and adjustment to life (Maddison and Kellehear, 1982).

Whatever depression is, it is an uncomfortable emotional and physical experience. The possibility of suicide is very real; the majority of suicidal patients are to be found among those who are depressed. The onset of depression is often so gradual that it may be difficult to ascertain from relatives when the patient became ill. The person often experiences difficulties in sleeping and a lack of energy and enthusiasm for any purposeful activity are common complaints.

The depressed person often engages in crying without being able to give a specific reason for his behaviour. He may feel anxious and irritable and suffer from feelings of guilt or remorse, often concerning things for which he has no real reason to feel responsible.

He may be indecisive and afraid or unable to make decisions; he may lack interest in what is happening in the world around him and spend a lot of time thinking about death.

The depressed person may sit for long periods of time, his eyes staring at nothing at all, his gestures minimised and his hands and arms playing little part in any conversation. In contrast the depressed patient who is also agitated cannot keep still and engages in stereotyped movements of pacing back and forth over the same territory. He moves his hands excessively, clenching his fists, rubbing his palms together and tapping his fingers restlessly on hard surfaces.

While one person presents with an attitude of resignation, the person who is agitated endeavours to cope through constant movements to ease the mind's unrest (Collins, 1983).

Sometimes a person will believe that he is physically ill because of the physical symptoms which accompany the depression such as poor appetite, aches, pains and general fatigue. Sometimes it is for these reasons that a person approaches his doctor and not because he recognises that he is suffering from depression.

The following nursing care studies illustrate the difference in the responses of individuals to a state of depression.

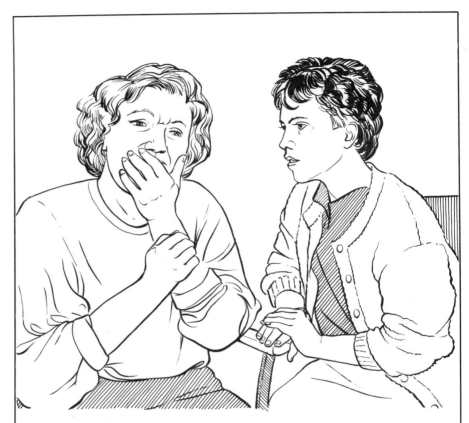

PATIENT PROFILE

Elle Johnson, aged 50, was referred to the community psychiatric nurse. Dr Hatton felt that his patient might benefit from some expert help.

For many years, Miss Johnson had cared for her elderly mother, who had died 18 months ago. In the months preceding her death, Mrs Johnson had been a most exacting and cantankerous patient. Miss Johnson had coped admirably, always exercising great patience and understanding towards her mother. Since her mother's death, Miss Johnson continued to live in the large Victorian house alone, despite advice from friends to 'get something smaller and more manageable'. Miss Johnson had worked in a local supermarket for many years and was highly thought of by the owners. Since her mother's death, Elle Johnson had told her friends that she was now really going to get on and to live her own life and to do all the things that she had always wanted to.

However, for the past few months, Miss Johnson had been feeling more and more depressed. Everything was too much trouble—going to work or even seeing friends.

NURSING ASSESSMENT INTERVIEW

Surname _Johnson_   **Forenames** _Elle Louise_

Name person likes to be called _Miss Johnson_

Address _12 Old Lodge Lane_
Willbury
WIL 2XX

Telephone number _4213_

Date of referral/~~admission~~ _12.9.86_

Next-of-kin

Name _Doris Roberts_   **Relationship** _Friend_

Address _Priory Cottage_
Warren End
Willbury

Telephone number _—_

Date of birth _____

General practitioner _Dr Hatton_

Single/~~married/divorced/widowed~~

Address _60 Links Road_
Willbury

Consultant _None_

Status under Mental Health Act _—_

Psychiatric diagnosis _Depression_

History of self-harm or harm towards others _None_

Occupation _Supervisor in a grocery store_

Occupational history
Worked in an office many years ago

Hobbies and interests _Theatre, golf, walking, embroidery_

Patient's perceived reason for referral/~~admission~~ _'Dr Hatton thinks that it may help me to talk to another woman.' Doesn't know whether it will do any good_

Relatives' understanding of patient's problems _____

NURSING ASSESSMENT INTERVIEW (continued)

Persons of significance in person's life

Family/friends/pets _Several friends closest to Doris – went to school together_

Spiritual needs

Used to go to church – but not lately. Hasn't wanted to be involved in 'social chit-chat' after church. Feels that she wants to avoid people

Problems causing concern at home

Not relevant

Community services involved/referred

Name _Helen Morse_   Status _Community psychiatric nurse_

Telephone number _7719_   Date of referral _2.2.86_

Mental status

History of present problems _Miss Johnson has felt quite low for some months_

Previous psychiatric history _None_

General appearance and behaviour _Neatly dressed. Clothes cared for. Pale lady. Sits erectly_

Speech and communication patterns _Quietly spoken. Polite; guarded_

Problems with perception _Wears glasses_

NURSING ASSESSMENT INTERVIEW (continued)

Affective state _Not overtly depressed. Gives brief nervous smile_

Disturbances of thinking or judgement _None apparent_

Orientation

Person _No problem with orientation_

Place

Time

Activities of living

Safety and mobility _Takes reasonable care_

Eating and drinking _Eats 'enough'. Never has been a big eater_

Elimination

Bladder _No problems_

Bowel _No problems_

Sleep patterns _Tends to get up at night but always has. Pattern established when mother was alive_

Personal needs _Needs social distance_

General health

Any medical condition for which the person is receiving treatment
Doctor offered anti-depressants. Miss Johnson doesn't believe in taking 'pills for this and that'

Doctor's instructions _Provide support and counselling_

Areas of concern to patient _Deferred_

NURSING ASSESSMENT INTERVIEW (continued)

Problems identified

Probably underestimates herself.
Feels that it's a bit late to plan positively for the future.
Says that there are some things she would find very difficult to tell someone else

Date of interview _1 . 6 . 86_   Signature _N. Morse_

History taken from _Miss Johnson_

by _Helen Morse_   Designation _Community psychiatric nurse_

Additional information   Date _____

Says that she has never thought of 'ending it all',
although she has felt pretty down at times

USE OF PEPLAU'S DEVELOPMENT MODEL

Helen Morse, the community psychiatric nurse, understood the importance of interpersonal relations as a therapeutic tool and decided to base her practice on Peplau's (1952) developmental model. (Chapter 7 gives an overview of this model.)

(a) Orientation phase

In the first phase of Peplau's developmental model, orientation, the nurse acquainted Miss Johnson with the purpose of the nurse–patient relationship so that she would understand from the beginning that the relationship was to be purposeful and goal centred. During the first few meetings the nurse had to show Miss Johnson that her concern was genuine and that she could be trusted. After all, trust is not something which is freely given or automatically owned by virtue of a person's professional position. To gain trust, a person must be worthy of it (Ruditis, 1979).

Trust in the relationship is essential to enable the patient to disclose things which are important to her. The patient must also perceive the nurse as being credible and able to assimilate the knowledge in such a way that it will be beneficial to the relationship (Curtin, 1981). Miss Johnson was not ready to reveal much about herself during the first few visits; the nurse was not concerned because she knew that rapport is best established with the depressed patient through shared time.

The nurse's visits indicated to Miss Johnson that she was perceived as a valuable person; the nurse's presence alone does not fulfil the requirement of *being there*. Being there and being available to the patient can only be conveyed through a genuine interest and attentiveness (Gregg, 1963).

(b) Identification phase

During the *identification* phase, Miss Johnson seemed more at ease with the nurse and they were able to work towards clarifying the problems.

The nurse took on the role of counsellor and conveyed an attitude of quiet acceptance. The creation of a therapeutic environment in which the patient could release emotion was not something which just happened. It depended very much on the kind of person that the nurse was and her own degree of self-awareness (Swanson, 1975).

PLAN OF NURSING CARE

Towards the end of the identification phase the nurse and patient were able to agree on a number of problems, goals and helping behaviour (*Table 12.1*), but Miss Johnson was still reluctant to reveal her true feelings.

Table 12.1   Patient's problems and goals, and nursing orders

Patient's problem	Patient's goal	Nursing orders
Poor self-esteem	To experience an increase in self esteem	To raise self-esteem by helping Miss Johnson to perceive and utilise her strengths
Lack of life goals	To establish positive life goals	To enable her to establish positive living goals through the helping relationship
'Feelings that I cannot share'	To express emotional feelings	To facilitate the expression of pent-up emotion in an appropriate and safe way

(c) Exploitation phase

During the *exploitation* phase the nurse helped Miss Johnson to develop her inner resources to increase her ability to cope. The nurse's acceptance of the patient as she was made it possible for her to explore her feelings and to uncover facets of underlying problems.

The nurse was prepared to listen to the patient, allowing her to communicate in her own time and without any pressure. The nurse adopted a listening posture by leaning slightly towards the patient and conveying a receptiveness to her messages with and without words. The nurse's willingness to listen conveyed through her body language encouraged Miss Johnson to share more of herself.

Miss Johnson had made it very plain to the nurse that there were some things that she would not share with anyone and yet, as Miss Johnson talked about her relationship with her mother, the nurse could sense her anger. Her voice was raised and she was trembling. She was desperately trying to control herself. The nurse reached out to Miss Johnson and conveyed verbally and non-verbally that it was alright to express feelings (*Table 12.2*); soon her anger was accompanied by tears.

Anger is a feeling of resentment that occurs in response to heightened anxiety when an individual perceives a threat. It is characterised by a feeling of tension; the nurse recognised the need for Miss Johnson to discharge this tension.

Table 12.2   *Factors associated with the nurse as a person which may either enhance or inhibit the release of pent-up emotions (catharsis)*

Enhancing factors	Inhibiting factors
Self-awareness	Uncomfortable with emotional expression
Well adjusted	
Acceptance of the patient	Feels threatened by situation
A non-judgemental attitude	Lack of appropriate therapeutic skills
Ability to empathise	Preoccupied with own unresolved problems
Comfortable with physical contact, e.g. touch	
Free attention	Over-involvement
Encouraging a verbatim description of past events	Immaturity
Encouragement of emotions	Poor understanding of facilitator role

Listening to another person expressing anger is not easy and can be a frightening experience. Encouraging a patient to express anger can have positive benefits in terms of learning, self-growth and increased self-esteem (Smitherson, 1981). The most important function of the nurse is to convey to the patient that he or she is there to help to deal with the anger safely and to teach the patient that such emotions need an appropriate outlet.

When the patient begins to express anger, the nurse must be prepared to hear her out, and this can take time. The nurse cannot leave the patient in a highly emotional state just because it is time to go home. The nurse must accept the anger as part of the patient's developmental process. The nurse will require some self-understanding of how he or she deals with his or her own angry feelings so that he or she will not be critical or take the patient's anger personally. Just by listening to the patient ventilating feelings of anger can have a powerfully supportive effect.

The feelings of anger which Miss Johnson had expressed to the nurse had stemmed from events which happened almost 25 years ago. When Miss Johnson was in her twenties, she had been planning to marry a Canadian. Her mother never liked her fiancé and, 2 weeks before the wedding, Mrs Johnson had been taken seriously ill and rushed into hospital. As there was no one else to care for her mother, Miss Johnson was forced to postpone the wedding and her fiancé had to return home alone. When Mrs Johnson came out of hospital, she seemed less able to care for herself and was very dependent on her daughter. Miss Johnson was torn between her duty to her mother and love for her fiancé in Canada. Tired of waiting, he eventually wrote and broke off the engagement. For years, Miss Johnson bottled up her feelings of resentment and many times she wished for her mother's death. Yet now that her mother was dead and she was free, she felt guilty and lacked the capacity to live her life to the full.

Miss Johnson also felt angry because she was not an only child. Her married sister had kept very much 'out of it' at the time. Her sister had no children and had died of leukaemia 9 years ago.

As the nurse–patient relationship continued, Miss Johnson began to see her old friends again and to return to work. She was able to formulate more positive plans for the future and the renewing of old friendships helped to provide others to fill the surrogate role that had been taken by the nurse.

(d) Resolution phase

In the last phase, *resolution*, the nurse and patient were able to evaluate the achievement of goals. Miss Johnson confessed that she had always been brought up to control her feelings, especially feelings of anger. She now felt as if she had been relieved of a great burden. Sharing her feelings and learning that the expression of anger in an appropriate manner is 'okay' enabled Miss Johnson to come to terms with her feelings. The nurse too had learned more about her fellow human beings and herself through helping Elle Johnson.

DEPRESSION FOLLOWING CHILDBIRTH

by *Helen Lewer*

For some individuals, life situations can act as a precipitating factor in the causation of mental illness. A small number of women develop a psychiatric illness following childbirth. When a woman's adaptive defences break down during the process of child bearing, it is often found that old unconscious conflicts related to the mother–child relationship have caused the arousal of anxiety (Maddison and Kellehear, 1982).

While it is not possible to pin-point any one cause of mental illness associated with childbirth, unhealthy reactions to motherhood, unsatisfactory marital relationships, unwanted pregnancy and other psychological and social stresses may act as contributory factors (Batchelor, 1969).

The illness behaviours related to childbirth will largely be determined by a person's constitution and may take the form of withdrawal, elation, being out of touch with reality, anxiety or depression.

PATIENT PROFILE

Jeanne Loader, aged 26, has been married for 3½ years. She and her husband Kevin were very happy when they learned that Jeanne was expecting their first child. Jeanne gave up her job as a receptionist and focused her attentions on preparations for the new arrival.

The second bedroom was soon transformed into a nursery, and Jeanne's mother, who was very excited at the prospect of becoming a grandparent, helped her daughter to crochet a beautiful christening gown and cot cover.

The pregnancy and birth went smoothly. Baby Robert Clyde Loader, who was born at the local general practitioner unit on 12 May 1986, weighed in at 3.7 kilograms.

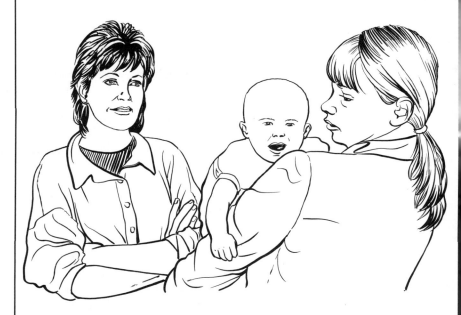

Jeanne coped admirably for the first 2 weeks but then began to cry for no apparent reason. She stopped breast feeding and decided to put the baby on bottle feeds. Robert began to cry a lot but Jeanne just shut the door of the nursery so that she could not hear him. Kevin thought the baby was crying because he was hungry. He became very concerned because Jeanne did not seem to care whether she fed him or not and would only do so when prompted. Kevin had great difficulty in taking time off from work because he was preparing for an important sales conference. Jeanne's mother had Jeanne's maternal grandmother to care for and was therefore unable to give as much support as she would have liked. Both she and Kevin were very concerned about Jeanne's behaviour and called Dr John. After a domiciliary visit by Dr Mencat, Jeanne and her baby were admitted to the mother and baby unit at the local psychiatric hospital (Robert was now 4 weeks old).

NURSING ASSESSMENT INTERVIEW

Surname _Loader_   Forenames _Jeanne Kyla_

Name person likes to be called _Jeanne (family call her Jenna)_

Address _141 Milfield Park_   Telephone number _5711_
Willbury   Date of referral/admission
WIL XJ6   _13.6.87_

Next-of-kin

Name _Mr K. Loader_   Relationship _Husband_

Address _As above_

                                                                  Telephone number _—_

Date of birth _2.5.60_   Single/married/divorced/widowed

General practitioner _Dr J. John_   Address _Claremont_
                                                                       9A High Street
                                                                       Middlesdown

Consultant _Dr S. Mencat_

Status under Mental Health Act _Informal_

Psychiatric diagnosis _Puerperal depression_

History of self-harm or harm towards others _No history_

Occupation _Housewife_

Occupational history
Receptionist / typist

Hobbies and interests _Travelling, sailing,_
plays in local hockey team

Patient's perceived reason for referral/admission _Too early to say_

Relatives' understanding of patient's problems _Very worried — all looking forward_
to the baby so much, especially Jeanne. Feeling
rather stunned by events

NURSING ASSESSMENT INTERVIEW (continued)

Persons of significance in person's life
Family/friends/pets _Husband, mother (Mrs Bonner)._
No pets. Several girl-friends

Spiritual needs
Has always attended church regularly

Problems causing concern at home _No_

Community services involved/referred
Name _Mrs B. Frain_   Status _Health visitor_
Telephone number _7414_   Date of referral _Has visited already. See_
whether Mrs Bonner can be given
more support by community staff.

Mental status
History of present problems _Very well after birth of baby, 'coping - as if she_
had cared for babies all her life'. Onset of depression was quite sudden.

Previous psychiatric history _None - never allowed herself to feel down. Was_
very cut up when father-in-law died a year ago - but didn't
talk about it very much

General appearance and behaviour _Remains on her bed, usually lying, but_
sometimes sits with her head bowed, looking down at her hands

Speech and communication patterns _Talks quietly to herself. Very little eye_
contact with others. Doesn't acknowledge baby

Problems with perception _Does not appear to want to listen to what others say_

NURSING ASSESSMENT INTERVIEW (continued)

Affective state _Depressed, flat, unresponsive_

Disturbances of thinking or judgement _Seems muddled_

Orientation

Person _Yes ✓_

Place _Knows that she is in hospital_

Time _Doesn't know time_

Activities of living

Safety and mobility

_—_

Eating and drinking

_—_

Elimination

Bladder _—_

Bowel _—_

Sleep patterns

_—_

Personal needs

_—_

General health

Any medical condition for which the person is receiving treatment

_No_

Doctor's instructions

Observe mother's reactions to baby

Areas of concern to patient

Mr Loader thinks that his wife is very anxious about handling the baby — she is an only child and has not had much contact with babies

NURSING ASSESSMENT INTERVIEW (continued)

Problems identified

_____

_____

_____

_____

_____

_____

_____

_____

_____

Date of interview ___13.6.87___   Signature ___P. McIntosh___

History taken from ___Husband and mother___

by ___Penny McIntosh___   Designation ___Staff nurse___

Additional information   Date ___13.6.87___

Mrs Loader's mother cares for her own mother who is
paralysed (Jeanne's father died some years ago). Mrs
Bonner is very apologetic because she cannot give
Jeanne more support at this time. The community
nurse calls every other day

NURSING ASSESSMENT INTERVIEW

Surname _Loader_   Forenames _Robert Clyde_

Name that parents like him called _Robert_

Address _141 Milfield Park_

Willbury

WIL XJ6

Telephone number _5711_

Age _4 weeks_   Date of Birth _12.5.87_

Religion _Church of England, not christened_

USE OF OREM'S SELF-CARE MODEL

Orem's (1980) self-care model has been chosen for Jeanne and baby Robert, to help to promote Jeanne's ability to provide infant care, thereby raising self-esteem and providing preparation for returning home (see Chapter 7).

The model is also in keeping with an infant's changing developmental requirements and the gradual acquisition of self-care skills. Orem accepts that self-care may need to be carried out by another and this is applicable where the infant is developmentally unable to provide his own care.

PLAN OF NURSING CARE

The plan of nursing care is given in *Tables 12.3* and *12.4*.

Table 12.3   Jeanne: universal self-care requisites, assessments, patient's goals, types of nursing action and evaluation

Universal self-care requisite	Assessment	Patient's goal	Type of nursing action	Evaluation
1. The maintenance of a sufficient intake of air	No evidence of respiratory problems			
2. The maintenance of a sufficient intake of water	Well hydrated			
3. The maintenance of a sufficient intake of food	Appetite good. Husband reports that Jeanne is eating more than she usually does			
4. The provision of care associated with eliminative processes and excrements	Shows no interest in own or baby's personal care. Not constipated. No urinary problems	To engage in personal self-care activities for self and baby	Wholly and partially compensatory self-care. Educative–supportive actions	Initially, Jeanne would attend to her own personal hygiene with prompting; she would not assume any responsibility for Robert's care. The nurse provided wholly compensatory self-care for Robert to correct the deficit which existed because of his mother's illness. While Jeanne seemed to show no interest in Robert, the nurse carefully explained each stage of his care and the rationale behind it. As Jeanne's depression lifted, she wanted to care for Robert; the nurse acted in a supportive–guiding role, increasing Jeanne's abilities to care for her son and building her self-confidence until such time that a self-care deficit between mother and child no longer existed
5. The maintenance of a balance between activity and rest	Lies on her bed most of the time. Appears to be detached from what is happening around her	To engage in post-natal exercises. To engage in interaction with her husband and family. To express feelings relating to her self and the baby	Educative–supportive actions	Jeanne was encouraged to do her post-natal exercises under the guidance of the physiotherapist. As she became more interested in her appearance, she also became more interested in maintaining her figure and carried out her exercises without prompting. Despite the pressures which Jeanne's husband had at work, flexible visiting times enabled him to see her every day. He also encouraged her to touch and talk to Robert and helped to increase her confidence in caring for him. As the nurse developed a relationship with Jeanne, she expressed her feelings of inadequacy as a mother. Jeanne responded to interventions which promoted her strengths and, in turn, her self-care capacities

Table 12.3 *(continued)*

Universal self-care requisite	Assessment	Patient's goal	Type of nursing action	Evaluation
6. The maintenance of a balance between solitude and social interaction	Reluctant to hold or cuddle baby. Makes little conversation with husband or nurse	To gain confidence in holding Robert and carrying out his self-care requisites. To interact with the baby while carrying out his care. To take increasing responsibility for baby's care. To talk about feelings with husband, mother and nurse	Educative–supportive actions	Eventually, Jeanne became more interested in the baby and more confident in managing his care and was gradually able to resume more responsibility for his well-being. Interaction between mother and baby was good. Has talked to the nurses about her feelings of depression but does not talk about her change in role or her expectations of parenthood. Nurse used positive reinforcement statements to enhance Jeanne's self-esteem
7. The prevention of hazards to human life, human functioning and human well-being	Not perceptive to potential dangers to self or baby. A potential problem could be that Jeanne has thoughts about harming herself and/or the baby	To demonstrate an understanding of the factors which promote safety for self and baby. To express thoughts and feelings in a non-judgemental accepting nurse–patient relationship	Educative–supportive actions	Says that she did not have suicidal thoughts—never felt 'that low'. Handles baby carefully, maintaining his safety
8. The promotion of human functioning and development within social groups in accord with human potential, known human limitations and the human desire to be normal	Feelings of depression, low self-esteem and inadequacy interfere with mother–infant bonding	To express feelings of confidence in roles of wife and mother. To develop normal bonds with Robert. To engage in small group diversional activities. To spend some time with husband and family without the presence of the baby	Educative–supportive actions	Coped very well in the occupational therapy group. Was quite proud of a clay pot that she made. A great improvement has been noted in the amount of time that Jeanne spends with the baby. Went out for a meal with husband and spent a successful weekend at home (18.7.87–20.7.87). Coped with baby, cooking meals and visited grandmother. *Discharged* 30.7.87. Is to be followed up by Mrs Train, the health visitor, who will contact the general practitioner if there are any further problems

Table 12.4   *Robert: universal self-care requisites, assessments, patient's goals, types of nursing action, nursing intervention and evaluation*

Universal self-care requisite	Assessment	Patient's goal	Type of nursing action	Nursing intervention	Evaluation
1. Maintenance of a sufficient intake of air	Robert is fair skinned, alert and healthy looking. His skin becomes blotchy red on crying. Robert can maintain his airway, except *when his nose becomes blocked by mucus* associated with crying and distress. Respiratory rate 40 per minute. Pulse rate 140 beats per minute (at rest)	Jeanne will demonstrate that she can maintain Robert's airway, especially when feeding, crying and sleeping	Wholly compensatory and educative–supportive	The nurse will show Jeanne how to position Robert, propped on his side, when putting him back to sleep after feeding. No pillow will be put in the cot. Jeanne will also be shown how to hold and comfort Robert when he is distressed and how to use moist cotton wool to clean his nostrils. (*Rationale:* infants unable to maintain airway if nasal passages blocked, as they do not coordinate mouth breathing)	Robert's nose ceased to block, once his feeding pattern and daily routine were established, thereby lessening periods of distress. Jeanne demonstrated that she could safely maintain Robert's airway
2. Maintenance of sufficient intake of food and water (all food in fluid form prior to 3 months of age)	*Robert is unable to provide food and fluid requirements—Jeanne is disinterested in feeding him.* Usual routine is 100 millilitres of modified (powdered and reconstituted) milk from a bottle, for six feeds during 24 hours. The night feed is still required	Jeanne will demonstrate that she is able: (a) To prepare an infant feed. (b) To maintain sterility of the feed and equipment. (c) To assess Robert's hydrational state. (d) To feed Robert correctly	Wholly and partly compensatory and educative–supportive	The nurse will observe Jeanne preparing Robert's feeds and the importance of maintaining sterility and correct feed dilution. The nurse will teach Jeanne how to assess Robert's fluid requirement, by checking his fontanelle, skin texture, mental alertness, urine and faecal output, and thirst. (*Rationale:* because an infant's fluid and electrolyte distribution differs from that of an adult, he is more susceptible to dehydration). The nurse can offer practical advice about feeding: (a) Warming the feed and testing warmth of milk on the back of the hand. (b) Positioning Robert comfortably and safely for feeding. (c) Keeping the bottle tilted and the teat full of milk to prevent air ingestion. (d) Positions for 'winding'.	Jeanne demonstrated after a short period of time that she was able to prepare a feed and to feed Robert correctly. Jeanne began to show interest in Robert's physical state. On a long-term basis, teaching would need to be continued, as changes in fluid and food requirements altered

Table 12.4 (continued)

Universal self-care requisite	Assessment	Patient's goal	Type of nursing action	Nursing intervention	Evaluation
		Jeanne will show that she can interact with Robert during feeding. Robert will gain 200 grams per week for the first 3 months of life and progress in growth and development as assessed by a centile chart		The nurse will sit with Jeanne and Robert through feed times and encourage Jeanne to look at, touch and cuddle Robert. Robert should be played with after the feed. Jeanne will be encouraged to weigh Robert (with supervision) on specified days and to note his weight in relation to development. She should continue to visit the health clinic on discharge and keep in contact with the health visitor	Jeanne slowly began to interact more with Robert. By discharge, she was playing with Robert after feed times and commenting on his facial alertness. Robert gained 150 grams in week 1 and then approximately 200 grams per week until he was discharged. In the long term the clinic and health visitor would continue to monitor weight
3. Provision of care associated with eliminative processes and excrement	Robert is unable to care for own elimination and Jeanne is disinterested in care. Urine output approximately 100 millilitres per day. Bowels open five times per day, faeces soft and yellow. Robert has a nappy rash on penile, scrotal and groin areas	Jeanne will demonstrate the ability to wash and clean Robert's nappy area, without prompting from nursing staff. Robert's nappy rash will heal without further skin breakdown or infection	Wholly and partly compensatory and educative–supportive	Jeanne will be shown how to wash and dry Robert's nappy area and how to apply barrier cream and a well-fitting nappy. She will be observed changing his nappy before and after feeds and encouraged to change it when Robert cries in distress between feeds. Robert's nappy area will be observed by the nurse for healing and for infection	Jeanne demonstrated her ability to care for Robert's elimination within a short time of hospitalisation. Nappy rash subsided by the end of week 2 and no infection was noted
4. Maintenance of a balance between activity and rest	Robert has developed in accordance with 'milestones'; at 4 weeks he can lift his head momentarily from bed when prone, look intently at the human face and demonstrate reflexes such as grasping, rooting, the Moro reflex and the tonic neck reflex. Robert sleeps only 1–2 hours after feeds and wakes crying. Jeanne ignores Robert's cries	Jeanne will show understanding of Robert's development. Robert will be assessed developmentally, by the paediatrician whilst in hospital and by the health visitor when he is discharged. Robert will sleep between feeds. Jeanne will be observed attending to Robert if he cries and Kevin will be encouraged to participate	Educative–supportive and partly compensatory	Jeanne will be shown Robert's developmental achievements and taught what to expect in 'milestones' in the next 2–3 months, i.e. social smile. Jeanne will be encouraged to adopt a routine for Robert, including a regular pattern of sleep between feeds. When he cries, Jeanne will be shown 'comforting' skills, including cuddling, 'winding', nappy changing and playing. Kevin will be involved in this care whenever present	By the end of week 3, Jeanne became interested in Robert's progress developmentally. Robert's routine was established by week 3, the sleeping pattern emerging as 2½–3 hours between feeds. He liked to waken and play before a feed, Jeanne slowly employed comforting skills and Kevin was always keen to assist

Table 12.4   (continued)

Universal self-care requisite	Assessment	Patient's goal	Type of nursing action	Nursing intervention	Evaluation
5. Maintenance of a balance between solitude and social interaction	*Robert had limited interaction with Jeanne during a 24-hour period. Robert frets when awake and alone, disinterested in playing. Jeanne ignores him.* Kevin visits and plays and interacts with Robert	Jeanne will demonstrate a closer relationship with Robert. Jeanne will love and comfort Robert, attend to his needs and provide play. Jeanne and Kevin will show a family relationship with Robert	Partly compensatry and educative– supportive	Jeanne will be assisted to interact with Robert during his planned routine. Interaction with touch, cuddling and talking to Robert will be encouraged. Robert's need to play will be shown to Jeanne and suitable safe, brightly coloured and soft toys will be put in his cot. Musical and mobile toys are also suitable. Jeanne and Kevin will be encouraged to keep in contact with their own family (phone, visits, etc.) and to interact with other families. Promotion of a 'life outside hospital' will be encouraged, such as shopping or an evening out together. Jeanne and Kevin were encouraged to communicate any concerns about Robert	Jeanne was observed touching and cuddling Robert towards the end of hospitalisation. Robert's development was enhanced by toys; he avidly watched a mobile above his cot and made primitive sounds when a musical toy was played. Jeanne and Kevin went home for a weekend before discharge. They visited the cinema on one or two occasions. Considerable discussion with staff was necessary prior to discharge
6. Prevention of hazards to human life, human functioning and human well-being	*Jeanne is not responsible for Robert's safety and could possibly harm him. Robert is unable to provide a safe environment.* He is dependent on Jeanne and Kevin for protection from environmental, mechanical, physiological and psychosocial hazards. Temperature 37 °C	Jeanne will understand the need for close observation from nursing staff until her depression has lifted. She will demonstrate that she is capable of providing Robert with a safe environment, initially under supervision, and in the long term by herself. In the long term also, she will contact the health visitor if she feels unable to cope safely and attend the health clinic for Robert's developmental checks and immunisations	Wholly and partly compensatory and educative– supportive	Jeanne will be supervised by a nurse until she feels safe to deliver care. She will be encouraged to verbalise any thoughts of harming Robert. Practical safety will involve: (a) How to hold Robert during handling, especially bathing. (b) Testing bath water. (c) Cleaning skinfolds, genitalia and umbilical areas to prevent infection. (d) Planning to have all items at reach when bathing, nappy changing or feeding. (e) Dressing Robert in soft non-restrictive warm clothes. Clothes which enhance his character. Fingers and toes need warmth, as does his head. Therefore, socks, mittens and hats are needed.	Jeanne did not show signs of or verbal thoughts about harming Robert and supervision was gradually reduced, Jeanne adopting safe self-care. Robert did not suffer any environmental, mechanical or physiological harm. However, evaluation of psychosocial hazards would need to be on a long-term basis and be followed up by hospital and community personnel

Table 12.4 (continued)

Universal self-care requisite	Assessment	Patient's goal	Type of nursing action	Nursing intervention	Evaluation
				(f) Regulating the environmental temperature so that he is neither too hot nor too cold. (g) Placing Robert in a safe position for sleeping and, if outside in a pram, that a cat net is used. (h) Placing cot sides fully upright. (i) Safe play toys. (j) Contacting health visitor prior to discharge to arrange for regular assessments. (Safety is involved in all universal self-care requisites, i.e. breathing, feeding, playing, mobility, etc.)	
7. Human functioning and development including social groups—in accordance with human potential, limitations and desire to be normal	Robert, as assessed using previous universal self-care requisites is developmentally 'normal' at 4 weeks old. *Jeanne is not functioning as a 'normal' mother*	Jeanne will show her ability to care for Robert in all self-care requisites and to understand the importance of her role in relation to Robert's normal development	Partly compensatory and educative–supportive	In all aspects of Robert's self-care requisites, the nurse will assist Jeanne to 'bond' with Robert, enhancing this by communication, love, security, play and provision of all his needs	Jeanne was discharged from hospital when she demonstrated that she could provide total safe care for Robert within a 'mothering role'

IMPLEMENTATION

The nurse's role whilst working with Jeanne, Robert and the family ranges from wholly compensatory to educative–supportive, sometimes doing for or providing psychosocial supportive or teaching as examples of nursing intervention. Ultimately, when Jeanne can provide for her own and Robert's self-care requisites, nursing intervention will not be required. However, the family will need continuing support from community personnel and services on returning home.

EVALUATION

Self-care was evaluated on the basis of Jeanne's increased knowledge and confidence in assuming responsibility for self-care.

Although Jeanne had never openly expressed any thoughts about harming herself or the baby, the possibility was always borne in mind by the nurse. Jeanne was not allowed to be alone with Robert and was observed for any change in mood through her verbal and especially her non-verbal facial expressions, body posture, use of eye contact and general behaviour. Any diurnal variations in her mood were noted, to see whether her depression was better or worse at particular times during the day and night.

The nurse adopted a quiet accepting manner in approaching Jeanne, allowing sufficient distance so as not to make her feel that her personal space was being threatened. The mere presence of the nurse helped to ease the loneliness of depression and communicated to Jeanne that she was perceived as a worthwhile human being.

When talking to Jeanne, the nurse allowed her time to respond, by adjusting her own pace to that of the patient. This meant learning to be comfortable with the long silences that occurred and using these silences therapeutically by not pressurising Jeanne to talk in order to relieve the nurse's own anxiety. The therapeutic use of self is an important aspect of caring for the patient who is depressed, particularly when the patient seems unresponsive, uninviting and not the most comfortable of people to be with.

The nurse appreciated that Jeanne's hospitalisation and illness provided a stressful situation for her family. Illness of one member of a family inevitably means that internal relationships and roles have to be adjusted to accommodate the illness (Miles, 1981). Many emotional feelings may be aroused, especially anxiety, as family members search their own consciences to see whether they are to blame in some way (Frost, 1970). The nurse provided support by being available to listen to their concerns and to answer their questions. The nurse's role in providing support for the family is important because the relatives of the mentally ill person often find it difficult to confide in others. While people are willing to talk about physical ailments, mental illness is a less comfortable subject for the lay person (Miles, 1981).

DISCUSSION

Deficits in Robert's ability to provide self-care exist mainly because of his developmental inability but are exacerbated by Jeanne's depressed post-natal state.

Jeanne was assessed as having the knowledge and skills to provide care and, once her depressive state has been overcome, the motivation necessary to provide Robert's care and to promote his development.

Initially, Jeanne's mental state caused concern with regard to Robert's safety; however, she clearly demonstrated that she did not intend to harm Robert. The environment in which Jeanne was nursed and the carefully planned nursing intervention assisted her to resume a normal mothering role.

REFERENCES AND FURTHER READING

References

Batchelor, I. R. C. (1969), *Henderson and Gillespie's Textbook of Psychiatry*, 10th edn, Oxford University Press, London.

Collins, M. (1983), *Communication in Health Care*, C. V. Mosby, St Louis, Missouri.

Curtin, L. L. (1981), Privacy: belonging to oneself, *Perspectives in Psychiatric Care*, **19**, Nos 3–4, 112–115.

Frost, M. (1970), Talking and listening to relatives, *Nursing Times, Occasional Papers*, **66**, No. 1, 36.

Gregg, D. (1963), The therapeutic roles of the nurse, *Perspectives in Psychiatric Care*, **1**, No. 1, 18 –24.

Maddison, D., and Kellehear, K. J. (1982), *Psychiatric Nursing*, 5th edn, Churchill Livingstone, Edinburgh.

Miles, A. (1981), *The Mentally Ill in Contemporary Society*, Martin Robertson, Oxford.

Orem, D. E. (1980), *Nursing: Concepts of Practice*, 2nd edn, McGraw-Hill, New York.

Peplau, H. E. (1952), *Interpersonal Relations in Nursing*, G. P. Putnam, New York.

Ruditis, S. E. (1979), Developing trust in nursing interpersonal relationships, *Journal of Psychiatric Nursing and Mental Health Services*, **17**, No. 4, 20–23.

Smitherson, C. (1981), *Nursing Actions for Health Promotion*, F. A. Davis, Philadelphia, Pennsylvania.

Swanson, A. R. (1975), Communicating with depressed persons, *Perspectives in Psychiatric Care*, **13**, No. 2, 63–67.

Further reading

Andrews, R., Jenkins, J. S., and Sugden, J. (1985), Origins of sadness as a response, *Nursing (UK)*, **2**, No. 34, 995–998.

Biley, F. (1985), Learn to believe in yourself, *Nursing Times*, **81**, No. 22, 40–41.

Blondis, M. N., and Jackson, B. E. (1982), *Non-verbal Communication with Patients*, John Wiley, Chichester, West Sussex.

Brammer, L. M. (1979), *The Helping Relationship*, Prentice-Hall, Englewood Cliffs, New Jersey.

Burgess, A. C., and Lazare, A. (1972), Nursing management of feelings, thoughts and behaviour, *Journal of Psychiatric Nursing and Mental Health Services*, **10**, No. 6, 7–11.

Burr, J., and Andrews, J. (1981), *Nursing the Psychiatric Patient*, 4th edn, Baillière Tindall, London.

Burton, G. (1979), *Interpersonal Relations*, 4th edn, Tavistock, London.

Campiello, J. (1980), The process of termination, *Journal of Psychiatric Nursing and Mental Health Services*, **13**, No. 2, 29–32.

Egan, G. (1986), *The Skilled Helper*, Brooks/Cole, California.

Gordon, V. (1986), Treatment of depressed women by nurses in Britain and the USA. In: *Psychiatric Nursing Research* (ed. Brooking, J.), John Wiley, Chichester, West Sussex.

Hale, S., and Richardson, J. (1963), Terminating the nurse–patient relationship, *American Journal of Nursing*, **63**, 116–119.

Hare, M. (1985), The physical problems of depressive illness, *Physiotherapy*, **71**, No. 6, 258–261.

Heron, J. (1975), Six category intervention analysis, Human potential research project, University of Surrey, 1975.

Hopkins, S., and Kumar, R. (1985), An identity crisis, *Nursing Times*, **81**, No. 34, 39–40.

Jasmin, S., and Trygstad, L. N. (1979), *Behavioural Concepts and the Nursing Process*, C. V. Mosby, St Louis, Missouri.

Kreigh, H. Z., and Perko, J. E. (1983), *Psychiatric and Mental Health Nursing*, 2nd edn, Reston Publishing, Reston, Virginia.

Murray, R. B., and Huelskoetter, M. M. W. (1983), *Psychiatric Mental Health Nursing: Giving Emotional Care*, Prentice-Hall, Englewood Cliffs, New Jersey.

Peplau, H. (1960), Anxiety in the mother–infant relationship, *Nursing World*, **134**, No. 5, 33–34.

Skinner, K. (1976), The therapeutic milieu; making it work, *Journal of Psychiatric Nursing and Mental Health Services*, **17**, No. 8, 38–44.

Stuart, G. W., and Sundeen, S. J. (1983), *Principles and Practices of Psychiatric Nursing*, C. V. Mosby, St Louis, Missouri.

Topalis, M., and Aguilera, D. (1978), *Psychiatric Nursing*, 7th edn, C. V. Mosby, St Louis, Missouri.

Watts, A. (1986), Living with depression, *Psychiatry in Practice*, **5**, No. 3, 19–21.

Williams, J. (1986), Not just the baby blues, *Nursing Times*, **82**, No. 20, 38–40.

Chapter 13

Nursing care of the person who is suicidal

'Communication is critical to the prevention of suicide. If there is no amnesty from stress and anxiety, the time may come in life when the client thinks nothing helps—nothing heals.' (Collins, 1983).

INTRODUCTION

Suicide is a direct purposeful action taken by a person to end his own life. The person who is suicidal demonstrates a wide range of moods, perceptions and behaviours; at one extreme, a person may attempt suicide on impulse and, at the other, he may meticulously plan his own death (Soreff, 1981). A person's aim may be actual self-destruction, or he may be attempting to bring about some change in his life; he may wish to hurt someone, perhaps a friend, parent or lover (Hoff, 1978). Self-destruction may be seen as the only way to escape from feelings of hopelessness, helplessness or what are perceived as insurmountable problems.

Jourard (1970) suggests that a person may choose to destroy himself in response to an invitation originating from others that he has stopped living. A person lives in response to repeated invitations to continue living and lives only as long as his experience of life has meaning and value and he has something to live for. A number of people who finally commit suicide feel isolated from significant people around them or feel that there are no significant people in their lives.

The plight of the suicidal person is often ignored by others; yet most people who commit suicide give specific verbal or non-verbal warnings. Sadly, in some cases the cues are not recognised until after death has occurred.

PATIENT PROFILE

Vernon Jensen, 19, has a history of mental illness. In the past, he has exhibited excited and bizarre behaviour. Over the past year, he has become quiet, solitary and resistive to interpersonal involvement.

From the age of 11 Vernon was under the care of the child guidance clinic. When he was 16, he was admitted to the adolescent unit after a severe suicidal attempt.

Efforts have been made to give Vernon and his parents support through family therapy, but they failed to keep appointments with the therapist at the clinic, and the sessions which were attended were viewed negatively.

USE OF ROY'S ADAPTATION MODEL
Roy's (1980) adaptation model (see Chapter 7) was used for Vernon's care.

NURSING ASSESSMENT INTERVIEW

Surname ___Jensen___   Forenames ___Vernon___

Name person likes to be called ___Vernon___

Address ___12A Church Street___
___Willbury___
___WIL 4XC___

Telephone number ___4711___

Date of ~~referral~~/admission ___13.3.86___

Next-of-kin

Name ___Mr and Mrs Jensen___   Relationship ___Parents___

Address ___As above___

Telephone number _____

Date of birth ___1.4.67___   Single/married/divorced/widowed _____

General practitioner ___Dr J. Yalom___   Address ___The Surgery___
___1 Moorfield Road___
___Willbury___

Consultant ___Dr S. Mencat___

Status under Mental Health Act ___Section 2___

Psychiatric diagnosis ___? Schizophrenia with depressive phases___

History of self-harm or harm towards others ___Severe suicidal attempt 3½ years___
___ago___

Occupation ___Shop assistant___

Occupational history
___Has worked in five different shops since leaving___
___school, but large proportion of time spent___
___unemployed___

Hobbies and interests _____
___Listening to music (records), collects posters___

Patient's perceived reason for referral/admission ___Wants to hurt himself but___
___doesn't know why___

Relatives' understanding of patient's problems ___Vernon has always been___
___a problem___

NURSING ASSESSMENT INTERVIEW (continued)

Persons of significance in person's life

Family/friends/pets _We don't know that he is really close to anyone_

Spiritual needs

Doesn't go to church but he's religious

Problems causing concern at home _None_

Community services involved/referred

Name _Gerald Whiting_   Status _Community psychiatric nurse at Pringle House_

Telephone number _4113 Ext 12_   Date of referral _29.4.86_

Mental status

History of present problems _Very solitary. Isolates himself from the family. Absent from work 3 days on four occasions. Given a verbal warning by the manager. No apparent reason for absence._

Previous psychiatric history _Under care of child guidance clinic since age of 11. Tried to end his life before – nearly made a good job of it!_

General appearance and behaviour _Always a loner – never brought friends home. Difficult to know what Vernon is thinking_

Speech and communication patterns _Not very communicative. Answers questions in monosyllables_

Problems with perception _Deferred for later assessment_

NURSING ASSESSMENT INTERVIEW (continued)

Affective state _? Depressed . ? Believes death will bring about some change in his life_

Disturbances of thinking or judgement

Orientation

Person _Deferred for later assessment_

Place

Time

Activities of living

Safety and mobility

Mental state poses threat to safety

Eating and drinking

Does not always want to eat in company

Elimination

Bladder _Not aware of any problems_

Bowel

Sleep patterns

Spends a lot of time sleeping

Personal needs

Deferred

General health

Any medical condition for which the person is receiving treatment

_No_

Doctor's instructions

Continuous observation.
Suicide precautions

Areas of concern to patient

Deferred

NURSING ASSESSMENT INTERVIEW (continued)

Problems identified

See model

Date of interview _____   Signature _M. Wong_

History taken from _Mr and Mrs Jensen_

by _Matthew Wong_ _____   Designation _Charge nurse_

Additional information   Date _13 . 3 . 86_

_Mrs Jensen was recently made redundant from her
job at Willbury Motors. Gets very short tempered
with Vernon 'because of the way he is — he won't
get up in the mornings — he has no go in him.'
Finds it hard having Vernon around the house
all day_

PLAN OF NURSING CARE

The plan of nursing care is given in _Table 13.1._

Table 13.1 Adaptive modes, assessments, patient's problems and goals, and nursing orders

Adaptive mode	First-level assessment	Second-level assessment			Patient's problem	Patient's goal	Nursing orders
		Focal stimuli	Contextual stimuli	Residual stimuli			
Basic physiological needs	Unremarkable				No maladaptive response		
Self-concept		Actively self-destructive. Poor self-image	Means of self-destruction available. Family do not seem close to Vernon	A previous failed attempt. May be more determined (see the boxed section entitled 'Causes of suicide' at the end of this chapter). Lack of positive feedback from peers, family?	Self-destructive thoughts. Poor self-image. Lack of life goals?	The patient will not engage in self-destructive actions. To experience increased self-esteem	Continuous observation. To provide a safe environment. To encourage Vernon to talk about feelings. To convey acceptance
Role mastery		Difficulty in fulfilling roles of son, brother and employee	Ward environment reinforces patient's role	Has been unable to engage in appropriate role learning within family. Previous hospitalisation	Role conflict	To talk about relationships at home	To provide supportive interventions by: (a) Being with. (b) Listening. (c) Showing interest. (d) Caring. (e) Being available
Interdependence		A loner. Does not socialise easily	? Poor interpersonal relationships at home	? Disappointment in past relationships	Loneliness	To increase interaction with others	To establish a relationship with Vernon based on trust. To help him to relate to others

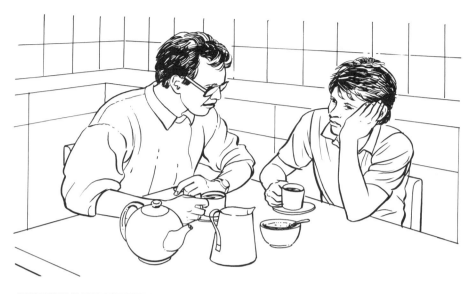

NURSING INTERVENTION

The immediate stimuli impinging on Vernon was his desire to end his life; the contextual stimuli provided self-destructive means and the residual stimuli took into account Vernon's previous suicidal attempt.

The nurse's first priority was to provide a safe environment for Vernon. When a patient is intent on ending his life, the nurse must consciously and conscientiously try to prevent the patient from committing suicide by his or her presence and actions (Blythe and Pearlmutter, 1983). His whereabouts must be known at all times; any lapse in observation may provide just enough time for him to inflict a fatal injury. It is better if one nurse is designated to be responsible for the patient; if this nurse has to leave the ward for any reason, information and responsibility regarding the supervision of the patient can be transferred to another member of staff (Schultz and Dark, 1982). Observation must continue throughout the day and the night. Darkness must never be allowed to obstruct the nurse's view of the patient. If the patient talks in his sleep, the content of his speech should be noted. This is particularly important when a patient is unwilling to discuss his suicidal intentions.

Any materials that could be used by the patient to harm himself should be withdrawn from the environment, and the nurse should maintain constant surveillance of any items brought into the ward. The patient who is suicidal may constantly test the physical layout of the ward to determine the availability of material for use in a suicidal attempt (Busteed and Johnstone, 1983) (see the boxed section entitled 'Maintaining a safe environment for the suicidal patient' at the end of this chapter).

One of the most important reasons for the nurse to observe the patient is that he or she may be able to pick up clues, to anticipate his behaviour and to prevent him from injuring himself (Hoff, 1978).

Communicating an understanding supportive attitude to Vernon was a most important act of intervention. Being with him, believing in him and showing a willingness to try to understand his problem can convey real concern and appreciation of him as a valued person. The nurse's responses, verbal and otherwise, to the patient will have a great deal to do with the establishment of a constructive helping relationship. Establishing rapport can be a powerful beginning for the non-communicative patient and can enable him to reach out and share his hidden fearful thoughts.

Vernon had had an unhappy life situation for some time. He saw himself as unloved and unlovable and he mistrusted others. He believed that death would be beautiful and relieve him from the pain of existence; contact with the nurse helped him to know that he was valued as a human being.

Vernon was not willing to talk at first and the nurse spent a great deal of time sitting with him in silence; it was important to convey acceptance, interest and a willingness to listen without pressurising Vernon or ignoring his need for privacy.

There is often a reluctance to talk about suicide—it may arouse feelings of uneasiness because the nurse's own feelings of security, personal philosophy and basic values are threatened (Collins, 1983). The question of suicide must be faced with frankness and take into consideration the patient's and nurse's differing views of the world.

Adaptation is promoted when the nurse helps the patient to explore death fantasies because he may have unrealistic ideas about his own death. He may believe that he will be present at his own funeral and be able to observe the reactions of survivors (Reubin, 1978). The patient will be more likely to disclose his thoughts and plans to someone who shows a genuine interest in him as a human being. Communication that enhances his self-esteem can diminish feelings of depression and foster hope (Collins, 1983).

As Vernon's condition improved, his position on the health–illness continuum changed in a positive direction. Observation was continued but carried out less obtrusively.

Gradually, Vernon began to talk about his feelings concerning his family. He did not feel particularly close to them and wanted to get away from home. The nurse had met Mr and Mrs Jensen once or twice—they behaved towards Vernon as if he was a very naughty boy and it was difficult to hold anything other than a very superficial conversation with them.

As Vernon became less withdrawn, his day was structured to enable him to participate in group activities and to have some time to engage in activities of his own choosing. Vernon liked watching television, but he tended to sit alone and adopt the same isolated lifestyle that he had at home where he spent a lot of time in his bedroom.

EVALUATION

The prevention of suicide was the highest priority for the multi-disciplinary team and of prime importance in Vernon's adaptation.

The decision to discontinue suicidal precautions was decided within the team when indicated by Vernon's verbal and non-verbal behaviour.

Vernon has shown some evidence of adaptation in the self-concept, role mastery and interdependent modes but needs the continued support of the nurse to achieve his full potential for adaptation.

The long-term goals in these modes will be to help Vernon to continue to improve his self-image, to work towards a suitable life plan, to develop other approaches and strengths to cope with problems rather than self-destructive behaviour and to find satisfactory supportive relationships.

The consultant feels that Vernon is now ready to be assessed for social skills training at a day centre and that a further attempt should be made to engage Mr and Mrs Jensen. This may enable them to learn to deal with their problems more effectively and to experience a decrease in family tensions. The community psychiatric nurse will play a vital role in supporting the patient and his family, in monitoring progress and in communicating with other professionals involved in Vernon's rehabilitation.

CAUSES OF SUICIDE

No one single cause or group of causes can account for the level of suicide rates. The following factors have been associated with a high risk (Stengel, 1970; Jasmin and Trygstad, 1979):

1. *Male sex.
2. Widowhood.
3. Increasing age.
4. *Single, widowed and divorced status.
5. Childlessness.
6. High-density population.
7. Alcohol and consumption of addictive drugs.
8. *Mental disorder.
9. Physical illness.
10. Residence in large towns.
11. A high standard of living.
12. Economic crisis.
13. A broken home in childhood.
14. Social class 1 and 2 (professional).
15. *Lack of support systems.
16. *Previous suicide attempts.
17. Masked depression.
18. *Low self-esteem; diminished judgement.
19. *Bizarre ideation on reality testing.

The factors indicated by an asterisk (*) related to Vernon and were taken into consideration when an assessment of suicidal risk was made.

MAINTAINING A SAFE ENVIRONMENT FOR THE SUICIDAL PATIENT

The following precautions should be basic to the patient's care:

1. 24-hour observation.
2. Removal of dangerous objects such as belts, ties, cords, string, razor blades, scissors, nail files, metal pins or glass objects.
3. Ensure that the patient *swallows* prescribed medication.
4. Instruct the patient to delay any self-destructive impulse and call for help (Frederick, 1973).
5. High risk times on the ward are those when the staff are occupied, e.g. change of shifts or staff meetings. Many suicidal attempts are made when the patient knows that the staff are busy (Grace and Camilleri, 1981).
6. Observe any particular circumstances in which suicidal behaviour occurs.
7. Nurse the patient in a ground-floor ward if possible to prevent injury from jumping (Frederick, 1973).
8. Never check the patient at regular intervals, e.g. every half an hour. He will quickly notice a pattern. Irregular checks are better (Grace and Camilleri, 1981).

Note: while the nurse endeavours to provide a controlled and safe environment, the patient who is desperate to end his life will use almost any article to aid his self-destruction.

FACT SHEET: METHODS OF COMMITTING SUICIDE

The methods of committing suicide are as follows (Sharpe, 1980):

1. Overdose of drugs.
2. Drowning.
3. Shooting.
4. Strangulation.
5. Starvation.
6. Suffocation.
7. Inhalation of poisonous fumes.
8. Jumping from a height.
9. Severing a major blood vessel.
10. Driving and crashing a vehicle.
11. Jumping in front of a moving vehicle.
12. Burning.
13. Drinking corrosive substances.
14. Electrocution.

FACT SHEET: CLUES TO SUICIDE

Clues to suicide can often be observed in four areas (Reubin, 1978):

1. *Verbal clues*, e.g. 'I won't be a problem much longer.'
2. *Behavioural clues*, e.g. putting affairs in order or giving away valued possessions.
3. *Somatic clues*, i.e. any symptomatic expressions of person's depressed effect, e.g. aches and pains.
4. *Psychodynamic clues*, e.g. hostility, apathy or agitation.

FACT SHEET: SUICIDE

1. A person with a well-thought-out suicide plan which includes the time, place and circumstances, with an available lethal method presents a high risk (Hoff, 1978).
2. If the patient says, 'Go away and leave me alone', he may be testing the sincerity of the nurse (Collins, 1983).
3. The patient may try to discharge himself so that he can leave a controlled situation to carry out his suicidal intent.

4. When the patient appears to be getting better, the nurse needs to be alert to what he is really feeling. If the nurse misses a clue, there may not be another chance (Grace and Camilleri, 1981).
5. Suicide may be the culmination of self-destructive tendencies that may result from a person turning anger inwards against himself (Schultz and Dark, 1982).
6. It is a mistake to believe that a patient will only commit suicide if he appears to be depressed (Frederick, 1973).
7. If a suicidal attempt does occur on the ward despite all precautions, an opportunity must be allowed for the nurse and patient to discuss their feelings about the incident. The situation should be approached as a learning situation in which suicidal precautions are reconsidered and amended if required (Margolis, 1965).

REFERENCES AND FURTHER READING

References

Blythe, M. M., and Pearlmutter, D. R. (1983), The suicide watch. A re-examination of maximum observation, *Perspectives in Psychiatric Care*, **21**, No. 3, 90–93.

Busteed, E. L., and Johnstone, C. (1983), The development of suicide. Precautions for an in-patient psychiatric unit, *Journal of Psychiatric Nursing and Mental Health Services*, **21**, No. 5, 15–19.

Collins, M. (1983), *Communication in Health Care*, 2nd edn, C. V. Mosby, St Louis, Missouri.

Frederick, C. J. (1973), The role of the nurse in crisis. Intervention and suicide prevention, *Journal of Psychiatric Nursing and Mental Health Services*, **11**, No. 1, 27–31.

Grace, H. K., and Camilleri, D. (1981), *Mental Health Nursing, A Socio-Psychological Approach*, Wm. C. Brown, Dubuque, Iowa.

Hoff, L. A. (1978), *People in Crisis, Understanding and Helping*, Addison-Wesley, Reading, Massachusetts.

Jasmin, S., and Trygstad, L. N. (1979), *Behavioural Concepts and the Nursing Process*, C. V. Mosby, St Louis, Missouri.

Jourard, S. (1970), Suicide: an invitation to die, *American Journal of Nursing*, **70**, 269–275.

Margolis, P. M. (1965), cited by Busteed, E. L., and Johnstone, C. (1983), The development of suicide. Precautions for an in-patient psychiatric unit, *Journal of Psychiatric Nursing and Mental Health Services*, **21**, No. 5, 15–19.

Reubin, R. (1978), Understanding suicide. In: *Mental Health Concept Applied to Nursing* (ed. Dunlop, L. C.), John Wiley, Chichester, West Sussex.

Roy, C. (1980), The Roy adaptation model. In: *Conceptual Models for Nursing Practice* (eds Riehl, J. P., and Roy, C.), Appleton Century Crofts, Norwalk, Connecticut.

Schultz, J. M., and Dark, S. L. (1982), *Manual of Psychiatric Nursing Care Plans*, Little, Brown, Boston, Massachusetts.

Sharpe, D. (1980), *Psychiatric First Aid—A Guide for the Lay Person*, Plain Facts.

Soreff, S. M. (1981), *Management of the Psychiatric Emergency*, John Wiley, New York.

Stengel, E. (1970), *Suicide and Attempted Suicide*, Penguin, Harmondsworth, Middlesex.

Further reading

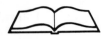

Divasto, P. V., West, D. A., and Christy, J. E. (1979), A framework for the emergency evaluation of the suicidal patient, *Journal of Psychiatric Nursing and Mental Health Services*, **17**, No. 6, 15–20.

Fallon, B. (1972), And certain thoughts go through my head, *American Journal of Nursing*, **72**, 1257–1259.

Hatton, C. L., and Valente, S. M. (1984), *Suicide Assessment and Intervention*, 2nd edn, Appleton Century Crofts, Norwalk, Connecticut.

Kreitman, N., and Dyer, J. A. T. (1981), Suicide and parasuicide, *Nursing, (UK)*, **30**, 1310–1312.

MacPhail, D. (1986), Skills in family therapy, *Nursing Times*, **82**, No. 26, 49–51.

Mellencamp, A. (1981), Adolescent depression: A review of the literature with implications for nursing care, *Journal of Psychosocial Nursing*, **19**, No. 9, 15–20.

Neville, D., and Barnes, S. (1985), The suicidal phone call, *Journal of Psychiatric Nursing and Mental Health Services*, **23**, No. 8, 14–18.

Peplau, H. (1955), Loneliness, *American Journal of Nursing*, **55**, 1476–1481.

Wilkinson, T. R. (1981), What about the family? Nursing young people in a psychiatric setting, *Nursing (UK)*, **30**, 1301–1302.

Chapter 14

Nursing care of the patient who is anxious

by *Neil Vermaut*

'*When a patient is given the opportunity to talk about his anxiety, he is able to clarify his own thinking and feeling to the point where he can give his own explanation. Furthermore, he is in a better position to accept the explanation of someone else.*' (Burton, 1977).

INTRODUCTION

Anxiety is a normal adaptive response of alertness to change or anticipated change in one's environment or circumstances. It is natural, for example, for someone to feel anxious before an examination or an interview for a job. On a more dramatic level, an impending threat or disaster increases mental alertness and produces physical changes throughout the bodily systems in preparation for confrontation or avoidance otherwise known as 'fight or flight'. In an acute anxiety state or panic, which is regarded as a psychiatric emergency, the patient appears bewildered and apprehensive and complains of palpitations, breathlessness, a choking sensation in the throat, sweating excessively, cold extremities and a feeling of impending collapse.

An anxiety state is a maladaptive condition of exaggerated and prolonged anxiety which is inappropriate to the situation. It is accompanied by physiological changes. The anxiety is not specific to an object or situation, unlike a phobia, but is 'free floating' and forms a background to the patient's behaviour and existence. Such patients complain of feeling tense, anxious and irritable. A persistent anxiety state can be very distressing, causing the patient to experience a prolongation of heightened alertness and increased tension. Whereas in normal anxiety the mind and body prepare for emergency action and then having dealt with it, resume normal functioning, in severe anxiety there is no reduction in this preparatory adaption and as a consequence the physical sensations of anxiety become the symptoms of which the patient first complains. These symptoms include tension, headaches, palpitations, sweating, restlessness, gastric disturbances, decreased libido, loss of appetite, insomnia, tight chest and tremulousness. These symptoms can themselves exacerbate the anxiety if the patient has no knowledge or idea of their cause or origin. The combined effects of these physical manifestations can be very tiring and exhausting, particularly if insomnia is present.

Those who develop severe anxiety tend to have a personality that inclines towards timidity, overconscientiousness, indecisiveness, hypochondria and oversensitivity. Their background tends to have been a domestic environment where the atmosphere is one of anxiety or the parents have been overprotective.

A number of theories have been suggested with regard to the aetiology of an anxiety state. Koshy (1982) refers to Freud's theory that incompletely repressed factors reach consciousness and evoke anxiety. Failure of defence mechanisms which protect us against anxiety is also theorised as a cause. Other factors include separation in infancy or childhood from the safe nurturing environment and emotional conflicts. Sometimes a change in a person's situation or way of life can precipitate an anxiety state if he is predisposed to its development. The prognosis of anxiety states is optimistic where there is a good pre-morbid personality.

PATIENT PROFILE

Karen James is a 22-year-old lady who worked as a clerical assistant in the Town Hall. Rather a timid and shy person, she attracted few friends and had a non-existent social life. At work, her colleagues who enjoyed teasing each other occasionally by seemingly innocuous references to one's 'love-life', regarded Karen as a 'dark horse' in a light-hearted sense. Recently, Karen was becoming easily embarrassed at their badinage despite the reassurance that their comments were in a jocular vein.

Living with her parents, who were very caring and overprotective at times, Karen regarded home as a haven in a psychological and a physical sense. Over recent weeks, however, Karen had experienced feelings of anxiety, tension and headaches although she was unable to pin-point the cause. Her sleep was restless also. Karen's mother, who was a firm believer in patent vitamin tonics as a remedy for tiredness and stress, assured her daughter that 'a bottle of medicine will soon make you feel better'. Karen's father, who suffered with stomach ulcers and asthma, suggested that a holiday would be useful. Despite both pieces of parental advice, Karen's anxiety continued, causing her to feel miserable and fatigued.

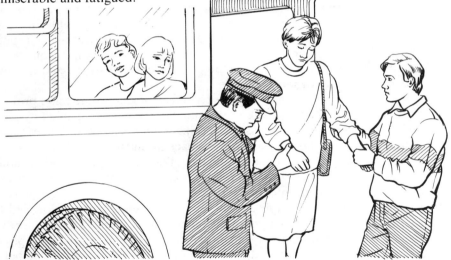

Her work colleagues noticed the change in Karen's behaviour, describing her as 'nervous and jumpy'. She was beginning to lose her appetite although she drank frequently because of a dry mouth. Easily upset by nature, she felt rather vulnerable and found difficulty in concentrating.

Without respite from her feelings of exhaustion and anxiety, Karen boarded the bus as usual one day to go to work. Within a few minutes of her journey, she was overcome by a feeling of panic, her heart was pounding fast and breathing became difficult as she broke into a cold clammy sweat. A passenger noticed Karen's distress and pale complexion and reported this to the driver, who stopped the bus at a convenient place. Karen's parents were contacted and they drove her home, extremely anxious themselves. An appointment was made with their general practitioner who after talking to Karen suggested a psychiatric opinion would be useful. Karen was referred to a day hospital for anxiety management therapy.

NURSING ASSESSMENT INTERVIEW

Surname* *James*   Forenames *Karen Sarah*

Name person likes to be called *Karen*

Address *152 Grange Road*   Telephone number *2215*
Willbury   Date of referral/admission *18.6.87*
WIL HX2

Next-of-kin

Name *Mrs E. James*   Relationship *Mother*

Address *As above*

Telephone number

Date of birth *15.4.63*   Single/~~married~~/~~divorced~~/~~widowed~~

General practitioner *Dr Hatton*   Address *60 Links Road*
Willbury

Consultant *Dr S Mencat*

Status under Mental Health Act *Informal*

Psychiatric diagnosis *Anxiety state*

History of self-harm or harm towards others *None*

Occupation *Clerical assistant*

Occupational history
Library assistant for 3 years before present job

Hobbies and interests *Reading, listening to records*

Patient's perceived reason for referral/admission *To overcome tension, headaches and tiredness*

Relatives' understanding of patient's problems *Parents feel that their daughter is 'under the weather' and needs a rest*

NURSING ASSESSMENT INTERVIEW (continued)

Persons of significance in person's life

Family/friends/pets _Parents and cat_

Spiritual needs
None

Problems causing concern at home _Parents are getting anxious about their daughter. Patient would like to go out socially_

Community services involved/referred _Not applicable_

Name _____   Status _____

Telephone number _____   Date of referral _____

Mental status

History of present problems _Has become more anxious over past 4 months_

Previous psychiatric history _None_

General appearance and behaviour _Anxious and tense. Blushes easily_

Speech and communication patterns _Talks quickly. Poor eye-to-eye contact_

Problems with perception _None_

NURSING ASSESSMENT INTERVIEW (continued)

Affective state _Apprehensive. Worries about future_

Disturbances of thinking or judgement _None_

Orientation

Person _Normal_

Place _Normal_

Time _Normal_

Activities of living

Safety and mobility
No problems

Eating and drinking
Poor appetite ; drinks copiously because of dry mouth

Elimination

Bladder _Frequency of micturition_

Bowel _Occasionally has diarrhoea_

Sleep patterns
Sleeps poorly

Personal needs
None

General health _Quite good_

Any medical condition for which the person is receiving treatment
_No_

Doctor's instructions
Anxiety management sessions with relaxations

Areas of concern to patient
Patient would like to know why she feels tense and tired and has headaches. Would also like to know why she panicked on the bus

NURSING ASSESSMENT INTERVIEW (continued)

Problems identified

1. Anxiety state with accompanying physical symptons.
2. Anxiety over physical complaints.
3. Unable to talk to parents without causing them anxiety

Date of interview ___18·6·87___　Signature ___S. Sayer___

History taken from ___Karen James___

by ___Sandra Sayer___　Designation ___Sister___

Additional information　Date ___19·6·87___

Patient is slightly asthmatic which is exacerbated in acute anxiety

ASSESSMENT

1. Karen has an anxiety state with accompanying physical symptoms.
2. She is anxious about her physical complaints.
3. She is unable to talk to her parents without causing them anxiety.
4. She feels that her current condition is preventing her from enjoying a healthy social life.

PLAN OF NURSING CARE

1. To treat Karen on a sessional basis at a day hospital.
2. To adopt a calm and sympathetic nursing approach.
3. To provide reassurance according to Karen's needs and to reduce any factors which may increase her anxiety during treatment.
4. To observe for any additional symptoms during treatment and to record these for medical investigation in case of an underlying problem.
5. To assess her level of anxiety and anxiety-evoking factors.
6. To help Karen to understand the relationship between anxiety and physical symptoms.
7. To instruct her in relaxation techniques.
8. To provide a supportive nurse–patient relationship.
9. To give opportunities for Karen to talk about her anxiety.
10. To reinforce her achievements.

IMPLEMENTATION OF PLAN OF NURSING CARE

Attendance at a day hospital for treatment on a sessional basis was considered to be more appropriate than an in-patient admission as the latter would, in all probability, increase Karen's feelings of insecurity after separation from her safe home environment. The nurse adopted a calm and sympathetic approach and was able to create a psychologically 'safe' therapeutic setting within which Karen would work towards a reduction of her anxiety by relaxation techniques and an understanding of the relationship between anxiety and physical symptoms. It seemed evident from the outset that Karen would need a great deal of reassurance. Initially, Karen was asked to describe her symptoms and to try to recall when she was particularly troubled by them. These were recorded and a physical examination was carried out to eliminate any organic disorder.

The nurse explained to Karen what her treatment would involve to achieve the goals of anxiety control. The nurse also explained the relationship between anxiety and physical symptoms. This helped to reassure Karen that her persistent headaches and tension were not due to a serious physical or organic condition. However, nurses were to observe Karen for any indication of a new symptom as this would need to be recorded and followed up.

Karen was taught relaxation techniques (see boxed section entitled 'Relaxation techniques') and advised to practise at home between sessions. The nurse stressed the importance of this skill which she would have to use regularly in order to cope with the anxiety arising from her day-to-day situations and circumstances. It was also explained to Karen that gaining self-esteem and confidence in being able to cope with anxiety problems would in themselves help to reinforce her ability to control her symptoms. After several sessions of learning to cope with anxiety by relaxation, reassurance, encouragement, reinforcement of her success at various stages of goal achievement and the provision of a supportive nurse–patient relationship, Karen was able to gain confidence and overcome a great deal of her anxiety and problems arising from it.

EVALUATION

From the outset, it was evident that Karen would need to be reassured a great deal. Her parents had mentioned Karen's reluctance to attend the day hospital and described how their daughter had felt sick with worry the day before. Acknowledging this, the nurse was able to plan the sessions accordingly using a calm, sympathetic and reassuring approach. Initially, Karen was unable to grasp the technique of relaxation and found difficulty in allowing her mind to concentrate on the various muscular exercises. This made her even more anxious about the success of her treatment. After practising at home between sessions, however, Karen eventually mastered the technique, which indeed was the first goal. She also began to understand the relationship between anxiety and physical symptoms. Her parents reported good progress and a reduction in Karen's headaches and tiredness. They were encouraged by her less intense facial expression. She seemed happier in herself and was able to converse more with her parents.

After nearly 3 months of treatment with sessions averaging 40 minutes, Karen was more confident in herself and her ability to reduce excess anxiety. She was given a relaxation tape to use at home if necessary and invited to attend a social skills group as an out-patient for weekly sessions but felt that she did not wish to become too dependent on the day hospital. An out-patient appointment was made with the psychologist for a month's time but Karen failed to attend. Her mother telephoned later to say that Karen's father had been admitted to hospital for treatment of his gastric ulcers and that Karen had 'gone to pieces' with worry.

RELAXATION TECHNIQUES

The session, which lasts about 30 minutes, involves the tensing and relaxing of large muscles throughout the body, accompanied by a comfortable and rhythmical breathing pattern the cumulative effect of which is intended to produce a state of relaxation.

To maximise the benefits of this technique, the patient should position himself comfortably, usually supinely, with his head resting on a cushion or pillow. Shoes can be removed and tight clothing loosened if desired. The room should be at a comfortable ambient temperature and away from possible interruption, distraction and excess noise.

The session begins thus: 'For the next few minutes I would like you to think about relaxation by closing your eyes and placing your arms by your side or on your stomach in a comfortable position and to try to empty your mind of problems as you concentrate on establishing a regular breathing pattern. Breathe in deeply—hold your breath—hold it—and then breathe out quickly. Once more, take a deep breath—hold your breath—keep holding—and then breathe out with a sigh. Now try to breathe regularly and comfortably as you feel some of the tension leaving you. Now concentrate on your feet and leg muscles as you place your legs and feet close together. Press your heels down firmly on the floor and push your toes forward away from you and feel the tension in your leg muscles as you hold them in that position—continue to hold—keep holding—and relax and appreciate the contrast. (Repeat exercise.) Now concentrate on your buttocks, waist and lower back by pressing your bottom firmly on the floor and hold it there—feel the tension—keep holding—and now relax and observe the contrast. (Repeat exercise.) Breathe comfortably and gently, and feel the tension leaving your body as you continue to relax. Now concentrate on the muscles in your arms by stretching out the fingers in your hands as you raise your arms from the floor. Feel that tension in your muscles—keep stretching and hold—hold that position—and now relax your hands and arms and notice the difference. (Repeat exercise.) Appreciate the effect of relaxation as your body begins to feel heavier and comfortable. Now concentrate as you press your elbows firmly onto the floor by your side and notice the muscles tensing as you hold—keep holding your elbows like that—feel that tension—and now relax and appreciate the contrast. (Repeat exercise.) Now for your shoulders. Pull your arms down towards your legs and feel the tension in your shoulders as you do so. Keep pulling in that position—and now relax. (Repeat exercise.) Now concentrate on your neck and press your head down firmly into the cushion until you feel the tension in your muscles—and hold it—hold that tension—and now relax and appreciate the contrast. (Repeat.) As your body feels more heavy and relaxed, think about your facial muscles, the forehead and scalp and tighten your eyes—keep your eyes tight—hold them—and relax and feel the difference in your face and head. (Repeat exercise.) As you continue to relax, concentrate once more on your breathing and take a deep breath—hold —and breathe out. Again, breathe in deeply—hold it and breathe out. Now make your breathing gentle and rhythmical again. As you lie there with your body relaxed and heavy, try to picture a secluded beach. Imagine yourself lying on that warm beach with the soft breeze blowing gently on your face. Listen to the sounds of the sea softly caressing the sand and the sea-birds flying overhead. As you lie there enjoying this feeling of warmth and tranquillity, your body is now totally relaxed.' (The introduction of soft music can enhance the effect.)

Allow the client to relax for several minutes before drawing the session to a close by asking him to open his eyes and to get up slowly and comfortably in his own time.

NURSING CARE OF THE PATIENT WHO IS PHOBIC

A phobia is an exaggerated or irrational fear of a specific object or situation. The individual who suffers with phobic neurosis realises the absurdity of his fear but is unable to control the distressing psychological and somatic symptoms of the anxiety produced by exposure to the object or situation. Symptoms include a feeling of panic, tremors, palpitations, excessive sweating and a dry mouth. Since the phobic sufferer is unable to confront the feared stimulus, he deliberately seeks to avoid it. The feared object or situation can be virtually anything from ants to aeroplanes although some phobias are more common than others. These include animal and insect phobias (e.g. spiders, cats and dogs), fear of darkness, social phobias (e.g. attending parties or dating) and claustrophobia (fear of closed spaces). Agoraphobia deserves particular comment here as its incidence appears to be increasing. 'Agora' is derived from the Greek word for market-place or place of assembly. The word agoraphobic is often misinterpreted to mean 'fear of open spaces' which is semantically and clinically incorrect (Vose, 1981). Married women in the age range 20–35 years appear to be the most acute agoraphobic sufferers. Such is the crippling effect of this phobia that it can literally confine the sufferer to a 'house-bound' situation for months or even years. In some instances it may appear that agoraphobia places a heavy burden on the family. However, prolonged contact with the family may reveal that one of the marital partners is using the agoraphobia to control the marriage (Hodgkinson, 1981a). Claustrophobia, the fear of closed places, is also a commonly recognised form. Indeed, some individuals may go to exhausting and elaborate lengths to avoid the possibility of becoming enclosed in a lift or a confined space, e.g. a person who climbs numerous flights of stairs to avoid the lift no matter how tiring this may be. Another example is the traveller who deliberately avoids the Underground and instead uses the bus to get round the town although it is much more time consuming.

Mitchell (1982) says that, the more anxiety prone and sensitive a person is, the more likely he is to develop a phobia, pointing out at the same time that there are no personality types who can be considered pre-phobic.

Several factors appear to contribute to the aetiology of phobia. Factors include the learned reactions of fear during child development, psychological conflicts, family stress, and the illness or death of a friend or relative.

PATIENT PROFILE

After a surgical operation for a back injury, Lesley Court, a 30-year-old married lady with two young children, was advised to rest for several weeks and to refrain from lifting and strenuous activity. This was sound practical medical advice but the necessity of managing a home with two demanding and energetic youngsters, together with daily domestic requirements and tasks, made her confinement less of a recuperative prospect. Lesley's self-employed husband envisaged a reduction in his business working hours to facilitate this new arrangement, a change that he could ill afford to make, particularly in the current competitive economic climate. Fortunately the neighbours, who were usually helpful, offered to take the children to school and to collect them if necessary. Additionally, they were helpful with local shopping for which Lesley was appreciative, although she sometimes felt a little embarrassed and guilty over their generosity.

After 2 months of convalescence during which Lesley had become accustomed to a more passive role in the day-to-day running of the home, she began to feel anxious and doubtful about her ability to resume a normal married life. When relatives and friends called round for social visits, Lesley made this one of the chief topics of her conversation which, perhaps, was her way of seeking reassurance.

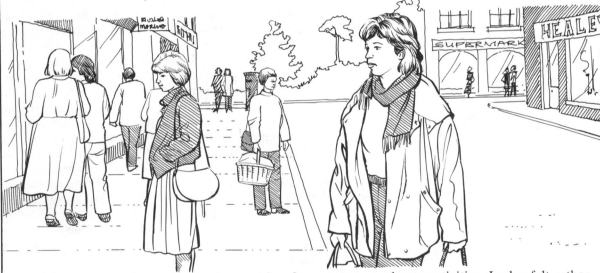

When her general practitioner declared her fit to resume moderate activities, Lesley felt rather lacking in confidence. On the morning that she was due to walk her children to the local school just ½ mile away, Lesley began to feel very anxious, her body tremulous with fear. Her daughter and son looked on with concern as she stood pale and shaking by the doorstep, unable to move. Sally, the eldest of the children, ran to the neighbour who came immediately and comforted Lesley as best she could. Discussing the episode with her husband later, Lesley realised how irrational and foolish her behaviour had been and felt embarrassed talking about it. She began to experience further self-doubt and apprehension in the ensuing days. When she thought about going outside to the shop or to the school, a feeling of extreme anxiety suffused her. Tension developed at home with Lesley's husband taking a less delicate and more insensitive attitude to his wife's behaviour by spending more time at work to avoid arguments.

When another crisis occurred just as Lesley was about to leave the house to go to the local shop, her husband, now extremely frustrated with all aspects of married life, contacted their general practitioner. After talking to Lesley, he suggested that she might be agoraphobic and referred her to a psychiatrist who subsequently suggested that a course of behavioural therapy would probably help to overcome the problem.

NURSING ASSESSMENT INTERVIEW

Surname .Court   Forenames   Lesley Anne

Name person likes to be called   Lesley

Address   15 Ash Road   Telephone number   5269
          Willbury   Date of referral/admission   22.3.87
          WIL CR6

Next-of-kin

Name   Mr D. Court   Relationship   Husband
Address   As above

                                   Telephone number

Date of birth   12.9.54   Single/married/divorced/widowed
General practitioner   Dr J. Yalom   Address   The Surgery
                                      1 Moorfield Road
                                      Willbury

Consultant   Dr J. Hinsie
Status under Mental Health Act   Informal
Psychiatric diagnosis   Agoraphobia

History of self-harm or harm towards others   None

Occupation   Housewife
Occupational history
     Shop assistant, receptionist, clerical work

Hobbies and interests   Gardening, cinema, knitting

Patient's perceived reason for referral/admission   To overcome fear of going outside

Relatives' understanding of patient's problems   Husband feels that she is
     overanxious. Blames her convalescence for her
     problem

NURSING ASSESSMENT INTERVIEW (continued)

Persons of significance in person's life

Family/friends/pets _Husband and children_

Spiritual needs

None

Problems causing concern at home _Tension and marital disharmony due to patient's anxiety and fear of going outside. Children get worried when (mother) patient panics_

Community services involved/referred _Not applicable_

Name _____ Status _____

Telephone number _____ Date of referral _____

Mental status _Not applicable_

History of present problems _Began during convalescence after patient's operation. Loss of confidence predated onset about 4 months ago_

Previous psychiatric history _Treated for depression after a miscarriage 2 years ago_

General appearance and behaviour _Appears tired and anxious. Slim build_

Speech and communication patterns _Speaks quietly. Feels unable to communicate fully_

Problems with perception _None_

NURSING ASSESSMENT INTERVIEW (continued)

Affective state _Feels a little low in mood_

Disturbances of thinking or judgement _None_

Orientation

Person _Normal_

Place _Normal_

Time _Normal_

Activities of living

Safety and mobility
No problems

Eating and drinking
Reduced appetite. Fluid intake within normal range

Elimination

Bladder _Normal_

Bowel _Regular_

Sleep patterns
Sleeps about 5-6 hours daily

Personal needs
None

General health _Fairly good_

Any medical condition for which the person is receiving treatment
Injury to coccyx, necessitating operation - has made good recovery

Doctor's instructions
Course of behavioural therapy

Areas of concern to patient
Patient wants to restore stability of marriage. Would dearly like to take children out again for walks

NURSING ASSESSMENT INTERVIEW (continued)

Problems identified

1. Unable to leave home because of fear.
2. Patient becomes panicky if she has to leave the house.
3. Patient feels cut off from friends and outside.
4. Has to rely on neighbours and husband for shopping and taking children to and collecting children from school

Date of interview   22.3.87

History taken from   Lesley Court

by   Peter Smith

Signature   P. Smith

Designation   Charge nurse

Date

Additional information

ASSESSMENT

1. Lesley is unable to leave home because of her fear of going outside.
2. She becomes panicky when she attempts to leave the house.
3. She feels cut off from friends.
4. There is some breakdown in normal marital relations because of tension between Lesley and her husband.
5. She has to rely on neighbours and her husband for shopping and for taking the children to school and collecting them.

PLAN OF NURSING CARE

1. To enable Lesley to overcome her fear of going outside by implementing a desensitisation programme.
2. To instruct Lesley in the technique of muscle relaxation.
3. To construct a hierarchy of anxiety-producing situations.
4. To create a good nurse–patient relationship.
5. To adopt a sympathetic and understanding approach to problems.
6. To praise and reinforce Lesley's positive achievements.
7. To be supportive throughout a treatment programme.
8. To encourage Lesley's social mobility outside the home.
9. To encourage her husband's support.

IMPLEMENTATION OF PLAN OF NURSING CARE

Lesley was referred to a day hospital in preference to an in-patient psychiatric admission as the programme of systematic desensitisation would be more effective and appropriate in overcoming the problem situations occurring in her daily life and local environment. Accompanied by her husband to the day hospital, Lesley felt less anxious travelling in the car which effectively served as an extension of the safe domestic situation. By this mode of transport, she was able to maximise her attendance.

The nurse who was trained in behavioural therapy techniques was able to reassure Lesley that the programme of systematic desensitisation was a safe method of treating phobias by the gradual and relaxed approach to the anxiety-producing situations.

It was important from the outset that a good nurse–patient relationship was established. This was best achieved by a sympathetic approach, an understanding of the obvious fear and anxiety that Lesley was experiencing and encouragement at each stage of her treatment. Explaining to Lesley how her irrational fears could have arisen and been magnified by her imagination were also important to the success of the programme.

Initially, Lesley was asked by the nurse to draw up a list of all the situations which aroused anxiety within her. From this, a hierarchy was constructed, ranging from those situations producing minimum anxiety to those causing maximum anxiety.

In order to facilitate a gradual elimination of anxiety-evoking stimuli, Lesley was instructed in the technique of deep-muscle relaxation. This involved tensing and relaxing muscles throughout the body and appreciating the contrast in sensation (see boxed section entitled 'Relaxation techniques' earlier in this chapter). In the first two sessions, each lasting 45 minutes, Lesley was asked to imagine herself in the least anxiety-producing situation, i.e. standing at the door of her home. When she reported feeling no anxiety during relaxation, the nurse moved on to the next situation in the hierarchy. By systematically encountering each situation in the hierarchy by imagination, Lesley would be able to eliminate her inappropriate anxiety. The nurse always praised Lesley's efforts and reinforced her achievements.

As Lesley gained more self-confidence, she was now ready in the fifth session to face the situations in reality. Unfortunately a feeling of panic arose within Lesley just as she was about to embark on a short walk. The nurse was very calm and supportive and was able to reassure Lesley, referring to her progress to date. With encouragement, Lesley was able to go for short walks, initially accompanied by the nurse but then allowed to go on her own.

The patient's beliefs and thoughts while in a feared situation are important; the agoraphobiac automatically thinks negatively in panic situations. Positive self-talk assists the patient to make his thoughts more positive (Hodgkinson, 1981b).

During the following three sessions, Lesley had progressed to walking from her home to the local shop, a distance of ½ mile. Eventually, she was able to take her children to school, now confident in her ability and free from the restricting grip that her anxiety and fear had forged.

EVALUATION

Lesley was able to grasp the technique of muscle relaxation very quickly, practising at home between sessions as suggested by the nurse. This enabled her to control her anxiety very effectively during the sessions when she was asked to imagine herself in the fear-provoking situations. Lesley demonstrated her anxiety prior to the realistic encounter of external stimuli, i.e. going for a short walk. However, the nurse was able to reassure Lesley by relating her success and achievement in the imaginal stages of treatment and reinforcing her ability to control the exaggerated anxiety and fear. This reflection was useful for Lesley who gradually overcame this initial uncertainty and subsequently her fear of the outside. As Lesley progressed through treatment, she reported that relations with her husband, who was very supportive and encouraging, had 'improved tremendously'. The achievement that gave Lesley greatest pleasure and satisfaction was being able to collect her children from school on her own. It also pleased her that she was not dependent on neighbours now for the children and shopping. Friends and relatives who visited Lesley and her family made diplomatic comments regarding her improvement.

During the following weeks, Lesley was visited regularly by the community psychiatric nurse who assessed her as a preventative measure against relapse. Lesley also attended the consultant psychiatrist's out-patient clinic at monthly intervals. 6 months later, Lesley remained free of phobic symptoms.

REFERENCES AND FURTHER READING

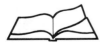

References

Burton, G. (1977), *Interpersonal Relations*, 4th edn, Tavistock, London.
Hodgkinson, P. E. (1981a), Far from the maddening crowd, *Nursing Mirror*, **153**, No. 1, 37–38.
Hodgkinson, P. E. (1981b), Learning to enjoy the great outdoors, *Nursing Mirror*, **153**, No. 2, 40–41.
Koshy, K. T. (1982), *Revision Notes on Psychiatry*, 2nd edn, Hodder and Stoughton, London, pp. 29–34, 170–173.

Mitchell, R. (1982), *Phobias*, Pelican, Penguin, Harmondsworth, Middlesex.
Vose, R. H. (1981), *Agoraphobia*, Faber and Faber, London.

Further reading

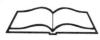

Agras, S. (1985), *Panic: Facing Fears, Phobias and Anxiety*, Freeman, New York.

Barker, P. J., and Fraser, D. (eds) (1985), *The Nurse as Therapist: A Behavioural Model*, Croom Helm, London.

Blenkinsop, J. (1986), There comes a big spider, *Nursing Times*, **82**, No. 2, 28–30.

Bond, M. (1982), The art of relaxation, *Nursing Mirror*, **155**, No. 14, 38–40.

Brockway, B. F., Plummer, O. B., and Low, B. M. (1976), Effects of reassurance on patient's vocal stress levels, *Nursing Research*, **25**, No. 6, 440–446.

France, R. (1986), Anxiety after tranquillizers, *Psychiatry in Practice*, **3**, No. 2, 11–12, 20.

Gomez, E. A., Gomez, G. E., and Otto, D. A. (1984), Anxiety as a human emotion: some basic conceptual models, *Nursing Forum*, **21**, No. 1, 38–42.

Johnson, P., Manchester, J., and Sugden, J. (1985), Anxiety, *Nursing (UK)*, **2**, No. 34, 1008–1012.

Koshy, K. T. (1982), *Revision Notes on Psychiatry*, 2nd edn, Hodder and Stoughton, London.

MacPhail, D., and McMillan, I. (1983), Fighting Phobias, *Nursing Mirror, Mental Health Forum 8*, **157**, No. 7, i–ii.

Mathews, A., Gelder, M., and Johnston, D. (1981), *Agoraphobia—Nature and Treatment*, Tavistock, London.

Mitchell, R. (1982), *Phobias*, Pelican, Penguin, Harmondsworth, Middlesex.

Mitchell, R. G. (1983), Anxiety states and phobias, *Nursing Times*, **79**, No. 7, 50–52.

Murdoch, W., and Newton, A. (1985), High anxiety, *Nursing Times*, **81**, No. 5, 26–28.

Neville, A. (1986), *Who's Afraid of Agoraphobia?*, Century Arrow.

North, N. (1985), Phobias—the misunderstood fear, *Nursing Times*, **81**, No. 1, 24–25.

Roach, F., and Farley, N. (1986), The behavioural management of neurosis by the psychiatric nurse therapist. In: *Psychiatric Nursing Research* (ed. Brooking, J.), John Wiley, Chichester, West Sussex.

Rycroft, C. (1968), *Anxiety and Neurosis*, Penguin, Harmondsworth, Middlesex.

Saucier, R. P. (1984), Panic attacks and generalised anxiety states, *Nursing Practitioner*, **9**, No. 8, 35, 37.

Stanworth, H. M. (1982), Agoraphobia, an illness or a symptom?, *Nursing Times*, **78**, No. 10, 399–403.

Thorpe, G. L., and Burns, L. E. (1983), *The Agoraphobic Syndrome*, John Wiley, Chichester, West Sussex.

Trick, L., and Obcarskas, S. (1976), *Understanding Mental Illness and its Nursing*, 2nd edn, Pitman Medical, London.

Wilson, L., and Barker, P. (1986), Behavioural therapy nursing: a new era?, *Nursing Times*, **82**, No. 1, 48–49.

Wolpe, J. (1973), *The Practice of Behaviour Therapy*, 2nd edn, Pergamon, Oxford.

Chapter 15

Nursing care of the patient who is obsessional

by *Neil Vermaut*

'*The adoption of ritualistic behaviour limits free choice of action. It reduces the number of experiences to which the individual must respond and therefore reduces the number of potential anxieties he must face; its sameness produces a certain form of security, and it becomes a defensive method of self-control.*' (Topalis and Aguilera, 1978).

INTRODUCTION

An obsessional illness can, in its intensity and protracted duration, be severely incapacitating for the sufferer and disruptive to family and social life. Its clinical features divide typically into two main categories:

(a) Obsessional thoughts.
(b) Compulsions.

Obsessional thoughts or ruminations are intrusive and repetitive and usually of a sexual, blasphemous or violent nature. Although the patient has insight into their nature, they differ from normal thinking in that they are alien to his personality and attitudes. The churchgoer, for example, may feel impelled to shout out blasphemies or the moralising individual have the urge to shout about promiscuity. These are characteristic of obsessional thoughts which tend to be bizarre, sometimes embarrassing and coarse in contrast with the patient's refined personality. Some individuals have obsessional doubts and anxieties such that they need to check and recheck to ensure that doors and windows of their home are closed or that they have turned off the gas even if they have a clear recollection of doing so. These doubts may be so severe that they have a crippling effect on the patient's life.

Compulsions are actions or rituals which the patient feels compelled to carry out any number of times during the course of the day. The completion of the act or ritual brings temporary relief from anxiety although it does not prevent him from repeating it subsequently.

Compulsive actions are recognised by the patient as irrational and futile but any attempts to divert or resist them may increase his anxiety to an intolerable or distressing level. Typical behaviour includes repeated hand washing sometimes until the skin peels off, arranging clothes in a particular manner before dressing, touching certain objects or avoiding others. In cases of obsessional fear of dirt or contamination, patients may wear gloves to protect their hands from germs. Others who are obsessional about knives will tend to lock them away for fear of harming others. Some individuals develop compulsions involving counting or numbers, e.g. counting steps or the rungs of a ladder or the number of paces when going for a walk. Others have to avoid using certain numbers (not necessarily 13). Although the obsessional realises the pointlessness of these acts, he feels compelled to carry them out as failure to do so may result in something terrible happening to himself or a loved one.

The incidence of obsessional neurosis in the psychiatric population appears to be relatively small and affects females slightly more than males. It is more likely to occur in individuals who have obsessional personalities although this is not always the case. According to Pollitt (1960), over 30% of cases in a study had no obsessional traits prior to breakdown. The seemingly obsessional action of children in play who avoid stepping on the cracks in the pavement is not necessarily an indication that obsessional behaviour will be manifested in adult life, the majority of them not developing this neurosis.

Aetiologically, there is evidence of genetic influence in obsessional disorder (Kringlen, 1965) and also environmental factors such as a harsh domestic atmosphere during upbringing with parental disharmony or a broken home. The relationship between the individual and a parent may have been rather rigid or affectionless. The pre-morbid personalities of those who develop an obsessional illness tend towards an excess of cleanliness, conscientiousness, rigidity, scrupulousness, proneness to self-criticism and indecisiveness. Many patients experience rapid mood changes, agitation, feelings of guilt, irritability, aggressiveness and suicidal ideation.

According to Kringlen (1965), his data seem to point towards a poor prognosis for the majority of patients. However, those conditions where an obsessional state is a secondary symptom in a depressive illness, the outlook is improved.

PATIENT PROFILE

George Chase, a 32-year-old teacher of English, was referred for treatment with a 1-year history of obsessional neurosis. In the 3 months prior to admission, his symptoms had become increasingly incapacitating and disruptive to his work. A single man, he would take a bath after breakfast and again in the evening; in addition, he would need to wash his hands up to 30 times per day to avoid what he felt were contaminants that would lead to an incurable disease. He avoided buses and other public transport, fearing they might be a source of infection. When shopping, a task which caused him great anxiety, George would pay by cheque so as to avoid handling 'contaminated' cash. This was embarrassing at times, particularly when the payment was for a trivial amount. At school where George had taught for 5 years and was recognised as a conscientious person, he began to wear thin gloves to protect his hands from the germs that he feared he would catch from pupils' textbooks. The library, which he had frequent access to, posed many problems with regard to handling books and caused him a great deal of anxiety when he was unable to avoid using it. This led to increased hand washing. George realised the irrationality of his compulsions but was unable to resist carrying them out. Although his bachelor lifestyle had allowed him the time and freedom to perform his rituals, more recently the additional need to check and recheck that the doors and windows of his flat were closed was interfering with preparation work for school and punctuality. On three occasions during the previous month he was late for attendance. This had not escaped the notice of the head teacher who made a friendly but firm suggestion about the good example that one should set for their pupils. George's rather sensitive personality led him to doubt his own ability to continue with teaching and, feeling rather anxious and depressed, he sought reassurance from his general practitioner. George was referred for an out-patient appointment with a psychiatrist who suggested a short course of behavioural therapy in hospital.

NURSING ASSESSMENT INTERVIEW

Surname _Chase_   Forenames _George Andrew_

Name person likes to be called _George_

Address _7A Brierly Avenue_   Telephone number _67192_
Willbury   Date of ~~referral~~/admission _15.3.87_
WIL JA2

Next-of-kin

Name _Mrs J. Chase_   Relationship _Mother_

Address _25 Grayson Avenue_
Willbury

Telephone number _2025_

Date of birth _19.8.52_   Single/~~married/divorced/widowed~~

General practitioner _Dr S. Kalkman_   Address _Dobbins_
Palmar Avenue
Willbury
WIL 4JJ

Consultant _Dr H. Kellehear_

Status under Mental Health Act _Informal_

Psychiatric diagnosis _Obsessional neurosis_

History of self-harm or harm towards others _None_

Occupation _Schoolteacher_

Occupational history
Trainee market research executive prior to attending teacher training college. Has held present teaching post for 5 years

Hobbies and interests _Crosswords, reading, photography, music_

Patient's perceived reason for referral/admission _To stop excessive hand washing and checking habits_

Relatives' understanding of patient's problems _Parents feel that George has been overworking_

NURSING ASSESSMENT INTERVIEW (continued)

Persons of significance in person's life

Family/friends/pets _Parents and two work colleagues_

Spiritual needs

None

Problems causing concern at home _Feels exhausted after work; has an uneventful social life; excessive hand washing; needs to check and recheck that windows and doors are closed and that gas is off_

Community services involved/referred _None_

Name _____   Status _____

Telephone number _____   Date of referral _____

Mental status

History of present problems _Began to get obsessional and felt insecure following the break-up with his girl-friend a year ago_

Previous psychiatric history _None_

General appearance and behaviour _Appears rather tense and overpolite. Tidily dressed_

Speech and communication patterns _Speaks rather quietly and hesitantly at times_

Problems with perception _None_

NURSING ASSESSMENT INTERVIEW (continued)

Affective state A little depressed and anxious

Disturbances of thinking or judgement None

Orientation

Person Normal

Place Normal

Time Normal

Activities of living

Safety and mobility

No problems

Eating and drinking

Reduced appetite. Drinks tea frequently at home

Elimination

Bladder Normal

Bowel Regular

Sleep patterns

Sometimes has difficulty in getting off to sleep

Personal needs

Improved social life

General health

Any medical condition for which the person is receiving treatment

Allergic rhinitis

Doctor's instructions

Short course of behavioural therapy — two sessions daily for 3–5 weeks. No medication. Use relaxation

Areas of concern to patient

Worried about the effect of his admission on his teaching career

NURSING ASSESSMENT INTERVIEW (continued)

Problems identified

1. Needs to wash his hands excessively and to bath.
2. Needs to check and recheck doors, windows and gas.
3. Feels anxious and insecure at home.
4. Unable to talk about his feelings to anyone.
5. Needs to wear gloves when handling books.
6. Unable to go into a shop and handle cash

Date of interview   15.3.87   Signature   P. Read

History taken from   George Chase

by   Paul Read   Designation   Staff nurse

Additional information   Date   16.3.87

   Patient is allergic to penicillin

ASSESSMENT

1. George needs to wash his hands and to bath excessively.
2. He needs to check and recheck doors, windows and gas.
3. He feels anxious and insecure at home.
4. He is unable to talk about his feelings to anyone.
5. He needs to wear gloves when handling books.
6. He is unable to handle cash.

PLAN OF NURSING CARE

1. To implement behavioural therapy using the techniques of (a) flooding, (b) modelling and (c) response prevention.
2. To assess level of anxiety and urge to ritualise, frequency and duration of rituals, anxiety-evoking objects and environments and to construct a hierarchy of problem situations.
3. To demonstrate a technique of relaxation to reduce anxiety.
4. To offer a simple explanation of the nature of his illness to George.
5. To establish a relationship of trust.
6. To adopt a stance of sympathetic understanding of George's genuine anxiety over his obsessional behaviour.
7. To encourage him to talk about his feelings.
8. To channel his energy into useful and creative activities.
9. To supervise George's activities between sessions according to progress.
10. To offer firm support throughout treatment.
11. To protect him from ridicule or embarrassment.
12. To evaluate efficacy of treatment by assessing degree of improvement.

IMPLEMENTATION OF PLAN OF NURSING CARE

George was admitted to a psychiatric hospital for a short course of behavioural therapy, a method of treatment commonly employed for obsessional disorders. Based on the learning theory that responses which lead to maladaptive habits can be eliminated and replaced with new and correct adaptive behaviour, the treatment evolved from this may be applied in various forms. That considered more appropriate for George's compulsive rituals consisted of three components: flooding, modelling and response prevention. Flooding involves exposing the patient to the situation and anxiety-evoking stimuli that he has previously avoided, which in George's case were the library, shops, buses, books and cash. The nurse acting as a model would demonstrate the adaptive or correct way of handling books or cash to George who would subsequently be encouraged to do the same. Response prevention refers to the restraining or prevention from carrying out the compulsive behaviour, i.e. hand washing following flooding and modelling between sessions.

After an initial interview with the therapeutic team, George was asked to provide details relating to his obsessional behaviour. Salient features of his neurosis were recorded, such as the number of obsessions and rituals, the situations and objects that elicited stimuli, his emotional response to the stimuli, what he avoided, the frequency and duration of his rituals, the emotional effect of performing his rituals, mood and social factors. Before therapy could commence, George was shown how to use rating scales to measure his level of anxiety and the urge to carry out rituals in a given situation. These would be useful quantitative ratings for evaluation purposes. George was also asked to provide a list of situations and objects that caused him problems. From this a hierarchy was constructed with those objects or situations

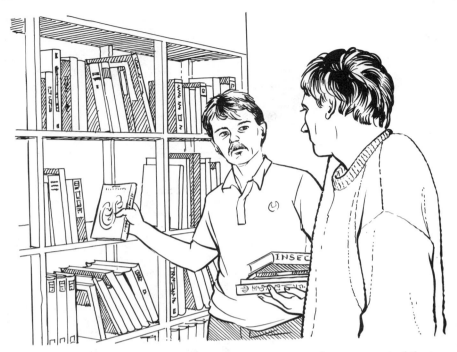

causing greatest problems at the top. The two nurses who were part of the team treating George showed warmth and sympathy, quickly establishing a relationship of trust and assuring him of their support throughout. A relaxation technique was also demonstrated to George to reduce anxiety between sessions (see boxed section entitled 'Relaxation techniques' in Chapter 14).

In the first session, George was asked to enter the library with a nurse and to remain there for 10 minutes. Reluctantly, he agreed to this, a situation that he usually avoided and at the top of the hierarchy. He reported very high anxiety and a strong urge to wash his hands and to take a bath. Supervision was needed to prevent this and by persuasion he was encouraged to engage in creative activities. George was also encouraged to talk about his feelings and reassured that the high level of anxiety that he had felt during the session would reduce appreciably with repeated sessions as would the urge to carry out his ritualistic behaviour.

After several more sessions involving modelling and flooding using the library books and paying for a newspaper with cash, George was able to refrain from washing immediately although a less intense urge was still present. Gradually after 5 weeks the compulsions diminished and the anxiety reduced to an appropriate level at which point George was discharged from hospital. Having assimilated the methods of flooding and response prevention, George was able to use these during the following months when he felt his symptoms were beginning to recur.

EVALUATION

Doubtful initially of the efficacy of behavioural therapy, particularly the component of flooding, George, nonetheless, participated well despite a high level of anxiety. The reassurance given by the nurse and the trusting relationship established were extremely important factors in George's progress. At the outset, George anticipated problems regarding his supervision by the nurse during response prevention, i.e. hand washing, but being engaged in other creative activities, e.g. artwork, helped considerably.

After discharge, George had monthly appointments with a psychologist to prevent any immediate relapse now that he was at home again. 5 months later, George remained free of symptoms, although at one point he began to experience anxiety after returning to school after summer vacation. A feeling of insecurity led him to recheck the windows at home which necessitated an urgent appointment with the psychologist. He was offered day hospital attendance for a short period but preferred to make a determined effort to overcome this problem by employing the relaxation technique instructed to him. George succeeded in preventing a recurrence of his obsessional behaviour.

He now planned to apply for a deputy head teacher's post in another county.

REFERENCES AND FURTHER READING

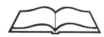

References

Kringlen, E. (1965), cited by Beech, H. R., and Vaughan, M. (1978), *Behavioural Treatment of Obsessional States*, John Wiley, Chichester, West Sussex.

Pollitt, J. D. (1960), cited by Rycroft, C. (1968), *Anxiety and Neurosis*, Penguin, Harmondsworth, Middlesex.

Topalis, M., and Aguilera, D. (1978), *Psychiatric Nursing*, 7th edn, C. V. Mosby, St Louis, Missouri.

Further reading

Barker, P., and Wilson, L. (1985), Behavioural therapy nursing new wine in old bottles, *Nursing Times*, **81**, No. 39, 31–34.

Farrington, A. (1983), Obsessive–compulsive disorder, *Nursing Mirror*, **157**, No. 7, vii–viii.

Chapter 16

Nursing care of the attention-seeking patient

'The kind of person each nurse is will make a considerable difference to what each patient will learn.' (Peplau, 1952).

INTRODUCTION

There are some people who simply thrive on being the centre of attention. Such people often have a whole range of accompanying personality problems which may include egocentricity, exhibitionism, suggestibility, superficiality and a tendency to overdramatise things. Consequently the person usually has poor interpersonal relationships, little consideration for other people and an inability to tolerate frustration. There may be angry outbursts particularly if the person does not get his own way. Mood fluctuations can mean that the person is crying one moment and laughing the next. While such behaviour is of course possible in either sex, the literature points to a higher incidence among females. Such females frequently dress and act seductively in relation to males. Heavy make-up is often worn and manipulation is quite common. Such people have generally suffered from some kind of emotional deprivation during formative years. Present behaviour is unconsciously motivated by anxiety and a desire to be loved and cared for. The individual may have been denied the opportunity to experience feelings of security and consistency during the process of growing up. Unfortunately for the person concerned, attention-seeking behaviour often arouses negative feelings in others.

PATIENT PROFILE

Marlene Speedman, aged 35, is an attractive woman with a long psychiatric history. Since her divorce 2 years ago, she has lived with several different men. Her present relationship with Terry Meadows seems relatively stable.

Marlene's ex-husband had custody of their two children Bibi, aged 12, and Guy, aged 9. Although Marlene had access to the children, she sees them infrequently. When Marlene was married, she had at one time been suspected of ill treating her daughter, and both children had been taken into care.

Marlene had recently been discharged from the district general hospital after taking an overdose of drugs. This it seems was brought about because she learned of her ex-husband's plans to remarry. Marlene has been a long-term patient of Dr Mencat and he suggested that she should attend the day hospital again. The staff, who know Marlene well, were not exactly overjoyed by the news. Marlene had attended the day hospital up to 3 months ago but had chosen to discharge herself. She always presented a variety of physical symptoms and was constantly requesting analgesics for headaches. She was also very manipulative. During her last attendance, she had several 'fits' in front of the other patients.

NURSING ASSESSMENT INTERVIEW

Surname _Speedman_   Forenames _Marlene Helena_

Name person likes to be called _Marlene_

Address _29 Station Approach_   Telephone number _7616_
Willbury   Date of referral/admission
WIL BJ1   _18.4.86_

Next-of-kin

Name _Mrs S. Baker_   Relationship _Mother_

Address _24 Melton Road_
Willbury
WIL CA2   Telephone number _____

Date of birth _12.6.51_   Single/married/divorced/widowed _____

General practitioner _Dr E. Sparly_   Address _Parkway Health Centre_
Old Barn Road
Willbury

Consultant _Dr S. Mencat_

Status under Mental Health Act _Informal_

Psychiatric diagnosis _Personality disorder_

History of self-harm or harm towards others _Has taken several overdoses_

Occupation _Cashier_

Occupational history
Hotel receptionist, waitress

Hobbies and interests _Dancing, wining and dining_

Patient's perceived reason for referral/admission _'Losing my kids'_

Relatives' understanding of patient's problems _Terry thinks that_
Marlene has had a lot to put up with

NURSING ASSESSMENT INTERVIEW (continued)

Persons of significance in person's life

Family/friends/pets _Terry Meadows (boy-friend), Bibi, Guy, Mother_

Spiritual needs _Church of England_

Problems causing concern at home

'Everything would be alright if I could get my kids back'

Community services involved/referred

Name _Betty Levis_   Status _Social worker_

Telephone number _2177 Ext. 319_   Date of referral _____

Mental status

History of present problems _Readmitted to day hospital after overdose_

Previous psychiatric history _Several previous admissions. History of vague suicidal attempts and acting-out behaviour_

General appearance and behaviour _Well dressed; feminine clothes. Immature behaviour. Can be demanding; sulky_

Speech and communication patterns _Sometimes, Marlene communicates by acting out rather than verbalising her needs_

Problems with perception _No_

NURSING ASSESSMENT INTERVIEW (continued)

Affective state _Mood changes quickly_

Disturbances of thinking or judgement _No_

Orientation

Person _No problem_

Place _____

Time _____

Activities of living

Safety and mobility

May pose a threat to own safety

Eating and drinking

Eats well; takes adequate fluids

Elimination

Bladder _No problems_

Bowel _No problems_

Sleep patterns

Late going to bed – late riser

Personal needs

Takes a pride in her appearance.
Means a lot to her

General health _____

Any medical condition for which the person is receiving treatment

_No_

Doctor's instructions

Set limits on patient's behaviour

Areas of concern to patient

Says that she would like to see her
children more often

NURSING ASSESSMENT INTERVIEW (continued)

Problems identified

_____

_____

_____

_____

_____

_____

_____

_____

_____

_____

Date of interview   18 . 4 . 86   Signature   C. Hallington

History taken from   Marlene

by   Celia Hallington   Designation   Sister

Additional information   Date   18.4.86

To attend day hospital 5 days and then to
reduce according to assessments

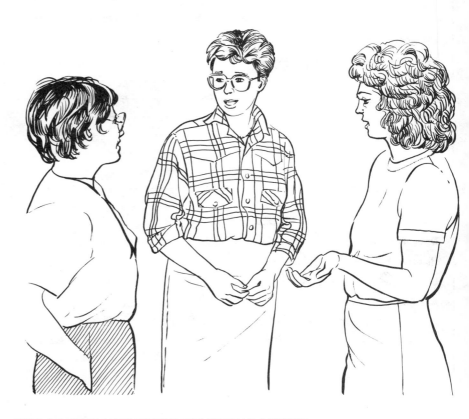

USE OF PEPLAU'S DEVELOPMENTAL MODEL

MacIlwaine's (1983) study highlighted the difficulties which nurses experience in interacting with patients who are not obviously sick or disturbed.

Peplau's (1952) developmental model was chosen for Marlene's nursing care. The decision to use this model was based on the fact that several of the nursing staff knew Marlene and admitted to a negative evaluation because of her previous history; previous enounters had led to a condemnation of her behaviour and a depreciation of her as a person. Such attitudes inhibited effective nursing interventions. Peplau's model may facilitate the development of more positive and constructive attitudes on the part of the nurses since both the nurses and the patient are participants in the process of maturation and human growth (see Chapter 7 for an overview of this model).

A meeting was held among the nursing staff so that feelings concerning Marlene could be expressed and shared. It was necessary for all the nurses to look at themselves and to explore the reasons for various feelings aroused by her behaviour. This required courage, honesty and a willingness to be open with one's self. One nurse had known Marlene for some time and recalled an occasion a year ago when she had taken an overdose of drugs while attending the day hospital; not only were the staff made to feel foolish, but also it probably made them look incompetent in the eyes of the consultant. Another nurse felt that Marlene's behaviour was 'a sham' and resented spending time with 'people like her' when there were patients who genuinely needed help. Other nurses felt that Marlene's behaviour caused disruption to the harmony of the ward, that her behaviour in front of other patients and visitors made it look as if the staff were not in control and that her suicidal attempts were merely gestures. Her past treatment towards her children also aroused some feelings of hostility and anger.

The nurses recognised that it was essential for them to come to terms with their own feelings and to examine why negative feelings are evoked by certain patients. Attitudes and feelings can only be examined in a supportive environment. The nurses themselves needed to recognise that they were not super-human beings. Like other people, each nurse had both strengths and weaknesses, which could only be understood through the process of self-discovery and peer assessment. It is only in the light of this self-discovery that the nurse is able to accept other human beings as they really are. If this self-awareness is lacking, then the nurse's behaviour may result from self-needs and anxieties. The nurse needs to be aware of the feelings that the patient arouses and to look closely to see which life experience is arousing these feelings. If the nurse fails to do this, the patient's behaviour may unwittingly be perpetuated.

(a) Orientation phase

Two key nurses were nominated to spend more time with Marlene in an attempt to get to know her really as a person. The key nurses and the other nurses tried to provide a continuity of approach by being kind and yet firm, realistic and consistent. Consistency among the staff was important because inconsistency provides an ideal setting for the patient to play one member of staff off against another. The nursing care plan was adhered to, and only agreed behaviours were reinforced by giving verbal praise and verbal and non-verbal approval.

Limits were set on maladaptive actions by ignoring inappropriate behaviour (see boxed section entitled 'Setting limits' and *Table 16.1*). The nurse must bear in mind that, if the patient acts out, she is *showing* the nurse how she feels rather than *expressing* her underlying fears and anxieties (Loomis, 1970). Acting-out behaviours may include temper tantrums, refusal to eat, suicidal threats or self-mutilation. The patient may actually find it very hard to understand that the nurse would be interested in her as a person if she did not behave in this way.

SETTING LIMITS

The nurse may fear that setting limits for the patient may interfere with the development of a nurse–patient relationship (Lyon, 1970). This will not be the case if the limit is perceived as necessary, beneficial and having some learning value for the patient. The setting of a limit on the patient's behaviour can actually communicate to him that someone cares for and is concerned about him.

The patient must be helped to understand the reasons for the limit. He is unlikely to adhere to the limit if he does not understand the reason for the limit in the first place. The limit must be realistic and meaningful, and the nurse must be very clear about what behaviour is being limited. The setting of a total limit is essential; if the limit is only partial, then the patient may become confused and unclear about the boundaries.

The patient must be provided with a consistent set of expectations which provide guidance towards self-control. The patient can be expected to test out the consistency of the limits.

Table 16.1　Setting limits on Marlene

Patient's behaviour on which limits are to be set	Limit set by nurse	Appropriate behaviour to be reinforced by praise or approval
Dressing seductively by wearing low necklines, revealing breasts, or tight clothing	The nurse will remind the patient that the mode of dress is inappropriate	The wearing of suitable clothing or clothing worn appropriately, e.g. blouse buttoned up or a less-revealing neckline
Falling around in front of an audience of visitors or patients	The nurse will ask the patient to refrain from behaviour	Behaviour that does not act out the need for attention
Monopolising the time and attention of other patients, visitors or professional workers	The nurse will ask the patient to remove herself graciously	Patient shows consideration for needs of others by withdrawing
Silent sulky behaviour	The nurse will ignore the behaviour	Give patient the opportunity to engage in interaction, e.g. discuss feelings

Source: Lyon (1970).

During orientation the nurse showed a willingness to listen to Marlene and conveyed acceptance of her as a person without being judgemental about her past behaviours. It was accepted by the nurses that caring for Marlene provided a learning experience as well as a challenge. It was made clear to Marlene that, while accepting her as a person, any maladaptive behaviour would be unacceptable.

(b) Identification phase

During the identification phase, it was necessary to try to clarify what Marlene's problems were.

The inappropriateness of her behaviour was discussed in a caring way together with the limits which were to be imposed. Her boy-friend Terry seems to be very concerned about Marlene and it was important that he was involved in the setting of goals and understood the reasons for them.

The actual setting of limits helped to convey to Marlene the nurse's interest and concern for her.

PLAN OF NURSING CARE

(a) Patient's problems

1. Immature attention-seeking behaviour.
2. Dependence on others.
3. Her history of vague suicidal attempts had to be borne in mind as a potential problem.

(b) Patient's goals

1. To verbalise anxieties rather than to engage in acting-out behaviours.
2. To explore reasons for present behaviour.
3. To learn more appropriate goal-seeking behaviour.
4. To display independence.

(c) Nursing goals

1. To get to know Marlene as a person.
2. To set limits on inappropriate acting-out behaviour by non-reinforcement.

3. To help Marlene to explore reasons for present behaviour.
4. To communicate clearly to other nurses and members of the multi-disciplinary team.
5. To demonstrate consistency towards the patient.
6. To encourage independence and belief in own decisions.
7. To recognise manipulative behaviour and to avoid being used as a tool.
8. To apply consistent expectations.
9. To praise Marlene's strengths to improve her self-concept.
10. To explore reasons for negative attitudes towards Marlene.
11. To be non-judgemental.
12. To demonstrate a genuine positive regard for the patient.

(c) Exploitation phase

During the exploitation phase, the nurse acted as a role model, guiding Marlene's personal growth towards self-awareness and independence.

Modelling is a process in which the behaviour of one person acts as a stimulus for another person who observes the behaviour. Pope (1986) suggests that a large proportion of a person's behavioural repertoire is developed not through personal experience but through observing other people acting in particular situations. In acting as a role model the nurse assisted Marlene to learn the behavioural skills necessary for her to function appropriately in social situations.

At first, as expected, Marlene tested out the nurse's consistency in maintaining the limits set for her but, in a very short time, Marlene was demonstrating a new level of functioning which allowed her to experience approval instead of disapproval. She told the nurse that she had often felt compelled to behave in a particular way to achieve what she wanted but could not really understand why she was doing it.

(d) Resolution phase

Marlene was prepared for the resolution phase of the nurse–patient relationship from the time of her admission to the day hospital. She was encouraged to join in the various activities and to learn to make her own independent decisions. The nursing goals were met. Setting limits and reinforcing approved behaviour eliminated the need for Marlene to act out. The staff were surprised about how well Marlene had adhered to the goals but felt that imposing limits on her behaviour had been beneficial in meeting her security needs. Furthermore, because each nurse had tried to examine their own negative attitudes towards Marlene and to get to know her as a person, nursing interventions were more effective. Rather than being viewed as a *nuisance*, she was perceived as a person with needs based on underlying anxiety.

Marlene was made aware from the time of her admission to the day hospital that the nurse–patient relationship was goal centred and would eventually be terminated. Her behaviour showed a marked improvement and she demonstrated a degree of maturity not previously seen. Marlene felt more secure and settled than she had for some time and was able to display new measures of independence and strength while participating in various planned activities. The number of days that she attended the day hospital was gradually reduced from 5 days to 1 day a week over a 6-week period. Marlene's relationship with Terry is going well. He has a new job and plans to move away soon. Marlene sees this as a chance to start afresh.

Marlene's altered level of functioning may enable her to change her self-concept and to cope with life's experiences more adequately. Dr Mencat, however, is less optimistic about her future behaviour.

REFERENCES AND FURTHER READING

References

Loomis, M. (1970), Nursing management of acting out behaviour, *Perspectives in Psychiatric Care*, **8**, No. 4, 168–173.

Lyon, G. G. (1970), Limit setting as a therapeutic tool, *Journal of Psychiatric Nursing and Mental Health Services*, **8**, No. 6, 17–24.

MacIlwaine, H. (1983), The communication patterns of female neurotic patients with nursing staff in psychiatric units of general hospitals. In: *Nursing Research: Ten Studies in Patient Care* (ed. Barnett, J. W.), John Wiley, Chichester, West Sussex.

Peplau, H. E. (1952), *Interpersonal Relations in Nursing*, G. P. Putnam, New York.

Pope, B. (1986), *Social Skills Training for Psychiatric Nurses*, Harper and Row, London.

Further reading

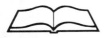

Burgess, A. C., and Lazare, A. (1972), Nursing management of feelings, thoughts and behaviour, *Journal of Psychiatric Nursing and Mental Health Services*, **10**, No. 6, 7–11.

Chitty, K. K., and Maynard, C. K. (1986), Managing manipulation, *Journal of Psychiatric Nursing and Mental Health Services*, **24**, No. 6, 8–13.

Efthymiou, G. (1976), Management of attention seeking patients—1, *Nursing Times*, **72**, No. 37, 1452–1453.

Efthymiou, G. (1976), Management of attention seeking patients—2, *Nursing Times*, **72**, No. 38, 1490–1491.

Frost, M. (1971), Acting out in psychiatric patients, *Nursing Times*, **67**, No. 19, 573–574.

Kumler, F. R. (1963), An interpersonal interpretation of manipulation. In: *Some Clinical Approaches to Psychiatric Nursing* (eds Burd, S., and Marshall, M. A.), Macmillan, New York.

Mooney, J. (1976), Attachment/separation in the nurse–patient relationship, *Nursing Forum*, **15**, No. 3, 259–264.

Richardson, J. I. (1981), The manipulative patient, *Nursing (US),* **11**, No. 1, 48–53.

Chapter 17

Nursing care of the elderly mentally impaired patient

'*Love is essential, because there is no other reason for the very helpless and especially the mentally impaired patient to live.*' (Terrington, 1985).

INTRODUCTION

Ageing is a normal part of the life cycle. Birth and death, childhood and senility, and adolescence and elderliness have mutual characteristics. Birth and death signify the beginning and the end (Robinson, 1983).

Lidz (1968) divides old age into three phases: the period of retirement when adjustment to a non-working life style takes place and independence is still possible; the period when some physical deterioration occurs and the person becomes dependent on others; finally the period when the brain ceases to function as an organ of adaption which enables a person to initiate appropriate responses to the environment. These periods may overlap and may not, of course, necessarily occur at all.

Because of an increasing elderly population, the nurse will encounter patients, both in hospital and in the community, who suffer from varying degrees of intellectual impairment accompanied by memory loss, poor judgement and personality change.

Wherever the patient is cared for it is important for her to be able to enjoy the years that she has left to the fullest capacity (Metz, 1976).

When a patient is severely mentally impaired, talking to her without getting much response can be very difficult for the nurse. However, although the patient may appear to be unresponsive and unaware of what is going on, she may well perceive far more of the nurse's feelings than she overtly indicates (Murray and Huelskoetter, 1983). Some nurses are inclined to be judgemental about the elderly, writing them off as senile, incontinent, obstinate or just plain difficult. Nurses must remember that the patient will judge them too; the one who is rough or in too much of a hurry to care; the one who says one thing but whose behaviour means something else (Davis, 1984). The patient will derive ideas about herself from what she reads into the behaviour of the nurse. The patient's attitude towards herself may be related to the respect, esteem and care shown by the nurse. If the nurse is bored or irritated or feels that work with the elderly mentally impaired patient is pointless, these feelings can be easily transmitted to the patient, making her feel anxious and insecure. If the nurse is primarily concerned with physical care, then there will be little time to get to know the patient as a person, and the patient may become merely an object to be fed, watered and maintained in existence. Furthermore, if the nurse is more concerned with acquainting the patient to hospital routines rather than with adapting nursing care to meet the patient's individual needs, then the patient's identity may be lost in a maze of procedures and treatments.

Caring for the elderly mentally impaired patient requires a large investment of self and a feeling of concern, regard and the respect that one human being has for another (Sobel, 1969). Every patient is entitled to humane treatment and to courtesy, gentleness and the preservation of dignity.

Caring requires an open heart as well as an open mind.

PATIENT PROFILE

Hannah Whitten, aged 80, had a history of minor bilateral strokes which had led to language impairment, facial weakness, poor intellectual ability and feeding problems.

For the past 2 years, Hannah had been successfully supported by the community psychiatric nurse and by attending a day centre. Recently the nurse had observed a deterioration in Hannah's memory and in her ability to care for herself. Periods of confusion and disorientation meant that Hannah now posed a risk to her own well-being and safety; she had been seen out in the road late at night wearing only her nightclothes. A neighbour who had persuaded Hannah to return home and go to bed reported this to the nurse.

As Hannah now required 24-hour care, she was admitted to hospital.

NURSING ASSESSMENT INTERVIEW

Date of admission _12.1.86_   Date of assessment _12.1.86_   Nurse's signature _Jane Sanderson_

Surname _Whitten_   Forenames _Hannah May_

Male ☐   Age _80_   Prefers to be addressed as _Hannah_

Female ☑   Date of birth _15.3.06_

Single/Married/Widowed/Other

Address of usual residence
37 London Road
Willbury
WIL S24

Type of accommodation (including mode of entry if relevant) _Bungalow (belongs to council)_

Family/others at this residence _No_

Next-of-kin

Name _Mr G. Palfry_   Address _Sandford Ward_
Relationship _Brother_   _St Mary's Hospital_
Bristol

Telephone number _____

Significant other (including relatives/dependants/ visitors/helpers/neighbours) _Mrs Monkford_
38 London Road
(Next-door neighbour – has been very good to Hannah)

Support services _Community psychiatric nurse / day centre_

Occupation _Retired teacher_

Recent significant life crises _Husband died 1981_

Patient's perception of current health status _Rather confused at present._

Family's perception of patient's health status _Brother (only remaining family). Also senile dementia_

Reason for admission/referral _Unable to care for self or to maintain safety_

Medical information (e.g. diagnosis, past history, allergies) _Senile dementia_

General practitioner _Dr V. Kalkman_   Consultant _Dr C. Spearman_
Address _Links Road_   Address _____
Willbury
Telephone number _0715_   Telephone number _____
Plans for discharge _None_

USE OF THE ROPER–LOGAN–TIERNEY ACTIVITIES-OF-LIVING MODEL

The Roper–Logan–Tierney activities-of-living model (Roper and Logan, 1985; Roper *et al.*, 1986) was adopted for her care so that her nursing needs and priorities of care could be readily identified. A description of this model can be found in Chapter 7.

Maintaining a safe environment

PLAN OF NURSING CARE

(a) Patient's problems

1. Poor memory for recent events.
2. Disorientated as to time, place and sometimes people.
3. Unable to make sound judgements.
4. Speech and language problems.

(b) Nursing goals

1. To provide a safe environment, by identifying actual and potential safety hazards.
2. To use reality orientation measures.
3. To supervise Hannah at all times, maintaining her safety in all aspects of living.

NURSING INTERVENTION

The nurse must ensure that the ward environment is free from dangerous hazards (*Table 17.1*). The decrease in perceptual abilities which accompanies the ageing process will mean that Hannah is less able to protect herself from harm. Reality orientation measures will help to decrease confusion (see 'Fact sheet: Reality orientation' and 'Fact sheet: More on reality orientation'). A safe environment has been maintained and Hannah remains free from injury.

Table 17.1   *Some examples of environmental safety hazards*

Safety hazards
Slippery floors
Poor lighting
Hot appliances
Unlocked bathrooms
Uneven floors
Unprotected radiators
Trailing cables
Stairs and steps
Worn carpet
Cleaning materials, e.g. bleach
Kitchen appliances
Obstructions and clutter
Untied laces

This list is not conclusive.

Communicating

PLAN OF NURSING CARE

(a) Patient's problems

1. Difficulty in speaking intelligibly. She seems distressed by this.
2. Difficulty in understanding spoken and written language.

(b) Nursing goals

1. To communicate with Hannah using clear verbal and non-verbal communication.
2. To refer to speech therapist.

NURSING INTERVENTION

Hannah was referred to the speech therapist for an assessment, so that the exact extent and range of her language problems could be ascertained. Hannah's history of strokes had left her with some weakness of the facial musculature, making her speech less intelligible. The speech therapist was able to engage Hannah in exercise involving the tongue, lips and palate to help this.

To communicate with Hannah, the nurse used a more total system incorporating pictures, signs, written language and gestures. Touch provided a particularly important means of providing human contact. Not only does touch help to provide a feeling of safety and security, but also it can decrease the elderly person's sense of isolation.

Touch and closeness can help the elderly patient to feel still loved and cared for. Burnside (1973) suggests that a simple warm human gesture such as placing a hand on the shoulder can do more for the elderly regressed patient than many more sophisticated techniques.

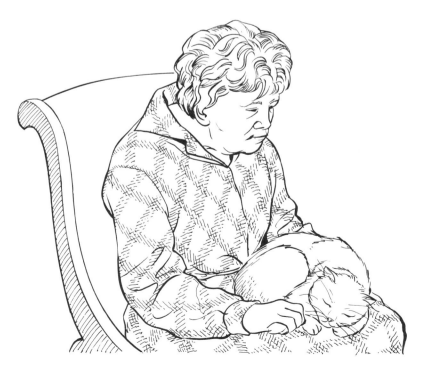

Hannah had never been particularly receptive to touch, but she seemed to fulfil her need for touch by stroking the ward cat Thomas Trouble. There was a special rapport, an unconditional acceptance, between Hannah and Thomas Trouble. Davis (1984) suggests that both are in need of physical contact and both are willing to respond to each other's need for affection. The nurse had noticed that contact with pets is positively beneficial to patients who are separated from their homes and loved ones.

EVALUATION

With the support of the speech therapist, there has been some improvement in Hannah's speech. When communications are directed through total input channels, Hannah's distress is reduced.

Breathing

Hannah breathes normally, and no respiratory problems are apparent.

Eating and drinking

Hannah is not malnourished.

PLAN OF NURSING CARE

(a) Patient's problems

1. Occasional choking and nasal regurgitation due to bulbar palsy.
2. Will not feed herself.
3. Unable to attend to oral hygiene.

(b) Nursing goals

1. To ensure that Hannah eats her food safely.
2. To seek advice of speech therapist.
3. Also to seek advice regarding problem of choking.
4. To provide regular mouth care.

NURSING INTERVENTION

The nurse was particularly worried about the choking and decided to approach the speech therapist for advice. The speech therapist suggested that Hannah should adopt a good feeding posture by sitting in a high-backed chair which has adequate support. The amount and consistency of the food needed to be considered and the size of the feeding spoon. The nurse needs to be positioned in front of the patient and should try to take note of any foods which Hannah does not seem to like.

Contrary to belief, many elderly people like food that is well seasoned and strongly flavoured because the decreased sensitivity of the taste buds causes food to taste less distinctive than formerly. Oral hygiene was practised after each meal to remove any food residue.

EVALUATION

An adequate amount of food and fluids were taken. Episodes of choking have been reduced by careful feeding.

Eliminating

While attending the day hospital, Hannah was continent of urine and faeces, but there was some faecal staining on her clothes. Rectal examination by the doctor indicated constipation.

PLAN OF NURSING CARE

(a) Patient's problems

1. Impacted faeces.
2. Incontinent of urine—occasional 'accidents'.

(b) Nursing goals

1. To give suppositories as prescribed; to observe and report the result.
2. To establish a routine so that bladder and bowel habits become regularised.
3. To ensure dietary fibre is included in diet.

NURSING INTERVENTION

If times of bowel and bladder habits are recorded, it will make it easier to establish the patient's pattern and to assist her to the toilet before a mishap occurs. Because of the patient's general confusion and disorientation, there may be times when accidents will happen. Remember that the patient's dignity can be either reinforced or shattered by words or deeds, and by attitudes or gestures in any place or situation and in any human encounter (Collins, 1983). Respect should be conveyed towards Hannah, however she presents herself.

EVALUATION

Regular bowel actions were recorded. The incidence of incontinence has been reduced through the establishment of a regular routine and reality orientation measures.

Personal cleansing and dressing

Hannah has always been meticulous about cleanliness and personal grooming. She liked good clothes when she was professionally and socially active.

PLAN OF NURSING CARE

(a) Patient's problems

1. Inability to engage in self-care of her own volition.
2. Clothing soiled and uncared for.

(b) Nursing goals

1. To assist Hannah to attend to her own personal hygiene needs by offering support and guidance.
2. To label her clothing and to send for cleaning.

NURSING INTERVENTION

Allow her to carry out her own personal care as far as she is able. Resist the urge to 'do' for her because it is quicker. Remember that, unless Hannah is allowed to maintain and practise the self-care skills that she has, she will become less independent and more dependent.

EVALUATION

She dresses slowly with assistance.

Controlling body temperature

Hannah's temperature is within the normal range, and her skin is warm to the touch. There are no problems in controlling her body temperature.

Mobilising

Hannah walks slowly but is steady on her feet.

PLAN OF NURSING CARE

(a) Patient's problem

1. Nails thick and long.

(b) Nursing goal

1. To refer to chiropodist.

NURSING INTERVENTION

The condition of her feet should be observed. Footcare is important as callouses and thick distorted toenails can lead to difficult and painful walking, thereby increasing the patient's accident-proneness. Regular visits from a chiropodist are desirable. The chiropodist is concerned with foot problems caused by ill-fitting shoes and stockings as well as those caused by poor circulation, skin diseases, abnormal gaits or other medical disorders. The services of the chiropodist are invaluable not only in promoting foot education but also in promoting comfort and mobility among patients and particularly the elderly.

EVALUATION

Hannah appears to walk more comfortably.

Working and playing

Hannah led a very active life until she became confused and disorientated. She always enjoyed activities in the day hospital.

PLAN OF NURSING CARE

(a) Patient's problem

1. Lack of activity exacerbated by failing sight, hearing and mental capacities.

NURSING INTERVENTION

It is important for the patient to feel wanted and useful, for time can hang heavily for the patient and the void is even greater if the patient is deprived of something to do (Davis, 1984). If there is an occupational therapist attached to the ward, her guidance should be sought, as she can usually suggest a programme of activities for even the most regressed patients. It is sometimes forgotten that each elderly person brings into hospital a wealth of experience gathered over the years. These experiences may not be apparent behind confused mumblings, incontinence and restlessness but they are still there (Norris and Abu El Eileh, 1982). As a person becomes older, the amount of reminiscing probably increases. It can be silent or spoken.

Reminiscence groups can provide a situation in which the elderly patient can discover a sense of worth and identity. Reminiscence is particularly useful for the patient who is beginning to experience memory loss. Such memory loss is often related to recent events which can make the present confusing and threatening. Concentrating on a time when memories are stronger and more certain can be more beneficial for the patient.

EVALUATION

Hannah was able to engage in simple planned activities, such as catching a large ball and doing movements to music. As her concentration is poor, she has required continuous prompting.

Expressing sexuality

Hannah always took a pride in her appearance and clothing. She likes to wear good perfume.

PLAN OF NURSING CARE

(a) Patient's problems
1. Inability to maintain previous standards.
2. Facial hair.

(b) Nursing goal
1. To assist the patient to maintain her appearance and femininity.

NURSING INTERVENTION

The patient should be helped to maintain her feminine appearance; therefore an appointment was booked with the beautician and hairdresser. Hannah should be assisted to wash and bath as part of an established routine. She should be allowed to take over these functions as far as she is able; she may respond to gentle prompting, such as placing the soap and flannel in her hand.

She will need special attention paid to her skin, particularly if she is not able to exercise good bladder and bowel control. As the skin is often dry, a soap with a cold cream or oil base may prove less irritating.

The patient should have her own clothes and, if possible, she should be allowed to indicate what she would like to wear. While this may seem like a very small area for the patient to govern, it will allow her to retain some autonomy.

Privacy should be ensured for all aspects of the patient's personal care; a lack of privacy can be degrading for the older person who grew up in times when modesty was highly valued.

EVALUATION

Hannah has retained her individual femininity and has been able to indicate her choice of clothing.

Sleeping

Hannah slept well up to 3 months ago.

PLAN OF NURSING CARE

(a) Patient's problem

1. Disorientation and confusion may cause Hannah to wander at night.

(b) Nursing goal

1. To promote restful sleep.

NURSING INTERVENTION

It should be ensured that Hannah follows her usual sleep habits as far as possible. Remember that, the more her lifestyle is disrupted, the more likely she is to become confused. If the patient wakes up, she should be offered the use of the toilet. She may be hungry or need a drink. She should be reassured by the use of touch and appropriate reality orientation.

EVALUATION

Hannah slept poorly the first 2 weeks but is now sleeping at least 8 hours, usually without waking.

FACT SHEET: ELDERLY PATIENTS

1. Establishing trust is basic to the nurse–patient relationship. It allows the patient who is in a very vulnerable position to feel secure in knowing that he can depend on the nurse.
2. The activities of the nurse have much to do with the quality of the patient's life.
3. Nursing practices which do not enable the patient to maintain or regain self-care skills can and do create unnecessary dependency. When nurses push patients towards unnecessary dependency, they may actually be 'nursing the patients to death' (Miller, 1985).
4. A person becomes human through the process of interacting with others and may also be dehumanised in the same way (Collins, 1983).
5. Add a kitten to the care plan of an elderly patient and something magical happens. The lethargic patient becomes alert and even the depressed patient may brighten up (Davis, 1984).

6. Some patients compensate for a lack of touch by rocking or swaying as a form of self-comfort (Davis, 1984).
7. The need for touch does not diminish as a person grows older and, during times of stress and illness, human contact becomes even more important (Davis, 1984).
8. Environments without planned activities other than daily routines can promote the symptoms of senility. The patient may become introspective and speak only when spoken to (Davis, 1984).
9. There are hospitals when patients are clothed from a common pool of laundry. To possess the clothes that you wear is a dignity so taken for granted by most people that it is hard to imagine the devastating implications of seeing someone else wearing the clothes that you wore last week (Snow, undated).

FACT SHEET: REALITY ORIENTATION

1. Colour coding can be used to enable the patient to find his way around the ward.
2. Sharply contrasting colours for door frames and walls enable the patient to see the door better.
3. The time of the year can be emphasised by letting the patient see and smell seasonal flowers.
4. Familiar objects, personal activities and pictures of the family can help to give the patient a sense of identity.
5. Visitors are an important link with the outside world.
6. When a patient does not have visitors, the nurse can always seek the help of the League of Friends who are usually only too willing to take a special interest in the patient.
7. Furniture can be arranged to facilitate small groups of patients. In this way, patients are encouraged to be aware of each other, whereas chairs arranged along walls restrict interaction.
8. Familiar routines and people contribute to the elderly patient's security.
9. All ward areas should be well lit to prevent fear and to promote safety.
10. A strict schedule for the patient's activities of daily living can help to maintain orientation even when the patient is inclined to be confused.
11. Little things such as ensuring that the patient's possessions are put away in the same place can assist orientation. Every interaction with the patient provides an opportunity for reality orientation.
12. Information given in a friendly supportive way can reduce the anxiety which is often experienced by the confused and disorientated patient.

FACT SHEET: MORE ON REALITY ORIENTATION

As age advances, and sensory abilities decrease, a person may find that he cannot detect many of the cues that he used previously to guide his everyday activities.

In hospital, *reality orientation* is an important method of treating confusion, disorientation and memory loss by helping the patient to relearn basic facts about himself and his environment. It helps to prevent a patient from withdrawing and cutting himself off from the reality around him.

A reality orientation programme should provide the patient with an environment in which he can receive benefit from all aspects of his surroundings over a 24-hour period.

For the elderly patient, recognition of his individual identity is just as important as having his physical needs met; therefore the patient's name should be used whenever the nurse approaches him.

If the patient cannot see or hear properly, the amount of stimulation that he receives will be reduced. This can lead to confusion because he is unable to make sense of his environment. If the patient needs glasses or a hearing aid, these should be worn because they help to give him contact with his surroundings.

The nurse should try to gain the patient's attention before speaking as he may be more attuned to his thoughts than to his environment. Touching him, using eye contact and requesting his name while standing in front of him can help to draw and maintain his attention. The use of brief concise statements is best, as long sentences will only serve to confuse the patient.

The 24-hour approach to reality orientation should be carried out whenever contact is made with the patient. The continuous feeding of information does not of course work miracles, but it has proved valuable in helping the elderly confused and disorientated patient to keep in touch with his surroundings.

'POETIC THOUGHTS OF AN OLD WOMAN'

What do you see nurses, what do you see?
Are you thinking when you are looking at me
A crabbit old woman, not very wise,
Uncertain of habit, with far away eyes
Who dribbles her food and makes no reply,
When you say in a loud voice 'I do wish you'd try'.
Who seems not to notice the things that you do
And forever is losing a stocking or shoe
Who, unresisting or not, lets you do as you will,
With the bathing and feeding, the long day to fill?
Is that what you're thinking, is that what you see?
Then open your eyes nurse you're not looking at me.

I'll tell you who I am as I sit here so still;
As I move at your bidding, as I eat at your will—
I'm a small child of ten with a father and mother,
Brothers and sisters who love one another;
A girl of sixteen with wings on her feet,
Dreaming that soon now a lover she'd meet;
A bride soon at twenty my heart gives a leap,
Rememb'ring the vows that I promised to keep;
At twenty-five now I have young of my own
Who need me to build a secure happy home;
A woman of thirty my young grow so fast
Bound to each other with ties that should last;
At forty my young sons now grown and will be gone
But my man stays behind to see I don't mourn;
At fifty once more babies play round my knee
Again we know children my loved one and me.
Dark days are upon me, my husband is dead,
I look to the future, I shudder with dread,
For my young ones are all busy rearing young of their own
And I think of the years and the love that I've known.
I'm an old woman now and nature is cruel
'Tis her jest to make old age look like a fool.
The body it crumbles, grace and vigour depart
There is now a stone where I once had a heart.
But inside this old carcass a young girl still dwells
And now and again my battered heart swells.
I remember the joys, I remember the pain
And I'm loving and living life over again.
I think of the years all too few gone too fast
And accept the stark fear that nothing can last.
So open your eyes nurses, open and see
Not a crabbit old woman, look close—see me.

REFERENCES AND FURTHER READING

References

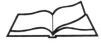

Burnside, I. M. (1973), Touching is talking, *American Journal of Nursing*, **73**, No. 12, 2060–2063.

Davis, A. J. (1984), *Listening and Responding*, C. V. Mosby, St Louis, Missouri.

Collins, M. (1983), *Communication in Health Care*, C. V. Mosby, St Louis, Missouri.

Lidz, T. (1968), cited by Robinson, L. (1983), *Psychiatric Nursing as a Human Experience*, W. B. Saunders, Philadelphia, Pennsylvania.

Metz, E. L. (1976), Assessing the older psychiatric patient. In: *Mental Health Concepts Applied to Nursing* (ed. Dunlap, L. C.), John Wiley, Chichester, West Sussex.

Miller, A. (1985), Nurse/patient dependency. Is it iatrogenic?, *Journal of Advanced Nursing*, **10**, 63–69.

Murray, R. B., and Huelskoetter, M. M. W. (1983), *Psychiatric Mental Health*

Nursing: Giving Emotional Care, Prentice-Hall, Englewood Cliffs, New Jersey.

Norris, A. D., and Abu El Eileh, M. T. R. (1982), Reminiscence groups, *Nursing Times,* **78**, No. 32, 1368–1369.

Robinson, L. (1983), *Psychiatric Nursing as a Human Experience*, W. B. Saunders, Philadelphia, Pennsylvania.

Roper, N., and Logan, W. (1985), The Roper/Logan/Tierney model, *Senior Nurse*, **3**, No. 2, 20–26.

Roper, N., Logan, W., and Tierney, A. J. (1986), *Elements of Nursing*, revised edn, Churchill Livingstone, Edinburgh.

Snow, T. (undated), cited by CIS Report, NHS Condition Critical Counter Information Services.

Sobel, D. E. (1969), Human caring, *American Journal of Nursing*, **69**, No. 12, 2612–2613.

Terrington, R. (1985), When can she come home?, *Nursing Times*, **81**, No. 7, 52–53.

Further reading

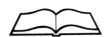

Allan, C., and Bennett, A. (1984), What year is it?, *Nursing Mirror, Clinical Forum*, **158**, No. 15, i-viii.

Armstrong, E. C. A., and Browne, K. D. (1986), The influence of elderly patients' mental impairment on nurse–patient interaction, *Journal of Advanced Nursing*, **11**, 379–387.

Ashwell, G. (1986), An independent mind, *Nursing Times*, **82**, No. 2, 25–27.

Baker, D. E. (1983), 'Care' in the geriatric ward: an account of two styles of nursing. In: *Nursing Research: Ten Studies in Patient Care, Developments in Nursing Research* (ed. Wilson-Barnett, J.), Vol. 12, John Wiley, Chichester, West Sussex.

Bergman, R. (1986), Nursing the aged with brain failure, *Journal of Advanced Nursing*, **11**, 361–367.

Biley, F. (1985), Put yourself in their shoes, *Nursing Times*, **81**, No. 34, 48.

Dick, D. (1985), The institutional trap, *Nursing Times*, **81**, No. 34, 47–48.

Farrant, E. (1983), The vital spark, *Nursing Times*, **79**, No. 19, 50–51.

Francis, G. (1981), The therapeutic use of pets, *Nursing Outlook*, **29**, No. 6, 369–370.

Goodykoontz, L. (1979), Touch: attitude and practice, *Nursing Forum*, **18**, No. 1, 4–17.

Hahn, K. (1980), Using twenty-four hour reality orientation, *Journal of Gerontological Nursing*, **6**, No. 3, 130–135.

Hayter, J. (1983), Modifying the environment to help older people, *Nursing and Health Care*, **4**, No. 5, 265–269.

Holden, U. P., and Woods, R. T. (1982), *Reality Orientation, Psychological Approaches to the 'Confused' Elderly*, Churchill Livingstone, Edinburgh.

Holderby, R. A., and McNulty, E. G. (1982), *Treating and Caring: A Human Approach to Patient Care*, Reston Publishing, Reston, Virginia.

Kempton, M. (1984), Keeping in touch, *Nursing Mirror, Psychiatry Forum*, **159**, No. 18, i-vi.

Kibber, P. E., and Lackey, D. S. (1982), The past as therapy: an experience in an acute setting, *Journal of Practical Nursing*, **17**, No. 9, 29–31.

Kroner, K. (1979), Dealing with a confused patient, *Nursing (US)*, **9**, No. 11, 71–79.

McIntosh, I. E. (1986), Mental failure in the elderly, *Psychiatry in Practice*, **5**, No. 3, 10–12.

Meekings, H. (1981), More than a helping hand, *Nursing Mirror*, **153**, No. 13, 20–23.

Mitchell, R. (1983), Four psychogeriatric disorders, *Nursing Times*, **79**, No. 3, 18–20.

Morris, M. (1986), Music and movement for the elderly, *Nursing Times*, **82**, No. 8, 44–45.

Pearson, J. (1984), The importance of touch. Just a touch, *Geriatric Nursing*, **4**, No. 2, 6.

Preston, T. (1973), When words fail, *American Journal of Nursing*, **73**, 2064–3066.

Reissmann, H. (1983), Make a conscious effort, *Nursing Mirror*, **157**, No. 24, 36–37.

Rimmer, L. (1982), *Reality Orientation Principles and Practice*, Winslow.

Rogers, R. E. (1982), The challenge of gerontological nursing, *Journal of Practical Nursing*, **17**, No. 9, 18–21.

Seers, C., Talking to the elderly and its relevance to care, *Nursing Times, Occasional Papers*, **82**, No. 1, 51–54.

Shaw, I. (1982), Coping with confusional states, *Nursing Mirror*, **154**, No. 21, 15–17.

Sugden, J., and Saxby, P. (1985), The confused elderly patient, *Nursing (UK)*, **2**, No. 35, 1022–1025.

Tobiason, S. J. B. (1981), Touching is for everyone, *American Journal of Nursing*, **81**, 728–730.

Watson, F. (1982), Quality of life in old age, *Nursing Times, Community Outlook*, 10 November.

Wells, T. J. (1980), *Problems in Geriatric Nursing Care*, Churchill Livingstone, Edinburgh.

White C. M. (1977), The nurse–patient encounter: attitudes and behaviour in action, *Journal of Gerontological Nursing*, **3**, No. 3, 16–20.

Chapter 18

Nursing care of the dying patient
by *Lynn Harris*

'*Communication with the dying patient is not limited to words. Many times words are insufficient. The most important activity for the nurse is to* simply be there.' (Drummond, 1970).

INTRODUCTION

When a patient is dying, treatment moves away from active efforts to cure the disease and concentrates instead on minimising distress and controlling symptoms. The nurse's aim in caring for a terminally ill patient is to provide personal support in maintaining an acceptable lifestyle and in enabling a peaceful death, having regard to the patient's culture and beliefs, values, preferences and outlook on life. For relatives and friends of the dying patient, the emotions connected with losing a loved one can be intense. The response to a loss may reflect the intensity of the previous relationship and the prospect of an impending loss can engender acute anxiety, distress and guilt at real or imagined past failings. An emotional response on the part of relatives to the impending loss and to the death when it occurs is a normal reaction and to be encouraged. Helping relatives through this experience is an intrinsic part of good nursing practice. Suppression of grief engenders tension, whereas expressing emotions and weeping, if this occurs, helps to reduce the stress of the situation (Lipe, 1980). The nurse's personal concern and support are often highly valued by both patients and relatives alike. Having someone to share the experience with them, explaining what is happening and acknowledging their psychological pain can help in coping with their distress. Just as relatives may find it helpful to express feeling verbally or to weep, so too may the nurse. She should not feel embarrassed to admit that she experiences an emotional reaction when a patient that she has cared for is dying and that she therefore finds her task upsetting at times. Although everyone has different ways of dealing with grief, it is often helpful to talk the experience through with caring colleagues who can help the nurse to come to terms with the situation, to express her sadness and to continue to care for the patient. Sadness when someone dies is an appropriate reaction and can be offset by the satisfaction obtained from knowing that patient and relatives have benefited from a high standard of patient care. The nurse's involvement in providing this means that caring for dying patients and their families is often one of the most satisfying and rewarding areas of nursing practice. A supportive ward environment is an essential prerequisite if this is to be achieved.

PATIENT PROFILE

Winifred Hastings, aged 74, was admitted to Rylands Ward 5 months ago for care and supervision. For the past 3 or 4 years, her family have noticed that her memory for both recent and past events has become increasingly muddled and defective. She has gradually lost interest in the local bowling club and her garden in which she formerly took great pride. A houseproud lady, she became disorganised and the house was chaotic and neglected. Although there have been periods when she seemed to regain some of her previous skills and interest, there has nevertheless been an overall deterioration in her ability to cope with running a household. Always a somewhat irritable and anxious lady, these traits have become exaggerated, with the addition of an overall depression. Minor household crises which she would normally take in her stride became a trigger for aggressive and tearful responses. Prior to admission, conversational ability had become limited to brief phrases, with frequent repetition and difficulty in recalling and pronouncing familiar words.

The admission was precipitated when Mrs Hastings was discovered by the village policeman huddled in a bus shelter shivering in her nightdress at 6 am. Mr Hastings was very agitated and upset by this incident. Married for 52 years, he had been aware of his wife's condition but had been afraid that, if he asked for help, they would be separated. A sufferer from bronchitis and emphysema himself, he had been unable to prevent the household's decline. Mr Hastings is now awaiting rehousing in a warden-controlled flat and in the meantime has a home help and meals on wheels. His son from Manchester comes to stay every weekend and Mr Hastings is well cared for physically, although he is very lonely.

Always susceptible to chest infections since she contracted tuberculosis in her teens, Mrs Hastings has suffered two bouts of bronchitis since her admission. 2 weeks ago, she developed a further chest infection. She was treated with antibiotics, but has gradually declined and is now bedridden and semiconscious. Mr Hastings has been told that his wife is dying and comes every day to sit by her bed and hold her hand when she will let him. She has not acknowledged his presence. He is quiet and sad and easily moved to tears but is embarrassed by this.

NURSING ASSESSMENT INTERVIEW

Surname _Hastings_ **Forenames** _Winifred Amy_

Name person likes to be called _Win_

Address _41 Pepys Way_
Willbury
WIL JJI

Telephone number _—_

Date of referral/admission _26 · 7 · 86_

Next-of-kin

Name _Jack Hastings_ **Relationship** _Husband_

Address _As above_

Telephone number _—_

Date of birth _12 · 4 · 11_ Single/**married**/divorced/widowed _____

General practitioner _Dr H. Sweeney_ **Address** _7 Park Road_
Old Town
Willbury

Consultant _Dr C. Spearman_

Status under Mental Health Act _Informal_

Psychiatric diagnosis _Senile dementia_

History of self-harm or harm towards others _None_

Occupation _Retired_

Occupational history
Housewife all her adult life. Occasional
cleaning jobs

Hobbies and interests _Garden, likes shopping, television,_
use to play bowls

Patient's perceived reason for referral/admission _Confused – thinks that_
she is at home

Relatives' understanding of patient's problems _'She just wasn't herself any_
more – her memory went. She went out
wandering. She couldn't cope with life'

NURSING ASSESSMENT INTERVIEW (continued)

Persons of significance in person's life

Family/friends/pets _Sister Beryl, aged 77. Son George lives in Manchester. Cat — Jimmy_

Spiritual needs

Goes to church on special occasions. No strong feelings about religion

Problems causing concern at home _Husband's adaptation to life on his own and social isolation. Ruth Smith has contacted Joanna McCaul, social worker to deal with finances and to arrange home help for Mr Hastings, social worker cannot undertake regular visiting. Health visitor to meet with a view to support_

Community services involved/referred _____ _and health education_

Name _Ruth Smith_   Status _Health visitor (Sorrel Lane_

Telephone number _2219_   Date of referral _____ _Health Centre)_

Mental status _____

History of present problems _Found wearing nightdress in bus shelter at 6 am_

Previous psychiatric history _Memory deteriorating 3 — 4 years_

General appearance and behaviour _Muddled and confused_

Speech and communication patterns _Brief phrases; repetitions Difficulty in pronouncing familiar words_

Problems with perception _Not sure of bearings; thinks that she is at home_

NURSING ASSESSMENT INTERVIEW (continued)

Affective state   _Anxious_

Disturbances of thinking or judgement   _Poor memory and judgement_

Orientation

Person   _Misidentifies people_

Place   _Thinks that she is at home most of the time_

Time   _Does not know time or dates_

Activities of living

Safety and mobility

Eating and drinking

Elimination

Bladder

Bowel

Sleep patterns

Personal needs

General health

Any medical condition for which the person is receiving treatment

Bronchitis 2 weeks ago. Treated with antibiotics

Doctor's instructions   _Observe for further chest complications_

Areas of concern to patient

NURSING ASSESSMENT INTERVIEW (continued)

Problems identified

_____
_____
_____
_____
_____
_____
_____
_____
_____

Date of interview   _26 . 7 . 86_   Signature   _C. Meredith_

History taken from   _Mr Hastings_

by   _Carol Meredith_   Designation   _Staff nurse_

Additional information   Date _____

_____
_____
_____
_____
_____
_____
_____
_____
_____
_____
_____
_____
_____
_____
_____
_____
_____
_____
_____
_____
_____
_____
_____
_____
_____

USE OF THE ROPER–LOGAN–TIERNEY ACTIVITIES-OF-LIVING MODEL

The nursing staff used the Roper–Logan–Tierney activities-of-living model (Roper and Logan, 1985; Roper *et al.*, 1986) (see Chapter 7) as a framework to enable them to meet the patient's total needs as she became more and more dependent.

Maintaining a safe environment

Although, when initially confined to bed, Win kept trying to get out, she is now immobile. Her ability to carry out this activity of living is impaired by both her mental and her physical illness.

PLAN OF NURSING CARE

(a) Patient's problems

1. Dependence on others for maintenance of a safe environment.
2. Susceptibility to pressure sores.

(b) Nursing goals

1. Ensure a safe environment.
2. To prevent pressure sores.

NURSING INTERVENTION

Because Win is unable to safeguard her own safety, the nurse must anticipate potential hazards.

Consideration should be given to the risk of transmitting further infection to Win via micro-organisms carried on the nurse's hands. Careful hand washing before touching food, drinks or medicines and before and after attending to the patient will reduce the risk of cross-infection. The possibility of errors in the administration of Win's drugs should also be borne in mind, and the hospital's procedure for checking drugs should be followed. Win is in danger of developing a pressure sore. When a patient is confined to bed and immobile, the pressure of the body on the capillaries restricts blood flow to the skin. In addition, she is incontinent and has to be lifted to change position in bed. This makes her susceptible to excoriation of the skin caused by contact with urine and faeces, and to shear forces damaging the integrity of the skin if she is dragged up the bed rather than lifted. Shear forces disrupt the tissue of the dermis and can thereby precipitate breakdown. It is possible to calculate the degree of risk of developing pressure sores. The Norton pressure sore rating scale was developed from studies involving elderly hospital patients. It is therefore an appropriate tool to use in assessing the degree of risk to Win (*Table 18.1*). It can be seen that Win's score is 5, indicating a high degree of risk.

Table 18.1   The Norton pressure sore risk rating scale

A Physical condition		B Mental condition		C Activity		D Mobility		E Incontinent	
Good	4	Alert	4	Ambulant	4	Full	4	Not	4
Fair	3	Apathetic	3	Walk with help	3	Slightly limited	3	Occasionally	3
Poor	2	Confused	2	Chair-bound	2	Very limited	2	Usually urinary	2
Very bad	1	Stuporous	1	Bedfast	1	Immobile	1	Doubly	1

Patients scoring 14 or less on this scale are considered to be in danger of developing pressure sores.
Source: Crow *et al.* (1981).

To prevent sores, it is necessary to reduce the likelihood of pressure, friction and shear forces. The nurse can relieve pressure by adopting a systematic turning schedule for the patient. In addition, devices such as a water bed or low-air-loss bed can be used if these are available. Friction can be minimised by keeping the skin clean and dry and protecting it with a barrier cream to prevent excoriation. Since Win is incontinent, the nurse will consider whether catheterisation would be helpful.

EVALUATION

Win is protected from cross-infection and medication errors. She has developed a small pressure sore on her sacrum but daily measurements show that this is not worsening and that further sores have been prevented.

Communicating

Had previously responded to simple requests and had sometimes been able to answer questions and to make her needs known. However, she now lies quietly and gives no obvious signs that she recognises those around her and does not respond to verbal communication.

PLAN OF NURSING CARE

(a) Patient's problems
1. Unresponsive.
2. Distress of husband who is upset that Win does not seem to know him.

(b) Nursing goals
1. To maintain communication and to utilise non-verbal means.
2. To offer support and comfort to Mr Hastings and to help him to utilise alternative communication channels.

NURSING INTERVENTION

Win is now confined to bed during the day when ordinarily she would be up and dressed and joining other patients in the day room. Her immediate environment has therefore changed. She is very ill and unable to move much or to respond to others but nevertheless may be anxious, not only because of her changed environment but also because she is feeling ill and does not understand what is happening to her. It is important that the nurses continue to talk to the patient and to maintain a warm calm presence, even though there is no response. Having familiar people and voices nearby may provide a link for Win with her familiar routine. Giving simple explanations of what is being done and remembering to tell the patient the day of the week and the time may help to overcome confusion and anxiety. It is difficult for the nurse to maintain a one-way conversation and to continue to sit with the patient who is unresponsive as there is no indication that her presence and actions are helpful. Nevertheless, the fact that the nurse is prepared to stay demonstrates that the patient is cared for and can help to alleviate any isolation which is felt. In addition to her verbal communication skills, the nurse should make use of her other communication skills in this situation. In particular, touch should be used to convey meanings and attitudes. Holding the patient's hand, stroking her arm or putting an arm around her shoulders communicates caring and understanding and lets the patient know that she is not alone. The meaning of a touch may be understood when the spoken word is not (Pratt and Mason, 1981). It is important that the nurse should keep Mr Hastings informed of events and procedures occurring not only while he is present but also when he is absent. He should be made to feel fully involved in his wife's care and should be encouraged, if he wishes, to participate in her physical care. The value of talking quietly to his wife and of holding her hand or touching her affectionately should be explained. Any embarrassment or discomfort that Mr Hastings may experience at communicating caring in non-verbal ways in an alien setting can be helped by the nurse demonstrating how to relate to Win in this way.

EVALUATION

In the absence of positive responses, the nurse assumes that Win is aware of her presence. She watches for signs of response such as eye movements or limb movements. Mr Hastings feels that, rather than being regarded as a visitor, he is seen as a full member of the caring team. He feels able to stay comfortably with his wife and to sustain efforts to reach her both verbally and non-verbally.

Breathing

Respirations are shallow and irregular, with an occasional weak cough. The chest is bubbly but no sputum is being expectorated. There is cyanosis of the lips and extremities.

PLAN OF NURSING CARE

(a) Patient's problems
1. Inability to expectorate.
2. Oxygen insufficiency.

(b) Nursing goals
1. To facilitate adequate air entry.
2. To clear secretions.

NURSING INTERVENTION

The nurse should note whether changing position has an adverse effect on the patient's breathing. If so, only those positions which do not embarrass respiration should be used. Administration of oxygen, as prescribed by a doctor, may help to alleviate cyanosis but this should be humidified to avoid drying up the respiratory passages. Careful explanation and reassurance is needed, since an oxygen mask can be frightening. The anxiety caused may have to be weighed against the benefits to be obtained for a dying patient, particularly when the patient has difficulty in understanding. The nurse should discuss such reservations with the prescribing physician if she feels that oxygen is having an adverse effect.

Gentle treatment by the physiotherapist can help in loosening secretions. However, as the patient cannot cough or use a sputum pot, the nurse must ensure that any secretions are wiped away gently or dealt with by using a catheter and gentle suction.

EVALUATION

The patient is kept in a comfortable position and free from distress. Unpleasant secretions are dealt with promptly.

Eating and drinking

Win is unable to take food or drink.

PLAN OF NURSING CARE

(a) Patient's problem
1. Dry mouth and lips due to reduced fluid intake.

NURSING INTERVENTION

If the patient is able, she can be given small pieces of ice to suck or teaspoons of cold water to moisten her mouth. Vaseline applied to the lips may prove soothing and prevent cracking of the lips.

Particular care is needed to observe whether the mouth becomes infected, for instance with a monilial infection since Win is weak and debilitated and therefore less resistant to infections.

EVALUATION

The patient is kept comfortable in spite of not eating or drinking.

Eliminating

Win is incontinent of both urine and faeces.

PLAN OF NURSING CARE

(a) Patient's problems
1. Discomfort due to soiling and dampness.
2. Susceptibility to pressure sores.
3. Husband's distress at his wife's inability to control these functions.

NURSING INTERVENTION

The nurse should act promptly to keep the patient clean and comfortable. She should check the bed often but be aware that an adverse reaction from her can be communicated to both the patient and her husband. The nurse therefore needs to ensure the patient's privacy and to be discreet and tactful in her management of the incontinent patient. The skin is washed and dried promptly, and clean bedclothes and nightclothes are supplied. The use of incontinent pads is inappropriate for a patient who is at risk of developing pressure sores since they are liable to crease and cause friction to the skin as will a creased drawsheet. The nurse decides to catheterise Win to assist in keeping her dry and preventing excoriation. The catheter used should be the smallest size which will allow adequate drainage. Aseptic technique is used for catheterisation and when the drainage bag is changed since this involves breaking the system. When emptying the bag, the nurse should ensure that both the container and her hands are clean. Frequent checks should be made to ensure that the system is not blocked or kinked and that urine is draining freely and there is no leakage. Blockages can occur, particularly if the fluid intake is low and a bladder wash-out using aseptic techniques may help to clean any debris obstructing the flow. Use of a silicone catheter makes this sort of blockage less likely.

EVALUATION

The patient is kept clean and comfortable and the risk of pressure sores is reduced.

Mr Hastings was relieved to see the nurse's tactful approach, and that his wife's dignity had been maintained.

Personal cleansing and dressing

Win was formerly fastidious in her personal appearance and is now dependent on others to maintain this activity of living.

PLAN OF NURSING CARE

(a) Patient's problem
1. Unable to participate in cleansing or dressing.

(b) Nursing goals
1. To ensure comfort.
2. To maintain well-cared-for appearance.

NURSING INTERVENTION

The nurse should ensure privacy for the patient's personal cleansing and dressing and should explain what is being done. The patient is washed in bed with her modesty protected and the limbs and trunk are handled confidently but gently. Since Win is unable to cooperate in lifting limbs or turning over, the nurse should assist her to do this, after explaining her intentions. Win's nails are kept clean and short as has been her custom, and her hair is brushed. The nurse should ensure that attention is paid to dentures and the mouth, dental plates being cleaned, and the mouth cleaned with foam sticks if necessary.

EVALUATION

Win's dignity is maintained and her comfort enhanced.

Controlling body temperature

Win's skin is warm and dry, and her temperature is 36.4 °C. There are no problems in controlling her body temperature.

Mobilising

Win was previously able to get up but is now confined to bed and dependent on others for assistance in moving.

PLAN OF NURSING CARE

(a) Patient's problem

1. Unable to alter position in bed.

(b) Nursing goal

1. To change patient's position regularly.

NURSING INTERVENTION

The nurse should ensure that the patient's position is changed regularly and in accordance with the schedule decided on to alleviate pressure and to help to prevent pressure sores. In doing this, she must have regard to the patient's comfort and sense of security when being moved in bed. The nurse should therefore explain beforehand what she intends to do and should only attempt to lift the patient if adequate help is available. Trying to drag the patient up the bed alone not only exposes the patient's skin to shearing forces and friction but also puts the nurse at risk of developing back injuries.

EVALUATION

The patient is moved efficiently and securely and does not experience the discomfort associated with lying in one position for too long.

Working and playing

Win is in bed and her physical condition is deteriorating.

Expressing sexuality

Win is unresponsive and immobile and does not seem to recognise her husband.

PLAN OF NURSING CARE

(a) Patient's problem

1. Unable to participate in marital relationship.

(b) Nursing goal

1. To enable husband to be alone with wife.

NURSING INTERVENTION

Sexuality does not relate simply to the act of sexual intercourse. For a couple such as this, it may be important that Mr Hastings is able to express his feelings for his wife and to tell her what she means to him before she dies, even though she cannot respond. The nurse should be sensitive to these needs. Mr Hastings may make only indirect references in conversation to this sort of need, or he may speak of it directly. The nurse should ensure that she is available to Mr Hastings to allow him to ventilate these feelings. She should ensure that he is left privately with his wife so that he can talk quietly with her and hold her if he wishes. In addition the nurse should be aware that this may cause him distress and should be available to support and empathise with him.

EVALUATION

Mr Hastings is enabled to spend time privately with his wife and to express his feelings for her.

Dying

Win's physical condition is very poor. Her husband remains at her bedside.

PLAN OF NURSING CARE

(a) Patient's problems
1. Control of physical symptoms.
2. Husband's distress.

(b) Nursing goals
1. To ensure a peaceful death.
2. To support Mr Hastings.

NURSING INTERVENTION

The nurse ensures the patient's comfort by attending to her activities of living. Distressing symptoms such as a death rattle can be relieved by asking the doctor to prescribe a drug such as hyoscine. Pastoral care is arranged if required. The nurse should stay near so that Mr Hastings will feel he can call someone if he is worried and will feel supported and that his wife is cared for. The nurse or the patient's husband should remain at the bedside and should talk to her and hold her hand so that she knows she is not alone. Dying patients are often frightened to feel that they are alone, and familiar caring people nearby will help to overcome this.

It is important that the nurse should feel able to stay close to a dying patient and the family. She may need to examine her own attitudes to death and dying in order to feel comfortable in this situation and to overcome her own fears and anxieties. The greatest need of the patient and family is to have someone to turn to who cares and who is able to offer them understanding and support. The nurse may have to comfort Mr Hastings in his distress, allowing him to weep without feeling embarrassed, as can happen if a man cries. Ventilating his feelings in this way is a positive action which can help to relieve the stress of this time (Lipe, 1980). Mr Hastings may be fearful of the moment of death, and anxious about how he will cope. The nurse should be sensitive to such feelings and help by careful explanations of what is happening and what can be

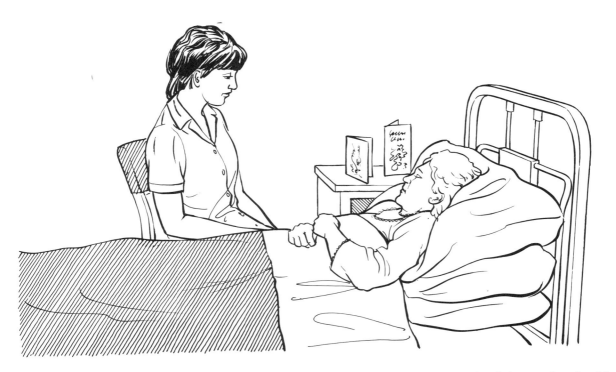

expected. Time to answer questions and to talk about what is happening should be made available, although just sitting quietly with Mr Hastings and showing concern and care in this way are equally valuable.

After the death, the nurse should help Mr Hastings to deal with procedures such as registering the death, collecting property and arranging the funeral.

Bereavement is a well-recognised process and is a normal response to the death of a loved one. The nurse can help the patient's relatives during this difficult time by listening and helping them to talk. Community services to aid bereaved relatives are also available.

EVALUATION

Win is enabled to have a peaceful death with her husband present. Mr Hastings will feel that his presence has been of value and will be helped in his bereavement by the concern and understanding shown to him.

The nurse has been able to provide a high standard of care and to explore and share her feelings about the experience. She has gained valuable insight into the effect which such a life event has on a family and will use this to continue to provide sensitive nursing care in the future.

REFERENCES AND FURTHER READING

References

Crow, R., David, J. A., and Cooper, E. J. (1981), Pressure sores and their prevention, *Nursing*, 26 June, 1139–1142.

Drummond, E. E. (1970), Communication and comfort for the dying patient, *Nursing Clinics of North America*, **5**, No. 1, 55–63.

Lipe, H. P. (1980), The function of weeping in the adult, *Nursing Forum*, **19**, No. 1, 24–44.

Pratt, J. W., and Mason, A. (1981), *The Caring Touch*, H.M. and M. Publishers, Aylesbury, Buckinghamshire.

Roper, N., and Logan, W. (1985), The Roper/Logan/Tierney model, *Senior Nurse*, **3**, No. 2, 20–26.

Roper, N., Logan, W., and Tierney, A. (1986), *Elements of Nursing*, revised edn, Churchill Livingstone, Edinburgh.

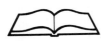

Further reading

Angeli, N. (1979), Special skills for special patients, *Nursing Mirror*, **148**, No. 14, 17–18.

Bayles, M. D. (1980), The value of life—by what standard?, *American Journal of Nursing*, **80**, 2226–2230.

Crow, R., David, J. A., and Cooper, E. J. (1981), Pressure sores and their prevention, *Nursing (UK)*, **26**, 1139–1142.

Cundey, B. (1981), A time of stress, *Nursing Mirror*, **153**, No. 23, 23–24.

Downie, R. (1981), Telling the truth, *Nursing Mirror*, **160**, No. 23, 43.

Earnshaw-Smith, E. (1981), Dealing with dying patients and their relatives, *British Medical Journal*, **282**, 1779.

Field, D. (1984), 'We didn't want him to die on his own'—nurses' accounts of nursing dying patients, *Journal of Advanced Nursing*, **9**.

Hinton, J. (1972), *Dying*, Penguin, Harmondsworth, Middlesex.

Howarth, H. (1977), Mouth care procedures for the very ill, *Nursing Times*, **73**, No. 10, 354–355.

Iveson-Iveson, J. (1985), A part of life, *Nursing Mirror*, **161**, No. 8, 43.

Jones, R., and Arie, R. (1982), The failing mind. In: *The Dying Patient* (ed. Wilkes, E.), M.T.P. Press.

Kubler-Rosse, E. (1969), *On Death and Dying*, Macmillan, New York.

Parkes, C. M. (1975), *Bereavement: Studies of Grief in Adult Life*, Penguin, Harmondsworth, Middlesex.

Parkes, C. M., and Weiss, R. S. (1983), *Recovery from Bereavement*, Basic Books.

Penson, J. M. (1979), Helping the bereaved, *Nursing Times*, **75**, No. 14, 593–595.

Pincus, L. (1976), *Death and the Family*, Faber and Faber, London.

Price, B. (1983), Facing death, *Nursing Mirror*, **156**, No. 3, 46–48.

Sawley, L. (1985), Preparing to die, *Nursing Mirror*, **161**, No. 9, 35–36.

Sheard, T. (1984), Dealing with the nurse's grief, *Nursing Forum*, **11**, No. 1, 43–45.

Shivnan, J. (1979), What happened to the man in bed 14?, *Nursing Mirror*, **148**, No. 14, 14–15.

Tyner, R. (1985), Elements of empathic care for dying patients and their families, *Nursing Clinics of North America*, **20**, No. 2, 293–401.

Zack, M. V. (1985), Loneliness: a concept relevant to the care of dying persons, *Nursing Clinics of North America*, **20**, No. 2, 403–414.

Chapter 19

Nursing care of the patient who is violent

'Violent behaviour is a source of concern to both patients and staff in health care settings. Anxiety escalates, adrenaline flows and the human responses of fright, flight and fight are often manifested; the therapeutic environment is suddenly challenged, loses stability and is temporarily thrown off balance.' (Boettcher, 1983).

INTRODUCTION

Violent behaviour involves ways of behaving which are harmful or hurtful to someone or something else. The patient who resorts to violent behaviour has not usually learned to meet his needs or to reduce his anxiety in a more appropriate manner.

BOETTCHER'S MODEL

Boettcher (1983) presents a theoretical model based on the premise that all human beings have innate potential for violence. She makes the following assumptions.

(a) The patient will experience an alteration in biopsychosocial need. One or more needs may be blocked, arousing feelings of discomfort and anxiety.
(b) A threat is posed to the patient's self-esteem.
(c) A state of arousal occurs and feelings of stress and tension will be present.
(d) Severe anxiety will narrow the patient's perceptual field, and learning will be inhibited.
(e) Feelings of helplessness and entrapment will occur and to overcome these the patient will resort to behaviours that have proved successful in the past as a means of controlling these feelings.

Boettcher defines an assaultive accident as 'any event in which a patient, struck, shoved, hit, yanked, grabbed, punched, kicked, bit, threw a potentially dangerous object, pulled hair, or tore at clothing of any person on the unit in an aggressive manner'. She proposes a need assessment tool which will enable the nurse to identify the patient's need or deficits in the following areas.

1. *Need for territoriality.* Each individual has a need for personal space, privacy and freedom from unwanted intrusions. Although the term territoriality has been used in relation to animals for a number of years, human beings are also strongly moulded by territorial drive. Territoriality enables a person to establish a comfortable degree of interaction with the

people and objects in his environment; it ensures a balance between privacy and community that minimises a psychological or physical threat to the self (Orland, 1978). Each individual's personal space forms an invisible boundary around the body. It is when this boundary is threatened by intrusion that a person's communication alters in response to it. The closer or more imminent the threat, the stronger the need to display defensive behaviour overtly (Pluckham, 1978).

2. *The need for communication* refers to the patient's need to talk to another person, e.g. the nurse. Communication is essential to life, and yet people are frequently discouraged by barriers that alienate individuals from one another. Most of these barriers are created by people. Identifying barriers to communication is a first step towards eliminating them but it is not enough. Each individual needs to learn about his own needs, values, bias and stereotypes and the ways in which his behaviour affects communication. Pluckham (1978) suggests that self-discovery is the only learning that really influences behaviour.

3. *The need for self-esteem.* Each person has a need for respect from others: freedom from insult, humiliation or the effects of stigmatisation. Self-esteem is the degree to which a person feels valued, worthwhile or competent. It is the feeling that an individual has about himself that makes him feel worthy of attention, recognition and honour. When a person has self-esteem, he has respect for himself and what he is, what he can do and what he has done (Hines and Montag, 1976). Generally a person tends to engage in interactions with people who sustain his self-esteem (Hollander, 1981).

4. *Need for safety and security.* A person needs protection from harm or physical injury and to feel free from danger. Maslow (1968) has suggested that needs for safety and security have to be met before a person can look for self-respect or group acceptance.

5. *The need for autonomy* refers to the need for a person to have control over his own life and to make his own decisions.

6. *The need for own time.* A person needs to move at his own pace, and not to be rushed or hurried by others. To have time to be alone to be himself and to be free from organised activity.

7. *The need for personal identity.* A person's identity is built on assured feelings of being one's self (Dennis, 1967). A person needs to retain his personal belongings and other items which have special significance for him.

8. *The need for comfort.* A person needs to be free from emotional or physical pain, from hunger and thirst, and from excessive heat or cold. Feelings of comfort evolve from an awareness that comfort needs will be met (Nissley and Townes, 1977).

9. *Need for cognitive understanding.* A person needs to be aware of his surroundings and free from confusion about what is happening to him. Boettcher suggests that the use of the nursing process and the theoretical model related to altered needs can provide the nurse with a methodology to reduce the incidence of violent behaviour.

PATIENT PROFILE

Frederick Silver, aged 49, has a long history of mental illness. He drinks heavily and has a low frustration threshold. He is sensitive and flies off the handle easily. In the past, he has been in trouble with the police because of his violent behaviour.

Since his wife divorced him 5 years ago, he has lived in a number of hostels and lodging houses. His two sons have refused to have anything to do with him since the break-up of their parent's marriage.

Mr Silver has held many different jobs and his work record is poor. At the present time, he is unemployed and has little prospect of obtaining another job.

Since 1972, Mr Silver has been admitted to the psychiatric unit 11 times. On this occasion, he was brought in by the police on Section 136 after creating a public disturbance.

NURSING ASSESSMENT INTERVIEW

Surname _Silver_   **Forenames** _Frederick Roy_

Name person likes to be called _Fred or Mr Silver_

Address _Church Mews Hostel_   **Telephone number** _3771_
Brancaster Lane   **Date of ~~referral~~/admission** _12.3.86_
Willbury
WIL 5IJ

Next-of-kin

Name _Mrs J. Lowe_   **Relationship** _Sister_

Address _141 Deep Street_
Aberdeen

                                   Telephone number _None_

Date of birth _20.5.37_   ~~Single/married~~/divorced/~~widowed~~

General practitioner _None_   **Address**

Consultant _Dr S. Mencat_

Status under Mental Health Act _Informal 15.3.86_

Psychiatric diagnosis _Borderline personality. History of alcohol abuse_

History of self-harm or harm towards others _Potential for violent behaviour_

Occupation _Unemployed for 3 months_

Occupational history _Casual labouring jobs, ex-policeman_

Hobbies and interests _Sport, television_

Patient's perceived reason for referral/admission _Complaints made about him by other residents at hostel_

Relatives' understanding of patient's problems _No one has visited_

NURSING ASSESSMENT INTERVIEW (continued)

Persons of significance in person's life

Family/friends/pets *'Some good blokes in hostel'*

Spiritual needs

Not religious

Problems causing concern at home *Hopes to return to hostel*

Community services involved/~~referred~~

Name *Delia Diers*

Telephone number *7743*

Status *Social worker*

Date of referral *1981*

Mental status

History of present problems *Violent and abusive after drinking according to the police. Mr Silver denies this*

Previous psychiatric history *Last admission 11 months ago*

General appearance and behaviour *Untidy appearance; unshaven; clothes very worn. Says that he's decided to grow a beard*

Speech and communication patterns *Defensive; guarded. Easily becomes argumentative and lashes out at others or environment*

Problems with perception *Does not perceive drinking as a problem. Says that he only drinks socially*

NURSING ASSESSMENT INTERVIEW (continued)

Affective state _Easily frustrated_

Disturbances of thinking or judgement _Impulsive – acts before he thinks_

Orientation

Person _Fully orientated_

Place

Time

Activities of living

Safety and mobility
Safety of others may be threatened

Eating and drinking
Not malnourished. Appetite fluctuates

Elimination

Bladder _No problem_

Bowel _No problem_

Sleep patterns
Sleeps for short periods. Reads if he wakes up

Personal needs
Mr Silver needs space. Teeth appear to be neglected – refer to dentist

General health

Any medical condition for which the person is receiving treatment
History of pulmonary tuberculosis. Clear now. Still monitored at chest clinic

Doctor's instructions
Will refer to the rehabilitation unit. Mr Silver can probably attend as an out-patient

Areas of concern to patient

NURSING ASSESSMENT INTERVIEW (continued)

Problems identified

Potential for violent behaviour. Main
problem and priority at present

Date of interview _13.3.86_   Signature _B. Smith_

History taken from _Fred_

by _Bobby Smith_   Designation _Staff nurse_

Additional information   Date _____

Does not keep in touch with sister. Mrs Diers
helped Mr Silver to get employment when
he was last discharged. She has been
informed of his admission and will see him
next week

PLAN OF NURSING CARE, NURSING INTERVENTION AND EVALUATION

The plan of nursing care is given in *Table 19.1*, together with the intervention and evaluation.

Table 19.1   Boettcher's assaultive incident assessment tool

Assessment area	Behaviour	Patient's problem	Nursing goal	Intervention	Evaluation
1. Need for territoriality	Tends to sit in the same chair in dining room and television lounge. Gets upset if someone else sits in 'his' place	Invasion of perceived personal space	To respect patient's need for privacy and personal space. Explain that some areas in the ward are for everybody's use	Remember that Man is territorial and needs space which he can call his own. Minimise invasion of territory. Teach other patients and staff to respect territorial space	Mr Silver shows a willingness to be more flexible in public ward areas
2. Need for communication	Extremely angry because a nurse promised to play Scrabble, but then went off sick. Patient was not told	Frustrated by a broken promise	The nurse should not make promises unless they can be fulfilled	If some unforeseen eventuality prevents the nurse from keeping a promise, the patient is entitled to an explanation as well as an apology	Explanations are received and understood by the patient
3. Need for self-esteem	Sensitive about people remarking on baldness	Sensitive about baldness	To show respect for patient	Accept the patient as he is	Patient feels accepted
4. Need for safety and security	Protects self from anxiety by outward manifestations of aggression	Reacts to perceived threats by outward projection	To ensure a safe and secure environment	Establish trust through the nurse–patient relationship. Promote safety and security and freedom from anxiety by giving adequate information and explanations	Safety and security maintained
5. Need for autonomy	Likes to be in control of himself	Reacts badly to bossy staff giving orders	To respect the patient's need for autonomy. To request rather than to instruct	Engage the patient in decision making to enable him to have some control over his own life	Patient feels able to make independent decisions
6. Need for own time	Dislikes being forced to do things by the clock	Dislikes routines	To appreciate that the patient is an individual who functions at his own pace	Allow as much flexibility as possible but explain that some fixed times, e.g. mealtimes, are necessary when catering for large numbers	Patient feels free to proceed at own pace

Table 19.1   (continued)

Assessment area	Behaviour	Patient's problem	Nursing goal	Intervention	Evaluation
7. Need for personal identity	Angry because another patient touched an ornament on his locker	Anxiety and anger aroused. Fear of loss of valued possession	To protect the patient's property	Ensure that the patient is provided with facilities for the care of valuables	The patient does not feel threatened by loss or interference with personal possessions
8. Need for comfort	Hot weather increased irritability	Does not tolerate extremes of heat	To help the patient to maintain homeostasis	Provide cool environment; avoid overcrowding. Ensure the patient has appropriate clothing and cool drinks	Patient's personal comfort is maintained
9. Need for cognitive understanding	Aggressive outbursts when medication was changed, and the patient was not consulted	Reacts badly to lack of information	To inform the patient of any changes in his treatment or medication	The patient will feel less anxious if he is provided with meaningful information. He should always be aware of what is happening	The patient understands what is happening

PREVENTION OF VIOLENCE

If the nurse is able to recognise potentially violent behaviour, then it will be possible to manage a situation to prevent actual violence from occurring.

Firstly, the nurse needs to be aware of his or her own behaviours in a situation and the effect that this is having on the patient. The nurse who has self-understanding can more easily distinguish between self-needs and those of the patient.

Stewart (1978) suggests that the actions of the nurse may have a great deal to do with the aggressive patient. The patient who lashes out at the nurse or his environment is asking for help, for limits and for control of his behaviour. Since he may be unable to express his needs verbally, he may know no other way of behaving other than acting out. It should be remembered that staff behaviour can provoke violent reactions among patients; inconsistency and conflicting responses from different nurses can cause escalation of violent behaviours.

Each person has his own unique characteristics when behaving aggressively, and for this reason it is important to assess those factors which influence the behaviour most significantly. The observant nurse will pick up cues when the patient's usual coping mechanisms are not working and his potential for violent behaviour is increasing. Non-verbal indicators of tension may include clenched fists, a wrinkled brow, jerky movements and lack of eye contact. Boettcher (1983) suggests that the patient should be taught and encouraged to recognise feelings of mounting tension and to report these feelings to the nurse. The nurse can then implement first-level interventions, providing the patient with

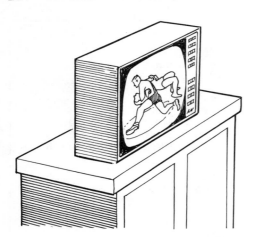
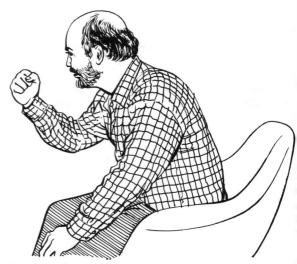

acceptable ways in which he can release his pent-up tension and aggressive feelings through physical means. The nurse can provide support by helping the patient to express his feelings of anger. It should be made clear to him that *destructive* anger is not acceptable. Limits must be imposed for the patient and he must be told that people or property must not be physically attacked. Activities which help to release aggressive feelings include those activities that involve punching, pounding, running, hitting, hammering, tearing and cutting. Watching boxing and wrestling matches while somebody else does the 'clobbering' can help the release of aggressive feelings. The patient must be made aware that the nurse is there to help him to deal with his feelings in an appropriate manner.

DEALING WITH VIOLENT BEHAVIOUR

There are times when a patient may engage in violent behaviour despite preventive measures.

An attempt should always be made to talk to the patient first by a nurse who knows him well and has a good rapport with him. However, if the patient is already physically aggressive, then he should not be approached on a one-to-one basis.

The starting point for controlling measures is when the patient can no longer be talked to, reasoned with, persuaded or contained.

Control must be established and the safety of the patient, other patients and staff the priority (Lenefsky *et al.*, 1978).

A brief discussion prior to restraining the patient will ensure that the staff make a coordinated effort to restrain the patient. The presence of a group of nurses is usually effective in controlling violence; the patient is more likely to submit to some control if he senses that he is going to be overpowered.

Smiling at the patient should be avoided because the patient may misinterpret the message and think that he is being laughed at. If the patient is noisy, the nurse needs to make sure that his or her voice can be heard, but the voice should not be raised in anger. The way in which the patient is approached is of the utmost importance. It is wise to react to the patient as though he is expected to do the right thing, because people have a tendency to behave in ways that they believe one expects of them (Stewart, 1978). The nurses should remove anything from their person which could get broken or cause injury either to themselves or to the patient.

If the patient is attempting to hit out, walking him backwards rather than forwards will reduce the force of his swing. Also, when walking with the patient, the stride should not be broken as momentum helps to maintain control (Nissley and Townes, 1977). If the patient is armed with a potential weapon, a mattress can be held in front of the nurses to give protection as the patient is backed into a corner. Restraint should never be more forceful than is necessary to control the patient, and it is preferable to hold the patient by his clothing to avoid injury to his body.

The patient needs to be taken to a quiet place away from the other patients. He needs some privacy in order to regain his composure. The nurses should try to encourage the patient to talk about his feelings and the reasons for his behaviour when he feels ready to do so. He may feel humiliated by the incident and so it is important for the nurse to maintain his self-esteem.

Information should be recorded as soon as possible after the incident occurred; otherwise the facts may become distorted and important details omitted. The nursing staff should try to identify any precipitating events. Discussion related to the incident can provide a useful basis for learning and may help to prevent further outbreaks of violence.

When one patient in the ward loses control, inevitably this will have a significant effect on the other patients and may arouse feelings of anxiety and uncertainty. At least one nurse should remain with the other patients while measures are being taken to control the patient who is violent. The physical presence of the nurse can provide stability and reassurance in a tense atmosphere. It is likely that the other patients will ask questions about the violent incident and the nurse should try to provide honest answers without breaching confidentiality.

FACT SHEET: THE PATIENT WHO IS VIOLENT

1. Whether aggressive behaviour is acceptable or valued is culturally determined. Inserting a knife into another person may be called surgery or assault with a deadly weapon. Surgery is acceptable and valued in our society; killing one's neighbour is not. In war time, killing the enemy is acceptable and valued (Jasmin and Trygstad, 1979).
2. Violence is a powerful way to communicate and is one of the most immediate and direct, albeit destructive, ways of communicating an intense human need. Identifying that need and addressing that need are paramount if violent behaviour is to be prevented (Boettcher, 1983).
3. The more excited a patient is, the more necessary it is for the nurse to show control.
4. A fear of injury may prevent a nurse from relating to the patient.
5. The nurse's perception of the patient may be distorted and he or she may be communicating to the patient that violent behaviour is the *expected* behaviour.
6. The patient should be provided with a full programme of stimulating activities so that boredom, frustration and resentment have less opportunity to build up.

REFERENCES AND FURTHER READING

References

Boettcher, E. G. (1983), Presenting violent behaviour, an integrated theoretical model for nursing, *Perspectives in Psychiatric Care*, **21**, No. 2, 54–58.

Dennis, L. B. (1967), *Psychology of Human Behaviour for Nurses*, 3rd edn, W. B. Saunders, Philadelphia, Pennsylvania.

Hines, A. R., and Montag, M. L. (1976), *Nursing Concepts and Nursing Care*, John Wiley, New York.

Hollander, E. P. (1981), *Principles and Methods of Social Psychology*, 4th edn, Oxford University Press, Oxford.

Jasmin, D., and Trygstad, L. N. (1979), *Behavioural Concepts and the Nursing Process*, C. V. Mosby, St Louis, Missouri.

Lenefsky, B., de Palma, T., and Locicero, D. (1978), Management of violent behaviour, *Perspectives in Psychiatric Care*, **16**, Nos 5–6, 212–217.

Maslow, A. H. (1968), *Towards a Psychology of Being*, 2nd edn, Van Nostrand Reinhold, New York.

Nissley, B. H., and Townes, N. (1977), Guidelines for intervention in aggressive behaviour. In: *Psychiatric/Mental Health Nursing; Contempory Readings* (eds Bacher, B. A., Dubbent, P. M., and Eisenman, E. J. P.), Van Nostrand, New York.

Orland, L. (1978), In: *Human Needs and the Nursing Process* (eds Yura, H., and Walsh, M. B.), Appleton Century Crofts, Norwalk, Connecticut.

Pluckham, M. L. (1978), *Human Communication: The Matrix of Nursing*, McGraw-Hill, New York.

Stewart, A. T. (1978), Handling the aggressive patient, *Perspectives in Psychiatric Care*, **16**, Nos 5–6, 228–232.

Further reading

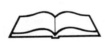

Barile, L. A. (1982), A model for teaching management of disturbed behaviour, *Journal of Psychiatric Nursing and Mental Health Services*, **20**, No. 11, 9–11.

Burrows, R. (1984), Nurses and violence, *Nursing Times*, **80**, No. 4, 56–58.

Castledine, G. (1981), Encounters of the violent kind, *Nursing Mirror*, **153**, No. 12, 18.

Cooper, K. H. (1984), Territorial behaviour among the institutionalized: a nursing perspective, *Journal of Psychosocial Nursing*, **22**, No. 12, 6–11.

Gluck, M. (1981), Learning a therapeutic verbal response to anger, *Journal of Psychiatric Nursing and Mental Health Services*, **19**, No. 3, 9–12.

Hein, E. C. (1980), *Communication in Nursing Practice*, 2nd edn, Little, Brown, Boston, Massachusetts.

Lathrop, V. G. (1978), Aggression as a response, *Perspectives in Psychiatric Care*, **16**, Nos 5–6, 202–205.

McFarland, G. K., and Waschinski, C. E. (1985), Impaired communication, a descriptive study, *Nursing Clinics of North America*, **20**, No. 4, 775–785.

Packham, H. (1978), Managing the violent patient, *Nursing Mirror*, **146**, No 25, 17–20.

Platzer, H. (1981), Jenny through the spy-hole, *Nursing Mirror*, **153**, No. 18 50–52.

Rix, G. (1985), Compassion is better than conflict, *Nursing Times*, **81**, No. 38, 53–55.

Self, P. R., and Viau, J. J. (1980), Four steps for helping a patient alleviate anger, *Nursing (US)*, **10**, No. 12, 66.

Selleck, T. (1982), 'Invasion'—a conceptual construct for nursing, *Nurse Education Today*, **2**, No. 4, 14–16.

Smeaton, W., and Field, R. (1985), The nature and management of hostility, *Nursing (UK)*, **2**, No. 35, 1033–1038.

Smith, A. E., and Brandt, S. H. (1979), Physical activity: a tool in promoting mental health, *Journal of Psychiatric Nursing and Mental Health Services*, **17**, No. 11, 24–25.

Chapter 20

The child, the problem and the family

by *Carl Dykes*

'A child's problems are manifested in behaviour that disrupts the routine of his daily living, his relationships with his parents and family, and sometimes the affairs of the community. The disturbance created by the child is his way of saying he needs help.' (Topalis and Aguilera, 1978).

INTRODUCTION

Dear Sir,

Referral: Michael Abbott—age, 11 years 9 months

Since starting at St Martin's Secondary School 6 months ago, concern h been growing among the teaching staff regarding this child's behavic and general performance. He is unpopular with his peers because of l argumentative and aggressive manner and has as a result become v isolated.

His attitude towards authority and general compliance with every-d limits and boundaries within the school is also poor.

He can be very stubborn and rude towards his teachers and lac positive motivation in his classwork. Michael's parents have had lit contact with the school and, although concern has been expressed them, they seem unable or unwilling to recognise the difficulties which is experiencing, saying that he does not give them any problems at hom

However, they have agreed to cooperate with a referral for assessmen

I would be grateful if an appointment could be arranged at your clir as soon as possible.

Yours sincerely,
Dr G. P. Barnes
School Medical Officer

The referral letter above will be one of a kind familiar to professionals who, a part of their daily work, come into contact with children who are exhibiti emotional and behavioural problems in a variety of contexts and who are call on to provide consultation, advice, intervention and solutions. The points which such referrals are dealt with may include child guidance clinics, chi psychiatric out-patient clinics in hospitals and health centres, residential ar day psychiatric assessment and treatment centres for children, etc. Assessme and treatment within these frameworks are most often provided by mult disciplinary multi-professional teams whose members may include child ps chiatrists, clinical and educational psychologists, social workers, psychiatr

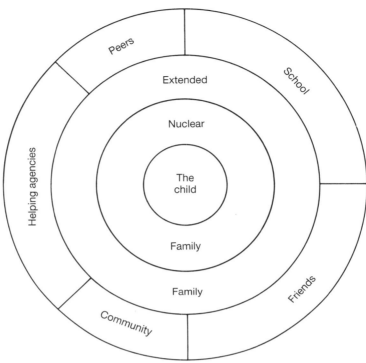

Figure 20.1   System boundaries

nurses, occupational therapists, child psychotherapists, teachers and others, whose skills are deployed individually and in combination to meet both the individual and the collective needs of this particular client group. Common to all these professionals, despite differences in experience, skills and role, is the likelihood that each will at some point come into contact with the family of the referred child.

A growing recognition and understanding of the importance of family life in the determination of individual emotional problems in childhood have led, particularly in the field of child psychiatry, to an increased emphasis on family involvement in both assessment and treatment.

THE FAMILY AS A SYSTEM

The family is one example of a natural group which, through the passage of its own history, has evolved complex patterns of interaction and relatedness between its constituting elements. These patterns of what are essentially modes of communication have coalesced through time to serve as rules or codes of behaviour whose functions are to bind the group together into a collective unit or *system* which is differentiated by those aspects of its own unique function from other natural groups in the environment, i.e. schools, work teams, clubs, societies, etc. These rules and patterns of interaction have the effect of maintaining the family system and preventing major change within it, creating a state of equilibrium or *homeostasis* both internally and in relation to the world beyond the boundaries created by them. They will also determine the quality of life experienced by all members of the family system and their ability to interrelate effectively with one another and with other systems beyond those circumscribed by the family boundaries (*Figure 20.1*).

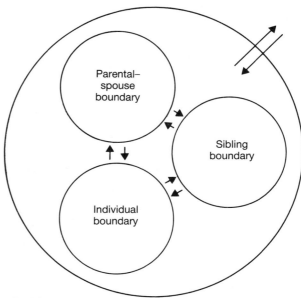

Figure 20.2   A healthy family system

Within a healthy family system the internal boundaries, codes of behaviou
and interaction are clearly defined and yet retain a flexibility and adaptability to
life events which will ensure the relative internal stability of the group.

Change within the family system is a normal and continuous process—
children are born and then grow through school towards independent live
outside their immediate family; parents and grandparents in old age remind u.
of the ever-present possibility of illness, enforced dependence and death; the
celebrations of life and the disappointments of life. Equilibrium within the
family system is therefore only ever a provisional state and the family's capacity
to cope with these changes in its life cycle will depend on factors such as:

(a) The existence of clearly defined identities within the family, providing a
mutually respected hierarchy, i.e. strong coalition between parents in
relation to both younger and older generations.
(b) Interpersonal trust and the ability to sustain appropriate, warm, caring
and mutually satisfying relationships with high levels of closeness and
intimacy, i.e. complementary marital roles, appropriate differentiation
between parental and children's roles, etc.
(c) Open clear spontaneous communication between individual family
members and with other individuals and systems beyond the immediate
family boundaries.
(d) Openness to new ideas generated both inside and outside the family
system and the ability to integrate and utilise new information effectively.
(e) Strong, varied and appropriate relationships outside the family, i.e.
friends, peers, work, etc.

Available research into family systems has identified a clear correlation
between the presence of these factors in combination and a low incidence of
individual symptomatic behaviour indicative of emotional disturbance
(*Figure 20.2*).

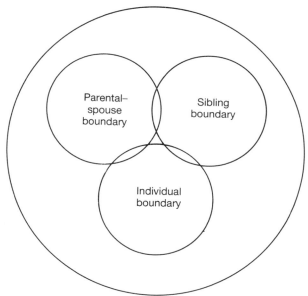

Figure 20.3   A dysfunctional family system

Conversely, within family systems presenting high levels of individual symptomatic behaviour, many of the following factors can be identified (*Figure 20.3*):

(a) Poor definition of identities within the family, producing blurred boundaries and shifting roles. Absence of a clearly defined hierarchy.
(b) Distrust in family relationships. Expectations within family of betrayal and desertion. Lack of marital satisfaction—competitive or dominant–submissive parental roles. Emotional distancing or invasiveness. Stereotyped roles.
(c) Communication may be rigid and unspontaneous. Vague, confused, evasive, contradictory and mystifying.
(d) Impervious to new ideas. Unable to cope with change in life events and loss.
(e) Relationships beyond family system poor. Defensive. Reliance on stereotyped, repetitive and unsatisfying modes of behaviour and interaction between family members.

THE SYSTEMIC CONTEXT OF THE SYMPTOM

Traditionally dysfunctional symptomatic behaviour has been viewed from a causal perspective (*Figure 20.4*). From this viewpoint, behaviour is seen as being the direct result of antecedent factors.

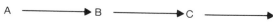

Figure 20.4   A linear causal view

Viewing the family from a systemic perspective, however, necessitates a shift in ways of thinking from one in which one individual's behaviour is defined as being the *cause* of another individual's behaviour to one which recognises the complex relationship between the behaviour of all members of the family system (*Figure 20.5*). One individual's actions within the family may well *influence* the actions of other family members but he will at the same time be influenced *by them*.

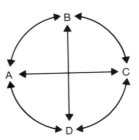

Figure 20.5   A circular systemic view

It follows that, when examining the behaviour of any single member of the family system, it would be an error to do so without at the same time exploring the systemic context, whether 'symptomatic' or not, of the behaviour under observation. When viewed in this way, dysfunctional symptomatic behaviour exhibited by one family member is indicative that dysfunction occurs within the family system as a whole. At a systematic level the symptom can be thought of as a 'solution' which has, in part, a protective function—protective in the sense of preventing a change which is perceived as potentially more threatening than the existing situation. The bearer of the symptom effectively sacrifices himself to, or is sacrificed by, the family to defend the relative stability of the system. In this way the symptom acts as a distance regulator between individual family members and represents an interactional conflict born out of the internal rules which determine the degrees of closeness and distance possible within the family.

If, for example, there is conflict between the parental couple which threatens the stability of the family the child may present with a problem or symptom, i.e. stealing, psychosomatic illness, behaviour problems, etc., which serves a dual function: bringing them closer together as parents to deal with the child's problem but also providing a potential focus for further disagreement and in this way preventing closer parental coalition.

The child is most often the family member who will become the symptom bearer; this is due largely to his greater vulnerability, in terms of both physical and emotional development, to stress and conflicts which occur within the family as a whole.

Despite its protective function of maintaining a tentative stability within the family the symptom can be seen, however, to be an inadequate and inappropriate solution whose roots can be located in complex dysfunctional patterns of communication and interaction which have developed and been repeated rigidly through time and often across several generations in the life history of the family concerned.

PATIENT PROFILE

Michael Abbott, the referred child considered at the beginning of this chapter, began to present with symptomatic behaviour shortly after commencing secondary school. During a family assessment arranged at a child guidance clinic the following story emerged.

Michael (aged 11 years 9 months) is the older child of two children of

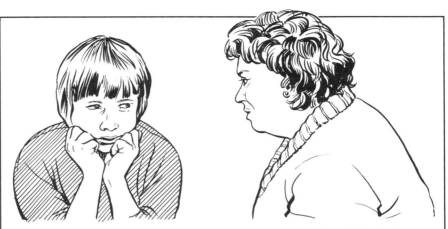

natural parents Mr and Mrs Abbott. His younger brother John is 6 years old and attends a local primary school where he appears to be doing well. The family live together in a two-bedroom flat, the parents sharing one room, the brothers sharing bunk beds in the other.

During the week, maternal grandmother also lives with the family, sleeping in a separate bed in the brothers' room. This arrangement has existed for the past 2 years since the maternal grandfather died following a long and painful illness. Grandmother spends weekends living in her own house which she does not want to give up. The family arrangement provides her with emotional and financial support whilst allowing her to retain a degree of independence and self-determination. At the weekends the brothers will often go to stay with grandmother at her house. Mr Abbott also lost his father following a stroke 3 years ago. Paternal grandmother now lives alone and the family have little contact with her because of the long journey involved.

Discussion about the effects of the loss of both grandfathers on the family is clearly painful. Mr Abbott in particular appears quite tearful when, in response to a question put to the the brothers, Michael talks animatedly about his memories of paternal grandfather. The double bereavement is something which is still being felt deeply by the whole family.

Mr Abbott works as a lorry driver and spends as much as 80 hours a week working away from home. As he is often home very late, 2 days can sometimes pass without his seeing the children at all. Mrs Abbott works part-time as a waitress but is able to spend more time with the children. She says that she sometimes finds it hard getting the boys to do as they are told at home and that they are more likely to behave when their father is home.

During the week, maternal grandmother plays a large role in looking after the children—getting them ready for school, cooking, shopping, cleaning, etc. Mrs Abbott says she finds this a big help.

During the interview, both parents appear tired and depressed. In reply to questions directed towards them as the parental couple, they rarely refer to one another in either support or disagreement. Both say that they do not understand why Michael should be behaving in the way that he is at school.

SYSTEMIC FORMULATION OF FAMILY PROBLEM

The loss of both maternal and paternal grandfathers within a space of 3 years is an event of huge importance in the Abbot family's life cycle (*Figure 20.6*). The threat to the stability of their family system has meant that substantial structural adaptive changes have had to be made across three generations in an attempt to cope with the effects of this double loss. This has involved a redefinition of roles and boundaries which the family have been only partially successful in achieving.

Although there are positive aspects about the maternal grandmother's helping–caring role within the family, it can be seen that Mrs Abbott's role as mother might have as a result lost definition for both her and her children. Mr Abbot's relative absence from the family home also lessens the possibility that emotional and practical support is available to his wife and the possibility of a strong parental coalition with regard to the care and management of the children. Father may also feel that his own role has lost definition within the family, given the potentially powerful mother–daughter coalition which is possible in the present family circumstances. Maternal grandmother can be seen in this case to be acting as a distance regulator between the parental couple and their children—helping at one level to maintain equilibrium within the family but at the same time preventing a more successful adaptation to painful and stressful life events.

Michael's symptomatic behaviour appears not only as a representation of wider dysfunctions within the Abbott family but also at an important time of change in his own life cycle, in this case the move upwards and out of the more protective environment provided by the primary school which he has recently left into the socially, emotionally and intellectually more demanding confines of a new secondary school.

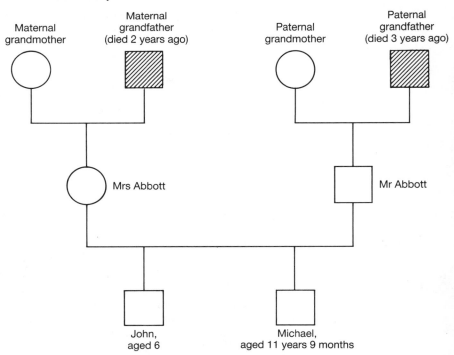

Figure 20.6   The Abbott family

PATIENT PROFILE

Alicia Lopez was referred for assessment to a day treatment centre for emotionally disturbed children by the school medical officer of the primary school which she had been attending for 4 months.

On commencing school it had been observed that Alicia (aged 5 years 6 months) had experienced great difficulty in separating from her mother. In the classroom, she had dramatic tantrums during which she would scream and cry and also often vomit. Her social and communication skills were poor and she was withdrawn and isolated from her peers. At break times and lunchtime, Alicia could not be persuaded to eat or drink anything. Efforts by teachers to persuade her resulted in further tantrums, tears and vomiting.

The parents were seen together by the assessment team to whom referral had been made. The family consisted of parents Mr and Mrs Lopez, both Spanish and their two daughters Maria, aged 12 years and Alicia, aged 5½ years.

Maria was attending a local secondary school and, although described as a 'quiet girl', did not appear to be presenting or experiencing any particular problems.

The parents had met and lived together initially in Spain where Maria had been born. When Maria was 3 years old, Mr Lopez travelled to England where he hoped to establish a small engineering firm. Mrs Lopez and Maria stayed behind, living together with maternal grandmother in Madrid for 2 years, after which they too travelled to England to rejoin Mr Lopez whose business had been successfully established by this time.

Alicia was born just over a year later. During Mrs Lopez' pregnancy, however, her mother became seriously ill with breast cancer and, although cared for by other members of the extended family in Spain, Mrs Lopez was unable to return to see her before she died. This was a particularly painful and distressing time for the whole family and was not made easier by the fact that Mr Lopez was having to spend long hours working away from home because of financial difficulties in his business.

Mrs Lopez experienced problems with Alicia's feeding from birth. She said that Alicia would not accept breast feeding and that she vomited back any milk taken in. The only way that the parents had been able to feed her at all was by spending hours in turn squeezing small amounts of milk from a bottle into her mouth in the hope that some of it would be ingested. They said that they had taken the child to several doctors all of whom had said that they could find no physical abnormality to account for the problem. The problem persisted as Alicia grew, as did the parents' management of the problem. A ritual had evolved around Alicia's feeding time suffused with anxiety that the child would die if she did not keep down at least some of the food given to her. The child had never been allowed to progress to eating solid food, both parents attesting that she was unable to swallow anything solid without choking and vomiting it back up again. Instead all her meals were liquidised in a food processor and spoon fed to her by mother or father, each mouthful being followed up with a sip of milk from a mug 'to wash it down'. Both parents were convinced that there was a physical basis for Alicia's problem and were angry with the medical profession for not having discovered and treated the cause.

This was the prevailing picture at the time of Alicia's referral and assessment. Paradoxically, when first seen by the team involved, Alicia presented as a grossly over-weight 5 year old, a picture which ran counter to the image that one had been led to expect by the parents' description of her eating behaviour.

Agreement was reached for Alicia to be treated as a day patient at the unit following further home-based assessment of the family's management of the problem. Three home visits were made during the following week to observe the family's behaviour, specifically at mealtimes. Alicia's meal was prepared separately by Mrs Lopez. One meal observed was a dinner consisting of a large piece of white fish boiled together with three or four potatoes and carrots which was then liquidised together with an egg and spoon fed to Alicia by mother interspersed with sips from two large mugs of milk. It was estimated from observations that, in addition to three large liquidised meals, Alicia was also drinking between 2 and 3 pints of milk a day. Both Mr and Mrs Lopez seemed oblivious to the grossly inappropriate amount of food which Alicia was being expected to consume each day.

Subsequent treatment at the day centre focused on two main areas. The first involved help with the severe difficulty in separating from Mrs Lopez in the mornings; at these times, Alicia would scream and cry and often vomit copious amounts of milky fluid. The second involved treatment of her feeding difficulties with a behaviourally orientated treatment programme which rewarded Alicia with social praise for a graduated intake of small amounts of solid food fed by herself.

Alicia made rapid progress at the day centre but it was clear that Mr and Mrs Lopez were having difficulty in implementing the programme at home and said that they were making no progress there; they said in fact that she was being more difficult with her eating behaviour than usual. As Alicia's feeding problem improved at the day centre, so too did her general behaviour and ability to relate appropriately to other children and adults. She enjoyed attending the centre and the separation difficulties seen initially with mother became far less pronounced. However, in her daily contact with the centre, it became evident that Mrs Lopez was becoming preoccupied with her own health as Alicia made progress. She said that she was having pains in her chest and it became clear that she was afraid that she too might develop breast cancer as her own mother had done. She also talked with the centre staff at this time about the difficulties that she had always experienced in relation to leaving home or her family and how she had often vomited herself because of anxiety at these times. Mr Lopez was also clearly concerned about his wife's health at this time and also made reference to how everything was 'affecting her nerves badly'. Mrs Lopez also mentioned that her own mother had also experienced the same problem and that she had never travelled more than a few miles away from home during her lifetime.

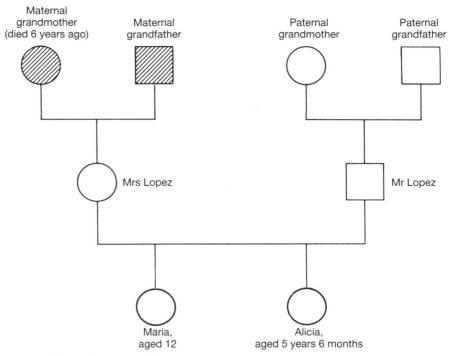

Figure 20.7   The Lopez family

SYSTEMIC FORMULATION OF FAMILY PROBLEM

The problem of separation from home, family and 'mothers' in particular can be seen to exist across three generations on the female side in this family (*Figure 20.7*). Mrs Lopez' separation from her own mother and home coincided sadly with her mother's illness and death and the birth of her own second child Alicia. Mrs Lopez may well have experienced some sense of responsibility and guilt for the loss of her mother and of being unable to return to see her during her illness.

These feelings, which are likely to have been present at the time of Alicia's birth and care during infancy, seem to be encapsulated in the child's symptomatic behaviour and may have been a contributory factor in the difficulty experienced at first with breast feeding and subsequently with any form of feeding.

Mr Lopez' involvement in the evolution and maintenance of the problem is likely to be related to a fear of what would happen to his wife in terms of her mental and physical health if the problem did not exist.

A great part of the family's life together is organised around Alicia's symptom. The soft diet, spoon feeding, enforced dependence and consequent difficulties in separation at a time when Alicia is moving outside the boundaries of the family for the first time amplifies the family's difficulty in allowing Alicia room for increased independence and maturational growth, for fear perhaps of what happens in terms of their own family history when a woman leaves home.

SOME IMPLICATIONS FOR A THERAPEUTIC APPROACH

Despite considerable development in the formulation and application of family therapeutic approaches to treatment during the past 20 years or so, family therapy can in many ways still be considered to be in its infancy. Its evolution has followed many different paths, relying on almost as many different conceptual frameworks within which to view family interaction and behaviour. Subsequently no single unified body of theory exists to guide us when we come to consider therapeutic work with families. Common to most approaches, however, is the view that, by definition, family therapy is something that should be directed towards the family system as a whole and not towards one part of that system in isolation, i.e. the identified patient.

Therapeutic approaches may be directed towards changing rigid patterns of communication and behaviour in the family which have contributed to and maintained specific individual problems over long periods of time. This may necessitate change in the behaviour of more than one member of the family, e.g. a father may need to become more assertive in his role and a mother less fearful and preoccupied about what may happen to their child during periods of normal separation if the child is to feel confident and able to move in and out of the family boundary into new relationships within the wider social system.

The elements of dysfunctional interaction which maintain the family in a state of 'no change' can often be seen to have qualities of a repetitive and ritualistic nature. Therapy may therefore need to be directed towards establishing new and more flexible modes of interaction and communication which will have the effect of allowing each member of the family to change those aspects of their own behaviour which have contributed to the maintenance of the existing family problem.

The formulation and negotiation of therapeutic goals between family and therapist will need to take into account the strong resistances to change which almost invariably arise as therapeutic work begins; change in the existing state of affairs is often perceived as a threat by some of, if not all, the family members. In defining and negotiating initial goals, family members may be unable to offer any suggestions themselves as to how to proceed in changing aspects of their own communication and interaction. They may strongly resist the view that family behaviour is in any way related to the existence of symptomatic behaviour in one individual member: 'It's not our fault that the child behaves badly.' They may also say that they have 'tried everything' to solve the problem or that they 'just don't understand why things should be the way they are'. Alternatively, families may come up with large, all-embracing and unrealistic solutions to the identified problem. In almost all these cases the therapist may need to help the family towards a solution through a series of small graduated steps over a period of weeks or months in regularly planned sessions.

Specific tasks may be suggested by the therapist for individual family members or for the family as a whole which will have the effect of challenging and changing rigid and redundant patterns of behaviour and interaction. For example, in a family where little time is spent engaged together in positive shared activity, the therapist may suggest that the family spend a short period of time each week doing something together as a group, i.e. going to the park on a weekend afternoon and playing a ball game together with the children or playing a board game chosen for its appropriateness to the developmental abilities of the children for half an hour each day after a family meal.

Some parents may need practical guidance in the management of their children's behaviour or in developing their own parental skills. The therapist in this case acts as a supportive teacher who, through the introduction of new information into the family system and the use of techniques such as modelling and role play, can help the family to learn new and effective ways of dealing with their own difficulties. The use of more than one therapist working in conjunction is common in family therapeutic approaches. Two therapists, perhaps one male and one female to parallel the parental couple, work jointly in engaging the family in therapeutic work. The roles of both therapists may have different emphases, e.g. one therapist may take a dominant active role working with the family while the second therapist acts as an observer whose role may be to help prevent his colleague from being drawn into the powerful collusive web which many dysfunctional families create as a way of preventing change.

The maxim 'two heads are better than one' has a tangible value when working together with dysfunctional families. Many therapists find it helpful to make a planned break during the course of the family session to discuss together details of strategy and approach before returning to the family with suggestions or directions regarding the next step in the therapeutic process.

The use, with family consent, of a one-way mirror or video monitoring system may also allow for valuable variations in therapeutic approach. For example, one therapist may work together with the family while one or more members of the therapeutic team observe the processes of communication and interaction enacted by therapist and family from a 'distanced' position. During a planned break in the course of the session the therapist and observers may again in this way join up to discuss the content of the session in detail and to plan therapeutic strategy.

For any professional considering entering into therapeutic work with families it should always be borne in mind that variations in social, economic, environmental and cultural status will play a very important part in determining the most appropriate therapeutic approach and that as a general principle the minimum necessary intervention to effect positive change should always be aimed for.

REFERENCE AND FURTHER READING

Reference

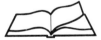

Topalis, M., and Aguilera, D. (1978), *Psychiatric Nursing*, 7th edn, C. V. Mosby, St Louis, Missouri.

Further reading

Haley, J. (1976), *Problem-solving Therapy*, Colophon Books, Harper and Row, London.
Minuchin, S. (1974), *Families and Family Therapy*, Tavistock, London.
Minuchin, S., and Fishman, C. H. (1981), *Family Therapy Techniques*, Harvard University Press, Cambridge, Massachusetts.
Palazzoli, M. S., *et al.* (1978), *Paradox and Counterparadox*, Aronson, London.
Pincus, L., and Dare, C. (1978), *Secrets in the Family*, Faber and Faber, London.

Chapter 21

Nursing care of the patient with anorexia nervosa

'*Always preoccupied with his or her physique, pubertal development and attractiveness, the adolescent today has an added worry, the fear of being a fat person in a society that values slenderness.*' (Schmidt and Duncan, 1974).

INTRODUCTION

Anorexia nervosa is an eating disorder that is characterized by severe and prolonged dieting. Self-imposed dieting results in severe weight loss, which threatens life and the individual's ability to function in society. The condition can occur in males or females usually within the age range 10–30 years. However, primary anorexia (i.e. anorexia occurring for the first time) is more common among females of adolescent age who predominantly come from middle class social backgrounds.

The physical picture is one of emaciation; amenorrhoea occurs and the body is covered in fine downy hair.

Anorexia is not usually a disorder that affects the patient alone; the patient may be expressing in a visible way a problem that affects the whole family. The dieting behaviour often begins during adolescence and may arise out of the person's inability to cope with the uncertainties of leaving childhood and becoming an adult. The patient's parents may be unduly rigid or repressive about sexual matters. Sexuality may be presented as something disgusting or frightening, or the vulnerability of women and the ill intentions of men may be emphasised.

Unconsciously, the patient may link eating with sexual behaviour. There may be an attempt to avoid adolescent sexuality by returning to an early stage of pre-pubertal development when the body was thin and child like. Food may be seen as a means of controlling sexual impulses, as a way of arresting sexual development and of achieving an identity.

Anorexic behaviour may also be a substitute for the usual adolescent behaviour of defying parental values and authority and moving towards independence.

The patient does not view the behaviour as self-destructive, and the concern with weight and body image is almost of delusional proportions. Despite the person's emaciated state the body is perceived as being fat and, when viewed in a mirror, parts of the body are seen rather than the whole. Thus the thighs may be seen as 'heavy' or the abdomen 'distended'.

The person is often quite euphoric about the ability to refuse food.

Some anorexics engage in periods of rigid starvation, alternating with binges of over-eating. Enormous amounts of food are consumed in response to pangs of hunger, sometimes with dangerous consequences. Because the idea of fatness fills the person with feelings of guilt, fear and disgust, vomiting is induced to relieve the guilt.

The person will often use diuretics, laxatives and enemas to help to achieve weight loss and to expend energy through vigorous exercise. It is not uncommon for the anorexic person to be very knowledgeable about the nutritional content and calorific values of food.

The anorexic person may be treated on an out-patient basis but, if there is a failure to achieve target weight, then hospitalisation may be necessary. Hospitalisation offers a controlled environment in which the food intake and output can be monitored. Furthermore, separation from the family may reduce factors that contribute to the condition.

Motivation and a willingness to accept treatment are of course important. In extreme cases, where the condition threatens a person's life, pressure must be placed on them to accept treatment. When the person achieves weight gain, many of their distressing symptoms disappear and they are able to view their problems from a more rational perspective.

PATIENT PROFILE

Gale Kogan developed anorexia nervosa at the age of 17. She became concerned about her weight while at college, where she was sometimes teased about her plumpness.

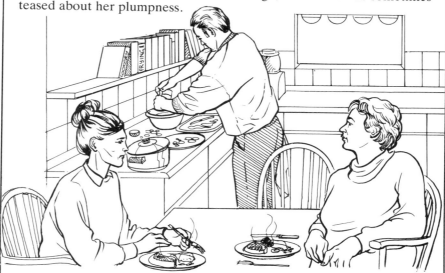

The Kogan family enjoyed their food but they tended to be 'fussy eaters'. Mr Kogan had always been a vegetarian and prepared his own food. Mrs Kogan read anything and everything about food that she could lay her hands on. She blamed her husband's peculiar eating habits for denying her the opportunity of trying out recipes from her enormous collection of cookery books. Despite her interest in food, Mrs Kogan was essentially a plain cook. Mealtimes were frequently used for the exchange of sarcastic comments between herself and Mr Kogan, and Gale was encouraged to take her mother's side in the subsequent arguments that arose.

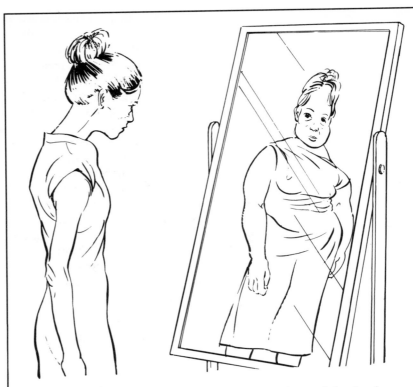

Sadie, Gale's elder sister, had largely stayed out of the food scene. At the age of 11, she had won a scholarship to boarding school and then had gone to train to be a nurse in Bath.

On admission, Gale whose height was 170.2 centimetres weighed 45 kilograms. She disguised her emaciated body with loose clothing.

NURSING ASSESSMENT INTERVIEW

Surname _Kogan_   Forenames _Gale Sharon_

Name person likes to be called _Gale_

Address _10 Manor Road_   Telephone number _1015_

Willbury   Date of ~~referral~~/admission _19 . 1 . 87_

WIL XII

Next-of-kin

Name _Mr and Mrs Y. Kogan_   Relationship _Parents_

Address _As above_

Telephone number _____

Date of birth _14 . 3 . 63_   Single/~~married/divorced/widowed~~ _____

General practitioner _Dr I. Yalom_   Address _Parkway Health Centre_

Old Barn Road

Willbury

Consultant _Dr S. Mencat_

Status under Mental Health Act _Informal_

Psychiatric diagnosis _Anorexia nervosa_

History of self-harm or harm towards others _Self-harm through starvation_

Occupation _Assistant at art centre_

Occupational history

Previously at art college

Hobbies and interests _Makes own clothes, embroidery, horse riding_

Patient's perceived reason for referral/admission _'Dr Mencat thinks that I'm underweight — I'm not — I'm fine'_

Relatives' understanding of patient's problems _Not stated_

NURSING ASSESSMENT INTERVIEW (continued)

Persons of significance in person's life

Family/friends/pets ___ Parents, sister, friend Patricia, Abigail (horse), Snow White (rabbit)

Spiritual needs

Neither Gale nor her family are churchgoers

Problems causing concern at home ___ Friend has promised to look after Abigail. Father will feed Snow White

Community services involved/referred ___

Name ___   Status ___

Telephone number ___   Date of referral ___

Mental status ___

History of present problems ___ Losing weight for several months, but only attended out-patient department for past 6 weeks

Previous psychiatric history ___ History of anorexia since age of 17

General appearance and behaviour ___ Thin; emaciated. Pale skin; fine downy hairs

Speech and communication patterns ___ Communicative — but voice betrays underlying anger sometimes

Problems with perception ___ Despite wasted appearance, perceives herself as 'chubby'

NURSING ASSESSMENT INTERVIEW (continued)

Affective state _Cheerful_

Disturbances of thinking or judgement _Thoughts are particularly related to food. Unable to judge accurately her own nutritional needs_

Orientation

Person _Fully orientated_

Place

Time

Activities of living

Safety and mobility

Eating and drinking
Anorexic – to be treated with dietary regime

Elimination

Bladder

Bowel _Usually constipated_

Sleep patterns
Sleeps alright

Personal needs
Hates resting and staying in bed

General health

Any medical condition for which the person is receiving treatment
Has been treated on an out-patient basis

Doctor's instructions
Nurses to ensure that Gale follows dietary regime

Areas of concern to patient
Wants to get home to pets

NURSING ASSESSMENT INTERVIEW (continued)

Problems identified

Grossly underweight.
Life centres around food (and avoiding it!)

Date of interview   20 · 1 · 87   Signature   B. Smith

History taken from   Gale

by   Bobby Smith   Designation   Staff nurse

Additional information   Date   21. 1. 87

USE OF BEHAVIOURAL APPROACH

A behavioural approach was adopted towards Gale's care, enabling her to receive privileges for specified weight gains.

PLAN OF NURSING CARE

(a) Patient's problem

   1. Severe weight loss and malnutrition.

(b) Patient's goals

   1. To adhere to the set dietary regime (*Table 21.1*).
   2. To receive privileges as specified for reaching target weights.

(c) Nursing goals

To ensure that the patient:

   1. Adheres to the dietary regime.
   2. Is weighed each morning on rising and after emptying her bladder.
   3. Is provided with specified rewards for reaching weight targets.
   4. Is encouraged to accept responsibilities for gaining and maintaining weight.
   5. Is encouraged to converse on non-food related topics.
   6. Is provided with a consistent and supportive atmosphere in which to explore problems.
   7. Is discouraged from engaging in manipulative behaviour.
   8. Is encouraged to relate to other young people of both sexes.
   9. Cared for by nurses who are themselves supported.

IMPLEMENTATION

Gale had been attending the out-patient clinic for some weeks. As she had failed to achieve an agreed weight target, Dr Mencat persuaded her to come in as an in-patient.

Dr Mencat had discussed the proposed treatment with her. Initially, she knew that she would be expected to remain in bed and to adhere strictly to a planned dietary regime. As she achieved the set weekly target weights, she would receive certain specified privileges for her efforts (see *Table 21.1*).

The doctor compared Gale's actual body weight with the desirable weight for her height.

At first, Gale was given a bland milk diet of 1500 calories. This was given in small amounts at 2-hourly intervals. This was increased over the next 2 weeks to 4000–5000 calories a day. Gale was encouraged to keep her weight chart beside her bed as an 'incentive'.

Sometimes, if a patient fails to cooperate with the dietary regime, the doctor will order tube feeding. This was not necessary for Gale but, if it is necessary, it should be carried out in the privacy of the patient's room and the patient should always be allowed the option of drinking the feed instead.

During the first few days, Gale displayed a good deal of anger towards the staff. This could have had the effect of alienating her and perceiving her negatively. Anger is difficult to deal with but, if the nurse understands some of the reasons why the patient is reacting angrily to her hospitalisation, then a more positive approach can be adopted. The anger could be a reaction to the patient's illness and the predicament that she finds herself in. For the nurse to react to anger with anger serves no purpose; in fact, it is more likely to ensure a continuation of the behaviour. The nurse should validate the patient's feelings

Table 21.1   *Dietary regime*

Phase	Total daily calorific values	Expected weight gain	Reward	Date achieved
1	1500	1.5 kilograms	To get up to toilet	
2	2000	1.5 kilograms	To have a bath and to get dressed	
3	3500	1.5 kilograms	To watch television for an hour	
4	4000	2.0 kilograms	To use the telephone	
5	5000	2.0 kilograms	To go outside for a walk	
6	5000	2.0 kilograms	To have a visitor	
7	5000	2.0 kilograms	To go home for a weekend	

The length of each phase will be determined by the patient's weight gain.
The dietary regime is graduated from light meals to ordinary meals. Complan or Build-up is given in addition to solid foods three times daily. This makes up the total daily calorific value.

with her and help her to express them. If the patient knows that she is being listened to and treated like an adult, it may help.

Supervision was essential, because the patient may find a means of disposing of food, and the nurse needs to be aware of the methods that can be used. The patient may drink water (even bath water if the opportunity arises) or conceal weights in or on the body prior to weighing. The patient may induce vomiting or take laxatives (smuggled in by patient). Food may be hidden in clothing, in furnishings, behind pictures or in other ingenious places that the patient will think of. When eating in company, others may be encouraged to share the food or food may be pushed around on the plate so that the patient looks to have consumed more than has actually been eaten. The patient may exercise vigorously, even while on bed rest. There is only one meaningful indication that the patient is eating satisfactorily and that is a steady weight gain. If the patient does not gain weight or loses weight, cheating must be suspected. The patient does not usually admit this and will deny any form of cheating.

Nursing the patient with anorexia nervosa requires a high degree of stability and emotional understanding. The patient is often manipulative and will try to influence the behaviour of others towards self-directed goals. One staff member may be played against another; there may be a tendency to bend the truth and attempts to cause confusion over the dietary regime. Some manipulative behaviour is quite obvious, but the patient usually engages in more subtle methods.

When entering Gale's room, the nurse was sometimes met with flattery and at other times silence. Because of the patient's tendency to manipulate, the staff must ensure that they communicate effectively and record nursing interventions accurately.

The nurse should try to develop a therapeutic relationship with the patient. If this is to be effective, there is often a need for self-examination in relation to feelings towards the patient and how these feelings can interfere with the relationship. The nurse tried to be sensitive towards Gale without being gullible and to show an interest in her but not to be taken in by her flattery or superficial charm. The nurse who is able to endure constant testing wthout feeling threatened or offended will probably be most successful.

The anorexic patient often focuses on food in conversation; this keeps verbal exchange at a superficial level and enables more threatening subjects to be avoided. If the nurse shows a willingness to listen actively to the patient, something may be learned about the underlying problems within the family. Nursing intervention should provide a supportive atmosphere for the patient's family, particularly in helping them to accept her movement towards maturity and independence.

The nurse can act as a role model, encouraging the development of self-confidence and the ability to relate to others on matters other than food. The patient is often confused about many things; social interaction can encourage the development of meaningful interpersonal relationships.

Gale was discharged from hospital when she had reached and maintained her final target weight for a week; she had by then spent a successful weekend at home.

EVALUATION

Gale achieved her weight targets quickly and earned the agreed privileges. She took over responsibility for gaining and maintaining weight, although on several occasions it was necessary to point out to her the number of salads that she was choosing.

Gale's earlier attempts to manipulate the staff were largely avoided by consistent approaches and sound communication between the staff. The nurses provided support for each other by showing a willingness to share and explore feelings.

Dr Mencat has given Gale an out-patient appointment for 4 weeks' time. He felt that, while Gale had responded well to treatment, there was a possibility that the problem would reappear as long as Gale continued to live at home. He did not recommend family therapy.

REFERENCE AND FURTHER READING

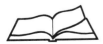

Reference

Schmidt, M. P. W., and Duncan, B. A. B. (1974), Modifying eating behaviour in anorexia nervosa, *American Journal of Nursing*, **74**, 1646–1648.

Further reading

Abraham, S., and Llewellyn-Jones, D. (1984), *Eating Disorders: The Facts*, Oxford University Press, Oxford.

Biley, F., and Savage, S. (1984), Anorexia nervosa, *Nursing Times*, **80**, No. 31, 28–32.

Blatch, P. (1980), An obsession with starving, *Nursing Mirror*, **150**, No. 4, 32–35.

Brockopp, D. Y., and Hall, S. Y. (1984), Eating disorders: a teen-age epidemic, *Nurse Practitioner*, **9**, No. 4, 32–35.

Claggett, M. (1980), Anorexia nervosa: a behavioural approach, *American Journal of Nursing*, **80**, 1471–1472.

Dally, P., Gomez, J., and Isaacs, A. J. (1979), *Anorexia Nervosa*, Heinemann Medical, London.

Grossniklaus, D. M. (1980), Nursing interventions in anorexia nervosa, *Perspectives in Psychiatric Care*, **18**, No. 1, 11–16.

Kalucy, R. S. (1973), Anorexia nervosa: a nursing challenge, *Nursing Mirror*, **1**, No. 36, 11–16.

King, D. A. (1971), Anorexic behaviour: a nursing problem, *Journal of Psychiatric Nursing and Mental Health Services*, **9**, No. 3, 11–17.

Lipkin, G. B., and Cohen, R. G. (1980), *Effective Approaches to Patients' Behaviour*, 2nd edn, Springer, New York.

McNelly, P., and Hickley, P. (1978), Anorexia nervosa: a challenge to the nurse, *Nursing Mirror*, **147**, No. 10, 32–34.

Richardson, T. F. (1980), Anorexia nervosa: an overview, *American Journal of Nursing*, **80**, 1470–1471.

Sanger, E., and Cassino, T. (1984), Eating disorders. Avoiding the power struggle, *American Journal of Nursing*, **84**, 31–33.

Wright, S. J. (1982), Altered body image in anorexia nervosa, *Professional Nurse*, **1**, No. 10, 260–262.

Chapter 22

Nursing care of the alcoholic patient

'*Progressing through the early, middle and late stages of alcoholism, the person lives and drinks, then lives to drink and finally drinks to live.*' (Mitchell, 1976).

INTRODUCTION

Alcohol is firmly established as a social drug within western society. It is consumed on many social occasions and is therefore an important part of social life and a symbol of hospitality (Plant, 1979).

When a person becomes dependent on alcohol, it can lead to major health and social problems. A person may begin to consume large quantities of alcohol to relieve tension and anxiety, to overcome feelings of loneliness or inferiority, to increase confidence or to relieve depression, discomfort or pain.

The choice of alcoholic beverage and the quantity that a person drinks will vary for each individual; a person may engage in compulsive drinking binges followed by periods of remission or may spread the consumption of alcohol more evenly.

When a person consumes alcohol regularly over a period of time, tolerance can develop, i.e. more alcohol is needed to achieve the same effects that were achieved when the person first started drinking. Tolerance can in turn lead to physical dependence, although a person may not experience any major symptoms to indicate what is happening to the body until drinking ceases; he will then experience the symptoms of withdrawal because of the body's reactions to the loss of a substance that it has grown used to. The most common sign of withdrawal is the tremor of the hands, which is experienced by the person in the morning, following a fall in blood alcohol levels during sleep (Plant, 1979). Hallucinations and fits may also occur.

Excessive drinking over a number of years can cause a wide range of physical problems including cirrhosis of the liver, nutritional deficiencies especially of vitamin B and peripheral neuritis. Chronic gastritis may lead to vomiting, poor appetite and digestion. There may be confusion, black-outs, memory loss and dementia. Some alcoholics engage in the cross-use of alcohol and other drugs. This can have a particularly dangerous effect, especially as alcohol potentiates the actions of many drugs.

Social problems commonly include absenteeism, road traffic accidents, outbreaks of violence and debt.

The alcoholic label threatens both the individual and the family, and the family may find it very difficult to seek help for the member who is dependent on alcohol. Furthermore, the family may minimise the problem and use numerous defences such as denial or rationalisation to justify the behaviour.

The nurse will encounter the person with problems of alcoholism in many different settings: in the community, in the psychiatric hospital or in the accident and emergency department or wards of the general hospital.

PATIENT PROFILE

Stefan Williams, aged 33, has always been a shy and rather anxious person. His parents have been the proprietors of The Willbury Arms since his father retired from the Army. Mr Williams senior looks younger than his 52 years and is a keen sportsman and physical fitness fanatic. Stefan has always felt overshadowed by his father and inadequate in his presence. Stefan has never enjoyed sports and, as the only son, feels that he has failed to live up to his father's high hopes. In his teens, he began to resort to alcohol to relieve his feelings of discomfort. Stefan has never had any sexual interest in girls and the one or two that he has taken home were merely an attempt on his part to live up to his parents' expectations. Stefan has known for a long time that he is homosexual. At first, he felt guilty but has learned to come to terms with his feelings; he once tried to confide in his mother, but she did not seem to grasp the significance of what he was saying and continued to ask him when he was going to get married and to settle down.

Stefan has had treatment for his alcoholism previously, but the break-up of an important relationship led him to resume his former drinking habits. Patterns of lateness and absenteeism also led to the loss of his job. He has now established a fairly stable relationship with Gregory and has been sharing a flat with him for 6 months. Their relationship is a stormy one, and many of the rows and beatings which occur are related to Stefan's drinking.

He was seen at the out-patient clinic by Dr Leininger and agreed to receive treatment because he is afraid of losing Gregory.

NURSING ASSESSMENT INTERVIEW

Surname _Williams_   Forenames _Stefan John_

Name person likes to be called _Stefan_

Address _Flat 4_   Telephone number _1470_
39 River Street   Date of ~~referral~~/admission _27·8·86_
Middlesdown
MID 44A

Next-of-kin
Name _Mr G. Williams_   Relationship _Father_
Address _Willbury Arms_
Market Place
Willbury   Telephone number _2182_
Date of birth _11·4·53_   Single/~~married/divorced/widowed~~
General practitioner _Dr I. Singh_   Address _44 Jamison Street_
Forest Wood
Middlesdown

Consultant _Dr B. Leininger_
Status under Mental Health Act _Informal_
Psychiatric diagnosis _Alcohol dependence_

History of self-harm or harm towards others _No_

Occupation _Unemployed for 6 months_
Occupational history
Carpet fitter, last job, Salesman

Hobbies and interests _Painting, reading_

Patient's perceived reason for referral/admission _'Drink has been giving me_
physical problems'

Relatives' understanding of patient's problems _Gregory thinks that_
Stefan uses alcohol as a prop

NURSING ASSESSMENT INTERVIEW (continued)

Persons of significance in person's life

Family/friends/pets   Gregory Silverton, Two cats Smudge and Smithy

Spiritual needs   Believes religion is about respecting others

Problems causing concern at home   Only wants to get home as soon as possible

~~Community services involved/referred~~   To be referred to Alcoholics Anonymous

Name _____   Status _____

Telephone number _____   Date of referral _____

Mental status _____

History of present problems   Has been okay until break-up of an important relationship about 13 months ago

Previous psychiatric history   Treated for alcohol dependency 3 years ago

General appearance and behaviour   Well dressed, Seems tense

Speech and communication patterns   Tends to let Gregory do the talking when he is here

Problems with perception   No

NURSING ASSESSMENT INTERVIEW (continued)

Affective state _Anxious if he can overcome problem._

Disturbances of thinking or judgement _Not when alcohol free_

Orientation

Person _No problem_

Place

Time

Activities of living

Safety and mobility

Eating and drinking

Elimination

Bladder

Bowel

Sleep patterns

Personal needs _Need to feel accepted_

General health

Any medical condition for which the person is receiving treatment
Peripheral neurosis

Doctor's instructions _Refer to physiotherapy_

Areas of concern to patient
Hopes that Gregory will not get fed up with him

NURSING ASSESSMENT INTERVIEW (continued)

Problems identified

_____

_____

_____

_____

_____

_____

_____

_____

_____

_____

Date of interview _28 . 8 . 86_   Signature _K. O'Neil_

History taken from _Stefan and Gregory_

by _Kate O'Neil_   Designation _Ward sister_

Additional information   Date _28 . 8 . 86_

_____

_____

_____

_____

_____

_____

_____

_____

_____

_____

_____

_____

_____

_____

_____

_____

USE OF OREM'S SELF-CARE MODEL

Orem's (1980) self-care model (see Chapter 7) was chosen for Stefan's care because the success of treatment will largely depend on his motivation and ability to carry out self-care requisites and to relinquish activities which have led to the need for health deviation self-care requisites.

PLAN OF NURSING CARE

The plan of nursing care is given in *Table 22.1.*

Table 22.1   Self-care requisites, patient's problems and goals, nursing goals and types of nursing actions

Self-care requisite	Patient's problem	Patient's goal	Nursing goal	Type of nursing action
Universal 1. Air	Potential for respiratory infection	To achieve adequate respiratory ventilation	To encourage Stefan to take exercise and fresh air	Guiding, teaching, supporting
2. Food	Has not been taking food regularly	To meet nutritional requirements	To encourage regular nutritious meals	Guiding, teaching, supporting
3. Water	Drinks insufficient water	To drink 1½ litres of water per day	To ensure that Stefan is offered a variety of drinks	Guiding, teaching, supporting
4. Elimination	Usually constipated	To take fruit and dietary fibre	To ensure that fruit and fibre form part of daily diet	Guiding, teaching, supporting
5. Activity and rest	Discomfort and numbness in legs, particularly at night	To experience reducton in lower limb discomfort	To ensure adequate rest and sleep. To refer to occupational therapist for assessment	Guiding, teaching, supporting
6. Avoiding hazards to life and well-being	Accident-proneness when drinking alcohol has led to physical effects on health	To function in a safe environment. To learn about the harmful effects of alcohol on health	To provide a safe environment. To educate Stefan about the harmful effects of alcohol	Guiding, teaching, supporting
7. Solitude, social interaction	Lacks confidence; never mixed with others easily	To be accepted by others	To help Stefan to feel part of the group	Guiding, teaching, supporting
8. Being normal	Does not feel equal to others. Problems of sexual orientation. Less guilt now	To experience increased self-esteem	To use goal achievement as a means of increasing his self-esteem	Guiding, teaching, supporting
Developmental 1. Effects of health on human development	Alcohol has dominated life. Has learned to use alcohol as a coping device when tense	To abstain from alcohol. To explore alternative coping methods. To initiate relaxation	To support patient's goals by encouraging, listening, accepting and confronting. To provide teaching of relaxation methods	Guiding, teaching, supporting
Health deviation 1. Adjustments made to ill health	Has begun to accept need to overcome dependency problem	To remain motivated and to complete treatment	To encourage him to talk about feelings. To ensure long-term support	Guiding, teaching, supporting

IMPLEMENTATION

Prior to admission, Stefan had agreed to accept treatment but, once in the unit, he denied the nature of his problem and frequently tried to focus attention away from his problem by introducing different topics of conversation. The treatment of alcoholism is aimed at helping the patient to live a sober, productive and satisfying life, and these aims cannot be achieved unless the patient is willing to recognise that he has a problem; therefore, in the first instance the patient has got to learn to be honest with himself. When Stefan denied his problem, the nurse had to confront him to make him face up to the reality of his situation. This was done in a direct way by giving Stefan objective feedback on his behaviour. Confronting the patient can be a supportive measure if it is carried out in a caring non-judgemental way and can help him to gain insight into the way that he uses his defences maladaptively. Self-insight can be a painful process and arouse feelings of anger. The patient will need the nurse's help to work through this anger by channelling the anger into constructive activities.

The nurse who helps the patient with dependence problems must have a genuine desire to help him; otherwise, negative attitudes will be communicated to the patient through body language (Meisenhelder, 1985).

The nurse encouraged Stefan to take regular meals and the vitamin supplement ordered by the doctor. He was urged to increase his fluid intake and attended physiotherapy for exercises to help to relieve the discomfort that he felt in his legs.

Throughout the treatment, the nurse helped to keep Stefan's motivation high by reassuring him that he was making progress. In this way, each small achievement was acknowledged, his self-care capacity was increased and the ultimate goals seemed less remote.

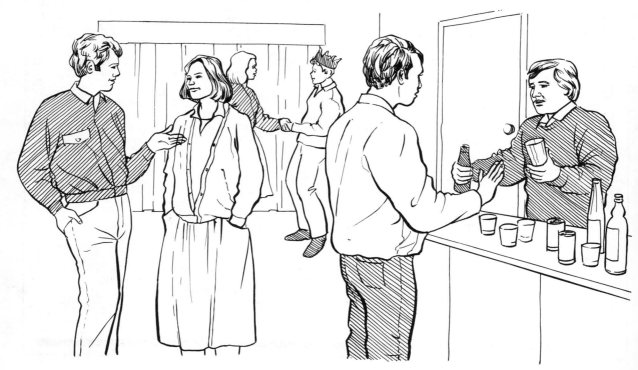

When a person's life has centred around alcohol, its removal can leave feelings of emptiness. Stefan had to be helped to come to terms with this loss by identifying the alternatives to alcohol. The nurse provided guidance and support to enable him to cope with social engagements by encouraging his participation in role play in which he was able to enact his role in social and problematic circumstances.

This helped Stefan to cope with situations in which alcohol was featured.

Role play sessions helped him to be more assertive and confident. He was also taught to initiate self-relaxation, thereby increasing his sense of self-control. He was helped to depend on his own resources and to reach out to others rather than to reach for the bottle. Stefan was encouraged to learn recreational skills in the occupational therapy department to help him to develop new interests and skills.

Group therapy enabled Stefan to share problems and to gain insight into not only his own behaviour but also the behaviour of others with similar problems. He was able to receive support when focusing on his own particular problems and to give support to others. This helped him to feel valued as a person and gave him a sense of belonging.

Stefan and his friend Gregory were homosexual. Although they had been in a flat together for 6 months, Stefan was concerned about Gregory's faithfulness; like any heterosexual couple, homosexual partners may have fears about promiscuity and sexual activity outside their established relationship.

The nurse is bound to meet patients whose sexual orientation is different and perhaps incompatible with his or her own definition of acceptability. The nurse who is able to accept his or her own sexuality is more likely to be able to accept the patient's sexuality even when his sexual habitation is different.

When the nurse is unable to resolve personal feelings about a patient's differing sexual practices, this may inhibit the development of a therapeutic relationship. Total nursing care cannot be given without considering the patient as a sexual being (Zalar, 1975). When the nurse is uncomfortable with sexual matters or lacks the appropriate skills to help the patient come to terms with a sexual problem, then it is better to be honest with the patient and to refer him to an appropriate person or agency.

Stefan frequently spoke of his feelings towards his parents, particularly his father because he felt he had not come up to his expectations. His relationship with his father was painfully negative and he felt that his father had very rigid views about gay people. He thought they were 'bent', 'effeminate' and 'limp wristed'. Stefan felt that his parents would never accept his homosexuality despite the fact that he had 'come out' and was quite open about it with most people. (The phenomenon of 'coming out' means that a person identifies himself (or herself) as gay. Through the coming-out process the individual learns that there are others with a similar sexual orientation with whom he can identify.)

Stefan was referred to Alcoholics Anonymous prior to his discharge and introduced to the support group held in the evenings at the unit, to increase his self-care capacity.

EVALUATION

Stefan has responded well to treatment and, with the continued support of Gregory, is determined to abstain from alcohol. He has gained weight, feels well and seems happier and more confident. He has met the goals of his universal self-care requisites through nursing actions which aimed to support, to guide, to facilitate learning and to strengthen his self-care capacities.

In overcoming the problems of dependence the supportive–educative system of care has been the most crucial aspect of nursing. The nurse, having sought to reduce the deficits in Stefan's self-care needs, must bear in mind that support will be required for some time after discharge from the unit. Stefan has been introduced to Alcoholics Anonymous and is to attend the self-help group at the unit. The community psychiatric nurse who is attached to the alcohol dependency unit and who has got to know Stefan well during his stay will continue to provide the supportive educative component of nursing care until Stefan is able to completely resolve his self-care deficit.

DETECTING THE EARLY SIGNS OF ALCOHOLISM

A problem in *one* of the following areas is insufficient cause for concern but four or five factors could signify danger (Calhoun, 1973; Bakdash, 1978):

1. A preoccupation with alcohol.
2. Drinking alone.
3. An increased tolerance to alcohol.
4. Using alcohol as a medicine.
5. Black-outs.
6. Morning drinking.
7. Drinking occupies time formerly given to other interests.
8. Overspending on alcohol.
9. Protecting the supply.
10. Gulping drinks, i.e. drinking quite fast.

REFERENCES AND FURTHER READING

References

Bakdash, D. (1978), Essentials that nurses should know about chemical dependency, *Journal of Psychiatric Nursing and Mental Health Services*, **16**, No. 10, 33.

Calhoun, B. (1973), Alcoholism, a challenge to nursing, *Journal of Practical Nursing*, **23**, No. 5, 24–27, 39.

Meisenhelder, J. B. (1985), Self esteem: a closer look at clinical interventions, *International Journal of Nursing Studies*, **22**, No. 2, 127–135.

Mitchell, C. E. (1976), Assessment of alcohol abuse, *Nursing Outlook*, **24**, No. 8, 511–515.

Orem, D. E. (1980), *Nursing: Concepts of Practice*, 2nd edn, McGraw-Hill, New York.

Plant, M. A. (1979), *Drinking Careers*, Tavistock, London.

Zalar, M. (1975), Human sexuality, a component of total patient care, *Nursing Digest*, **3**, No. 6, 40–43.

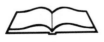

Further reading

Betts, V. T. (1976), Psychotherapeutic intervention with the addict–client, *Nursing Clinics of North America*, **11**, No. 3, 551–558.

Carruth, G. R. (1982), Grieving the loss of alcohol: a crisis in recovery, *Journal of Psychiatric Nursing and Mental Health Services*, **20**, No. 3, 18–20.

Dobson, M. (1984), Problem drinking, *Nursing Times*, **80**, No. 12, 57–60.

Flowers, J. V. (1975), Simulation and role playing methods. In: *Helping People Change* (eds Kanfer, F. H., and Goldstein, A. P.), Pergamon, Oxford.

Gareri, E. A. (1979), Assertiveness training for alcoholics, *Journal of Psychiatric Nursing and Mental Health Services*, **17**, No. 1, 31–36.

Goldsborough, J. D. (1970), On becoming non-judgemental, *American Journal of Nursing*, **70**, 2340–2343.

Heinemann, E., and Estes, N. (1976), Assessing alcoholic patients, *American Journal of Nursing*, **76**, No. 5, 785–789.

Minardi, H. (1986), One day at a time, *Nursing Times*, **82**, No. 10, 34–36.

Morton, P. (1979), Assessment and management of the self-destructive concept of alcoholism, *Journal of Psychiatric Nursing and Mental Health Services*, **17**, No. 11, 8–13.

Reed, S. W. (1976), Assessing the patient with an alcoholic problem, *Nursing Clinics of North America*, **11**, No. 3, 483–492.

Silverberg, R. A. (1984), Being gay. Helping clients cope, *Journal of Psychosocial Nursing*, **22**, No. 2, 19–25.

Thorley, A. (1983), *Problem Drinkers and Drug Takers: Theory and Practice of Psychiatric Rehabilitation*, John Wiley, Chichester, West Sussex.

Chapter 23

Nursing care of the patient who abuses drugs

by *Neil Vermaut*

'*The attitudes of the nurse often influence the care given to the drug-dependent patient.*' (Lancaster, 1980).

INTRODUCTION

Drug abuse is recognised as a major problem in society, particularly as more younger people are becoming involved. Strang (1983) notes the increase in the illicit use of opiates, cocaine, amphetamine and barbiturates in recent years. Opioids (opiates and their synthetic equivalents) are used medically for analgesia. However, this group, which includes heroin, has increased in illicit use and availability over the last few years with 10 200 opioid addicts notified to the Home Office in 1983, although the actual number using opioids regularly may be up to 50 000. Of those notified, almost half were under 25. Recreational use of heroin also appears to be developing amongst teenagers, the practice of heating the drug on foil and inhaling its smoke through a tube being known as 'chasing the dragon'. Notified addicts are those users who have been attended by doctors for medical or other treatment and who display evidence of dependence on heroin, methadone, cocaine or one of a number of synthetic opioids including Diconal which are controlled by the Misuse of Drugs Act 1971. Recently, health authorities have been directed to give high priority to the expansion of its services for drug misusers.

Drug abuse and drug misuse are terms that connote illicit and indiscriminate drug use. Drug misusers may experience detrimental consequences, resulting in problem drug use. Thorley (1982) defines a problem drug taker as a person who experiences psychological, physical, social or legal problems related to intoxication, and/or excessive consumption and/or dependence as a result of his own drugs or chemical substances. As Dobson (1984) suggests, an exploration of the physical, psychological, social and legal factors is necessary in the examination of the difficulties of the problem drug user. The outwardly-manifested difficulties may be symptomatic of an underlying personality problem and it is towards this that treatment is ideally orientated through detoxification, support and rehabilitation. Thorley describes the heterogeneity of problem drug users who are likely to come from any social class.

There is no single causal factor of drug misuse amongst young people; adolescence can be a problem-laden stage of development for some teenagers. It can also be a time of curiosity and experimentation. If for the newly acquainted user a drug produces a subjectively pleasurable experience which to some extent transiently erases worries or problems, then the desire to achieve the effect again may be a sufficient inducement for its repeated use. Other members of the user's peer group may be similarly involved. Cannabis, which has the most widespread illicit use, is often the drug of initiation when it is smoked in the form of a cigarette or 'joint'. Sometimes, relatively excessive alcohol consumption is a concurrent feature amongst early drug takers. However, of those who initially experiment with drugs, only a minority become regular users. The regular use of a drug may lead to physical and/or psychological dependence, the latter being more widespread. Physical dependence describes a state whereby the user requires a repeated administration of the drug to avoid the unpleasant effects of withdrawal. Psychological dependence refers to the user's compulsion to continue to take the drug in order to maintain the pleasurable effects and to mask or erase reality. Many drug misusers are dependent on not only one drug. Some opioid users also take tranquillisers, alcohol, amphetamine or hallucinogens.

A further consequence of regular drug use is that the body develops tolerance so that a higher dose is needed to achieve the same effect. The physical and psychological problems associated with drug misuse include accidental overdose (perhaps fatal through interaction with alcohol or the inhalation of vomit during sleep), hepatitis, drug-induced psychosis and self-neglect (e.g. dietary deficiency). There are also legal implications. Since there are laws prohibiting the illicit use of certain drugs, e.g. cannabis, opiates and cocaine, the possession of these renders the user liable to prosecution. A further consequence is the possibility that the user is unable to finance the purchase of drugs on the illicit market, when he may resort to criminality, e.g. stealing or burglary to meet his monetary needs. Immersed in a drug-orientated lifestyle, the user's social relationships may be narrowed to association with those of similar habits. Maintaining or obtaining employment and being financially able to keep accommodation may be difficult in some cases.

Treatment for drug misuse can be a lengthy process requiring medical, psychological and social support to help the individual to identify and understand his problems and to involve him in making decisions regarding his future plans.

Oral methadone is used in some clinics in reduced doses for heroin withdrawal although an alternative drug clonidine, which is non-addictive, is also effective in reducing the stresses of withdrawal.

PATIENT PROFILE

After the divorce of his parents, Mark Cater, a 19-year-old college student, who lived with his father, a successful bookmaker, began to experience feelings of depression and disenchantment with life. A moderate drinker of alcohol for 15 months, he would meet regularly at night with fellow students at a local public house where they would theorise, philosophise and idealise about matters of life. Next day, in the cold dawn of reality, he would often feel flat and disillusioned. His father showed only a distant concern in Mark's mood changes, being too immersed in his string of betting shops. However, what he lacked in parental affection and comfort, Mark's father tried to compensate for in other ways. Mark suffered no financial hardship.

During an end-of-term party at a friend's house, Mark consumed more alcohol than usual, perhaps hoping it would serve as a psychological panacea, but it had the reverse effect and only exaggerated his depression. Temporarily diverting himself from the main activities, he found by chance in an upstairs room a friend evidently deriving pleasure from smoking heroin. Impressionable and suggestible by nature, Mark felt stunned to sobriety. The discovery released in him a curiosity which his friend was only too pleased to satisfy by demonstrating how to 'chase the dragon' and invited Mark to try it, which he did.

In the ensuing months, Mark became a regular smoker of heroin, financially able to purchase supplies, the sources of which became readily known to him and other drug users with whom he was associating in his narrowing field of social relationships. Almost 7 months after first trying heroin and now familiar with drug terminology and methods of use, Mark's increasing tolerance and growing dependency, to which his father was oblivious, were beginning to strain his pocket as he sought increased supplies of heroin. When a friend suggested the economic and practical advantages of using the drug by injection with its heightened effect, Mark decided to give it a try with his friend's syringe. It produced a mixed but decidedly pleasant reaction. 2 weeks later Mark was found unconscious in his bedroom by his father, a syringe on the floor.

Mark's heroin dependence was medically confirmed as he lay in hospital, his stunned father learning of the tell-tale signs of needle tracks, pin-point pupils and incipient withdrawal symptoms. The suggested treatment at an out-patient clinic involved Mark's having to take reduced doses of oral methadone. Although given every opportunity for counselling sessions which at this stage would have been invaluable, Mark failed to take advantage of these. He became rather disillusioned and guilty after his first heroin use and failed to keep his appointments. Before long he was using ½ gram of illegal heroin daily as before.

Mark began to run into financial difficulties. The only means that he knew of obtaining money without resorting to criminality was to take it from his father's drawer and hope that it would go unnoticed. However, the suspicion aroused in his father by Mark's odd behaviour following the discovery of the missing money led to a confrontation in which Mark was told in no uncertain terms that, if he did not stop taking heroin, he would have to leave home. Mark's father, anxious to seek a cure for his son's addiction, reapproached the clinic. He was told that the failure of Mark to comply with withdrawal in the community meant that the only option open to him was admission to the clinic's in-patient unit. With some fear and reluctance, Mark eventually agreed.

NURSING ASSESSMENT INTERVIEW

Surname _Cater_   **Forenames** _Mark Peter_

Name person likes to be called _Mark_

Address _48 Hadleigh Avenue_   **Telephone number** _5225_
Willbury   **Date of referral/admission** _17·8·86_
WIL 66P

Next-of-kin

Name _Mr S. Cater_   **Relationship** _Father_

Address _As above_

Telephone number _____

Date of birth _12·6·66_   **Single**/~~married/divorced/widowed~~

General practitioner _Dr Lever_   **Address** _60 Links Road_
Willbury

Consultant _Dr B. Leininger_

Status under Mental Health Act _Informal_

Psychiatric diagnosis _Drug abuse_

History of self-harm or harm towards others _None_

Occupation _Full-time student_

Occupational history
None

Hobbies and interests _Playing guitar, visiting pub with friends_

Patient's perceived reason for referral/admission _To withdraw from heroin_

Relatives' understanding of patient's problems _Drug abuse due to Mark's dissatisfaction with lifestyle. Appears to get bored easily and likes change and excitement_

NURSING ASSESSMENT INTERVIEW (continued)

Persons of significance in person's life

Family/friends/pets ___ Father and mother

Spiritual needs

___ None

Problems causing concern at home ___ Mark's stealing from father to finance purchase of drugs. Mark's not being prepared to give up drugs

Community services involved/referred ___ None

Name _____   Status _____

Telephone number _____   Date of referral _____

Mental status _____

History of present problems ___ Has been abusing heroin and other drugs for past 9 months and drinking heavily. Abortive attempt at withdrawing in community recently

Previous psychiatric history ___ None

General appearance and behaviour ___ Slim build; pale complexion. Anxious and appears drowsy; slight tremor of hands

Speech and communication patterns ___ Quiet; communicating little

Problems with perception ___ None

NURSING ASSESSMENT INTERVIEW (continued)

Affective state   Appears low in mood

Disturbances of thinking or judgement   None

Orientation

Person   Normal

Place   Normal

Time   Normal

Activities of living

Safety and mobility
No problem

Eating and drinking
Poor appetite; drinks coffee mostly

Elimination

Bladder   Normal

Bowel   Regular

Sleep patterns
Sleeps erratically

Personal needs
Would like to see mother

General health

Any medical condition for which the person is receiving treatment
No

Doctor's instructions
For withdrawal from heroin using oral method
in reducing doses; restricted visiting; supervised
collection of urine specimens

Areas of concern to patient
Feels guilty about letting family down.
Does not know how he will be able to cope
without drugs

NURSING ASSESSMENT INTERVIEW (continued)

Problems identified

1. Feelings of depression, low self-worth and disillusionment.
2. Difficulty in focusing on short- and long-term plans.
3. Unable to envisage marriage and future employment.
4. Cannot fully appreciate reason for support after drug withdrawal, feeling that he will be able to sort out his problems eventually.
5. Misses his mother and unable to discuss problems with father.
6. Apprehensive over the anticipated discomfort of withdrawal and particularly afraid that he will be unable to sleep without night sedation.
7. Would like to withdraw but feels that he may lose motivation.
8. Some weight loss and diminished appetite

Date of interview _____ 18.8.86 _____   Signature _____ T. Dale _____

History taken from _____

by _____ T. Dale _____   Designation _____ Charge nurse _____

Additional information   Date _____ 18.8.86 _____
_____ Patient has been sleeping very badly recently.

ASSESSMENT

1. Mark has feelings of low self-worth and disillusionment.
2. He has difficulty in focusing on short- and long-term plans.
3. He is unable to envisage marriage and future employment.
4. He cannot fully appreciate the reason for support after drug withdrawal, feeling that he will be able to sort out his problems eventually.
5. He misses his mother and is unable to discuss problems with his father.
6. Is apprehensive over the anticipated discomfort of withdrawal and particularly afraid that he will be unable to sleep without night sedation.
7. He would like to withdraw but feels that he may lose motivation.
8. He has some weight loss and diminished appetite.

PLAN OF NURSING CARE

1. To adopt a non-judgemental, sympathetic and understanding approach.
2. To ensure that Mark is not in possession of drugs on admission and that he takes prescribed medication only.
3. To supervise the collection of urine specimens.
4. To explore Mark's attitudes to drug taking.
5. To restrict visiting to next-of-kin only.
6. To create a relationship of mutual trust.
7. To create realistic goals with Mark.
8. To assess continuously Mark's perception, understanding and attitude regarding treatment to ensure that his needs are being met as he works towards the attainment of goals and an ultimate improvement in lifestyle.
9. To observe closely Mark's response to test doses of withdrawal medication for any changes in physical and psychological state and its effect on social interaction.
10. To maintain Mark's motivation to achieve goals by positive reinforcement of his progress.
11. To allow Mark the opportunity to ventilate his negative feelings and to reassure him and to increase his sense of self-worth.
12. To encourage his attendance at group meetings and occupational therapy.
13. To encourage family support.
14. To improve appetite and to restore weight loss by providing and encouraging adequate diet.
15. To be supportive throughout treatment.
16. To evaluate treatment and to provide information on community supportive agencies.

IMPLEMENTATION OF TREATMENT

For Mark, whose history of drug dependence was relatively short, treatment was directed at the identification of his problems and the provision of a supportive framework within which he could work towards the achievement of realistic goals through understanding and self-awareness. Creating a nurse–client relationship of mutual trust was an important factor, particularly in the early stages, for it laid the firm foundation for the consolidation of positive achievements. When Mark arrived at the unit, he was feeling apprehensive about the anticipated physical discomfort of heroin withdrawal. Acknowledging this, nurses reassured him that the prescribed medication would reduce these unpleasant features considerably and that he had made a wise and positive decision in agreeing to come off drugs. Mark was a little more relaxed although he admitted that he could not guarantee that he would be able to complete the course if his motivation diminished. He was again reassured that he would be supported throughout and was to report any problems should they arise.

A relationship of mutual trust and understanding now created, a search revealed that Mark was not in possession of drugs. Mark also appreciated the importance of a supervised collection of urine specimens and the need to restrict visiting to next-of-kin only as these measures would respectively detect and prevent the use of non-prescribed drugs.

An initial assessment enabled Mark to identify the significant problems in his life. The breakdown of his parents' marriage had been a catalytic factor in his disillusionment and, although he realised that drugs provided only a temporary abandonment from these depressive feelings, they did, at least, give him some spiritual uplift. He admitted to being easily led at times but, perhaps wrongly, felt that it showed that he was not narrow minded in his thinking or attitude. Having now reached a juncture, Mark needed to steer a corrective course by maintaining a realistic and healthy attitude towards his goals and an improved lifestyle. Nurses, who were able to observe Mark's response to medication, reported only minor physical problems and, as they were given control within a range of doses, they were able to adjust the oral methadone when necessary. Mark's appetite, poor at first, improved gradually.

Group meetings received mixed responses from Mark. At times, he displayed an argumentative streak and considerable capacity to justify his behaviour. On occasions, he was at variance with the views of some patients who, themselves, had experience of previous failure and suggested that Mark should stop associating with old school friends who had become drug users. However, there was no ill-feeling.

With good nursing support and visits from his parents, who came independently, Mark was able to achieve significant short-term goals.

EVALUATION

Mark was able to withdraw from physical dependence on heroin because of compliance with the treatment programme and good nursing support. Psychologically, he felt anxious about the future but, on discharge, he planned to work towards a social work qualification. The feelings of low self-worth that Mark had experienced improved a little while undergoing treatment at the clinic. Although Mark's drug dependence had drawn attention to his problems, it did not prove a reconciling factor for his parents. Mark planned for regular visits to his mother. His father, for whom divorce had meant that he could invest more time and effort into his business, now gave greater consideration to maintaining the stability of his son's lifestyle. Although given information about community supportive agencies, Mark felt no need for them. Having accomplished his goal of drug withdrawal, he was prepared to 'go it alone' as far as possible and make a fresh start. Within the following 3 months, having failed to gain a place on a social work course, Mark's disillusionment returned. He sought consolation with his circle of acquaintances and began to use heroin again. He has no plans yet to seek treatment.

FACT SHEET: ACTIONS AND EFFECTS OF SOME DRUGS

Table 23.1 Actions and effects of some drugs

Drug	Other names	Pharmacological action	Effects
Cannabis	Pot, Hash, Dope, Blow, Joint (as cigarette)	Alters perceptual function	Heightened perception, elevated mood, talkativeness, relaxation
Cocaine	Coke, Snow, Charlie	Stimulant	Increased alertness euphoria, feeling of optimism. After-effects—fatigue, depression
Heroin	H, Junk, Smack, Skag	Narcotic	Feeling of warmth and contentment. Tolerance soon develops
Benzodiazepines	Diazepam, lorazepam	Minor tranquillisers that depress nervous system	Relieves anxiety, sedating, helps with sleep problems. Very addictive
Solvents	Cleaning fluids, butane gas, glues	When inhaled, the effect is similar to being drunk on alcohol. Feeling of 'being merry'. Feelings of dizziness and unreality are common or nausea and fatigue. Very long-term solvent abuse can cause brain damage	

FACT SHEET: DRUG ABUSERS

1. Young people start to take drugs for a number of reasons including boredom with life, curiosity, depression, resentment towards their parents, school or work problems, as a 'cry for attention' or poor self-esteem.
2. Indications that someone may be using drugs are rapid changes in mood from cheerful to sullen, drowsiness or sleeplessness, unusual aggression or irritability, loss of appetite, loss of interest in hobbies, sport, school or friends, telling lies or furtive behaviour, pin-point pupils (from heroin use), money missing from home, unusual stains, smells or needlemarks on the body or the discovery of tablets, powders or scorched tinfoil. Needles or syringes are also causes for suspicion.

3. A number of agencies and clinics are available over the country, offering help for drug users. Narcotics Anonymous is a self-help society which meets every day and is run by former addicts. Anyone with a drug problem can attend a Narcotics Anonymous meeting. Families Anonymous is an organisation formed for the benefit of the relatives of drug users. Sometimes, by changing the attitude of relatives, the drug user may also improve. See 'List of useful addresses' at the end of this book.

REFERENCES AND FURTHER READING

References

Dobson, M. (1984), Responding to problem drug users, *Nursing Times*, **80**, No. 47, 57–58.

Lancaster, J. (1980), *Adult Psychiatric Nursing*, Medical Examination Publishing, New York.

Strang, J. (1983), *Problem Drug Taking*, Medical Education (International) Ltd.

Thorley, A. (1982), *What is Meant by Rehabilitation?*, Advisory Council on the Misuse of Drugs, HM Stationery Office, London.

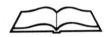

Further reading

Bethune, H. (1985), *Off the Hook: Coping with Addiction*, Methuen, London.

Childs-Clarke, A., and Cottrell, D. (1984), An eleven-year follow-up of drug clinic attenders, *Nursing Times, Occasional Papers*, **80**, No. 20, 52–53.

Corrigan, J., Bessant, A., and Eastland, M. (1985), Habit disorders, *Nursing (UK)*, **2**, No. 24, 1004–1007.

Faugier, J. (1986), The changing concept of dependence—in the drug and alcohol field, *Nursing Practice*, **1**, 253–256.

Freedom from the needle (1986), *The Times*, Friday 4 July, p. 11.

Gay, M. (1986), Drugs and solvent abuse in adolescents, *Nursing Times*, **82**, No. 5, 34–35.

Hodgkinson, L. (1985), *Addictions*, Thorsons, Wellingborough, Northamptonshire.

Institute for the Study of Drug Dependence (1985), Drug abuse briefing.

MacLennan, A. (1986), Taken over by heroin, *Nursing Times*, **82**, No. 7, 45–47.

Chapter 24

Nursing care of the patient who is overactive

'*The overactive patient loves the world and tries to incorporate everything into his environment.*' (Lipkin and Cohen, 1980).

INTRODUCTION

The person who is overactive can be amusing, likeable and full of fun. His witty remarks and puns have an infectious quality about them. Thoughts flow through his head in rapid succession, one pleasurable idea being replaced by another. He usually speaks so quickly that he misses words out of sentences completely or he may use words which rhyme.

He may dress in the brightest colours, in clothes that bear no relation to the weather. He is just as likely to be found wearing a beach outfit in the middle of winter as a thick woolly sweater on a hot summer's day.

He is highly active and bursting with energy. He is impulsive, moving from one thing to another; various activities receive fleeting attention and he leaves a trail of unfinished pursuits wherever he goes. Reams of letters may be forthcoming, addressed to the most eminent people in the land. Plans are made for important deals and, unsupervised, the person may squander large amounts of money or make unwise commitments.

The person's behaviour is meddlesome and domineering. He readily interferes in the affairs of other people, and yet he resents interference in his own transactions. He can be sarcastic, hostile and aggressive. He is sexually promiscuous and can cause others embarrassment by his crudity.

While he appears to be in control of his faculties, logic and rational thinking are not within his scheme of things and his attention span is brief. Because he has grandiose ideas about his own power and wealth, he may believe that there is simply nothing that he cannot accomplish.

The overactive elated person is generally viewed as being in jolly good spirits. It is only when he becomes a nuisance at home or in the community that illness is recognised and hospitalisation considered necessary.

PATIENT PROFILE

George Jackson, aged 47 and divorced, had become increasingly elated and noisy over the past few weeks. His general sense of well-being, his rapid ideation and excessive energy led him into trouble at the garage where he worked. George, who could be relied on to tell the most outrageous jokes, gradually assumed a demeanour of great importance, refused to serve petrol to customers, borrowed money from the till and was consequently sacked.

On admission, George was very demanding and wanted to throw a party for all the patients. He said that he would soon get everyone sorted out. George had had psychiatric treatment on several previous occasions, but this was his first admission to Willbury Hospital.

USE OF ROY'S ADAPTATION MODEL

Roy's (1980) adaptation model was chosen for his care (see Chapter 7).

PLAN OF NURSING CARE

The plan of nursing care is given in *Table 24.1*.

NURSING ASSESSMENT INTERVIEW

Surname _Jackson_   Forenames _George Arthur_

Name person likes to be called _George_

Address _14 Barn Road_   Telephone number _0701_
Warren End   Date of referral/admission _13 . 3 . 86_
Willbury
WIL 1XE

Next-of-kin

Name _Mrs I. Jackson_   Relationship _Mother_

Address _As above_

       Telephone number _At work 8855 Ext. 127_

Date of birth _6 . 2 . 38_   Single/married/divorced/widowed

General practitioner _Dr J. John_   Address _Claremont_
9A High Street
Middlesdown

Consultant _Dr J. Hinsie_

Status under Mental Health Act _Section 2_

Psychiatric diagnosis _Hypomania_

History of self-harm or harm towards others _Potentially aggressive when mood is elevated_

Occupation _Unemployed_

Occupational history
Last job motor mechanic. Has worked as a salesman, plumber's mate, lorry driver

Hobbies and interests _In local darts team, television, gardening, 'do-it-yourself'_

Patient's perceived reason for referral/admission _'I'm on top of the world — I suppose that the hospital needs me'_

Relatives' understanding of patient's problems _The old problem — George would have been okay if he hadn't married that woman_

NURSING ASSESSMENT INTERVIEW (continued)

Persons of significance in person's life

Family/friends/pets _Cats — George is mad about cats. Has a girl-friend Janet (she doesn't know about George's illness)_

Spiritual needs

Non-conformist — he'll go anywhere. Usually to weddings and funerals

Problems causing concern at home _Hope that he'll be able to get another job when this lot is over_

Community services involved/referred

Name _Gerald Whiting_   Status _Community psychiatric nurse_

Telephone number _4113, Ext. 12_   Date of referral _based at Pringle House_

Mental status

History of present problems _Elated; interfering behaviour over several weeks_

Previous psychiatric history _Long history of manic depressive illness but has only been depressed once — usually 'blows up'_

General appearance and behaviour _Inappropriately dressed for March. Wearing a straw hat and a sarong_

Speech and communication patterns _Talks rapidly; changes topic before completing sentence. Uses words that rhyme and popular sayings ('Pop goes the weasel!')_

Problems with perception _Grandiose ideas interfere with perception of self and others. George believes that he is exalted and powerful_

NURSING ASSESSMENT INTERVIEW (continued)

Affective state _Very elated ; happy ; jolly ; touchy ; easily irritated if others don't agree with him_

Disturbances of thinking or judgement _Thoughts are rapid and disjointed. Judgement is impaired_

Orientation

Person ⎤ _Misidentification and misinterpretation_
Place ⎬ _interfere with normal orientation_
Time ⎦ _processes_

Activities of living

Safety and mobility
Illness imposes threat to safety

Eating and drinking
Looks well nourished ; not dehydrated

Elimination

Bladder _No problems apparent yet — observe_

Bowel _No problems apparent yet — observe_

Sleep patterns
Normal sleep pattern disrupted. Deficit in sleep and rest

Personal needs
Body odour — encourage to attend to personal hygiene needs

General health

Any medical condition for which the person is receiving treatment
Inguinal hernia repair 3 years ago

Doctor's instructions
See Medicine sheet

Areas of concern to patient
Deferred

NURSING ASSESSMENT INTERVIEW (continued)

Problems identified

See attached nursing model

Date of interview ___13.3.86___   Signature ___B.J. Conroy___

History taken from ___Mrs Jackson___

by ___Barbara Conroy___   Designation ___Enrolled nurse___

     Date ___13.3.86___

Additional information

Table 24.1   Adaptive modes, assessments, patient's goals and nursing goals

Adaptive mode	First-level assessment	Second-level assessment			Patient's goal	Nursing goal
		Focal stimuli	Contextual stimuli	Residual stimuli		
Basic physiological needs	Attention deficit interferes with need state	Short attention span. Unaware of need state	All environmental stimuli interferes with attention to activities of living	Unconscious wishes. Unfinished developmental tasks. History of mental illness	To meet needs for: 1. Fluids. 2. Elimination. 3. Nutrition. 4. Rest and sleep. 5. Freedom from danger. 6. Personal hygiene. To take prescribed medication	To enable the patient to meet his physical needs through persuasion and opportunistic interventions. To promote rest and sleep. To prevent him from harming himself. To anticipate and remove or control potential hazards. To ensure that George takes his medication
Self-concept		Grandiose ideation	Attitudes of others. Faulty judgement	Unconscious wishes. Unfinished developmental tasks. History of mental illness	To base statements on reality	To accept the patient's statements but only to reinforce those based on reality
Role mastery		Lacks insight into own roles and roles of others	Present roles based on unreality	Unconscious wishes. Unfinished developmental tasks. History of mental illness.	To function considerately and harmoniously with others	To recognise irritation and increasing tension as sign of potentially aggressive behaviour. To use distractability to reduce effects of patient's behaviour on others. To provide outlets for aggression. To demonstrate self-control and consistency
Interdependence		Lacks normal social constraints. Overfamiliar	Easily irritated. Sensitive to remarks of others	Unconscious wishes. Unfinished developmental tasks. History of mental illness	To engage in acceptable social behaviour	To recognise George's need to be needed. To be sensitive to his body language. To be tactful and persuasive, and not authoritarian

NURSING INTERVENTION

The nurse's primary task was to assist George to make the transition from maladaptive behaviour towards adaptive functioning by altering the stimuli which fell within his adaptive modes.

George would not conform to the more usual patterns of daily living, and so his needs for food, fluids, elimination and personal hygiene had to be met when he was amenable. Overactivity can lead to weight loss and a general deterioration in the patient's health, and so every effort was made to promote George's physical status.

He was easily stimulated by loud sounds, bright colours and the presence of other people. Therefore, he was sedated and nursed in a single room. Contextual stimuli were minimised as far as possible by day and by night; this included reducing the number of nurses involved in his care. One nurse was assigned to care for the patient at a time; this reduced the number of people that he was able to interact with and enabled the nurses to adopt a more consistent approach towards him.

The nurse did not promote conversation with George, although a willingness to listen was conveyed. When speaking to George, short simple sentences were used; ambiguous statements were avoided. The nurse used a tone of voice that was kind and yet firm and low pitched. Demanding or authoritative tones of voice were avoided since this approach to the patient could easily have provoked a hostile or aggressive reaction.

Quiet persuasion is one of the most important interventions in gaining the patient's cooperation in all aspects of his care, especially when trying to urge him to take his medicine and he maintains that he is not ill or that he has never felt better in his life.

The nurse's attitude towards George was as permissive as the hospital environment would permit; limits were provided to prevent him from harming himself or others. It is as well to bear in mind that the patient feels so 'on top of the world' that he believes that he can do anything. He pays no heed to danger; he is unable to anticipate or perceive potential hazards in the environment and must therefore be protected. George's distractability was something that the nurse was able to use to his advantage by diverting his attention away from harmful activities.

Because the patient is so overactive, the nurse must not think that he has endless reserves of energy. Every effort must be made to prevent him from becoming exhausted by nursing interventions which reduce irritation, tension and stimulation. His fluid and nutritional needs must be met by using opportunities as they present themselves.

The nurse must accept the patient's argumentative behaviour as part of his illness and should not be offended if he makes some very personal or cutting remark. Undoubtedly, the nurse's patience and tolerance will be severely tested and so it is essential to be realistic about self-strengths and limitations.

The patient does not observe the usual social constraints; he is highly perceptive and may discover areas of sensitivity in others with some accuracy. To become angry or argue with him serves no purpose. It is in fact contrary to the nursing objectives and could increase the patient's maladaptive behaviour. A calm non-threatening approach is best adopted, using an open body posture and showing respect for the patient's body space.

When George made a delusional statement, the nurse accepted the statement but was careful not to reinforce his grandiose ideas by going along with

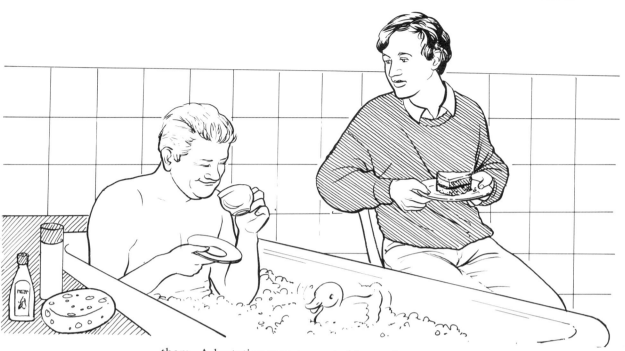

them. Adaptation was promoted by paying more attention to the statements that he made which were based on reality rather than the statements that he made which were not. In this way the nurse helped the patient to adapt towards a more realistic self-concept.

When George's mother arrived to visit him, he would frequently give her a cursory peck and then go and seat himself among another patient's visitors, whom he would greet like long-lost friends. They seemed to accept George's behaviour with good humour. However, the nurse was always ready to intervene tactfully to prevent embarrassment or a nuisance being caused to others.

EVALUATION

Caring for George required the utmost patience and tolerance on the part of the nurses. Nursing intervention played a vital part in promoting his adaptation towards more positive and acceptable behaviour. His physiological needs were met by the intervention of the nurse at opportune moments. In this way, George's attention was drawn to his needs for adequate food, fluids, personal hygiene and elimination. Rest and sleep were promoted by reducing all stimuli and by ensuring that George took his medication. It was often difficult to persuade George to take his medication, simply because he believed he did not need it. The task was usually accomplished after much perseverance and a great deal of tact.

The nurse accepted George's grandiose ideas with good humour; his mood was so infectious that it was often impossible not to laugh with him. After 2 weeks he became less gregarious, but he was still tending to interfere with other people's business and possessions. Usually, he could be distracted before any real harm was done. Adaptation towards reality and the formulation of sound judgements took several weeks. The nurse had helped George to respond to reality by reinforcing only statements based on reality.

Role mastery was achieved as George gained insight into social role co[n]straints. This was indicated through his behaviour and he no longer ask[ed] personal questions or made provocative remarks to other patients or sta[ff]. Interdependence was achieved as he learned to act in accordance not only wi[th] his own wishes but also with those of others.

George was discharged to the day hospital after 6 weeks in the ward. He [is] receiving support from the community psychiatric nurse, who has promised [to] keep the staff informed of George's progress.

FACT SHEET: THE OVERACTIVE PATIENT

The nurse should:

1. Always observe the patient.
2. Anticipate potential safety hazards.
3. Use tact, suggestion, persuasion and distractability to help the patient to meet his goals.
4. Always be honest with the patient.
5. Avoid arguments with the patient.
6. Exercise self-control and consistency in own behaviour.
7. Not be offended by, or sensitive to, personal remarks made by the patient.
8. Protect the patient and others from the patient.
9. Monitor the patient's mood, particularly for signs of tension, irritability and depression.
10. Use opportunities as they arise to meet the patient's needs for food, fluids, elimination, sleep and personal cleansing.

REFERENCES AND FURTHER READING

References

Lipkin, G. B., and Cohen, R. G. (1980), *Effective Approaches to Patient. Behaviour*, 2nd edn, Springer, New York.

Roy, C. (1980), The Roy adaptation model. In: *Conceptual Models for Nursin[g] Practice* (eds Riehl, J. P., and Roy, C.), Appleton Century Crofts Norwalk, Connecticut.

Further reading

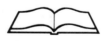

Barker, P., Hume, A., and Robertson, B. (1984), Within you—without you[?] An alternative approach to affective disorder, *Community Psychiatri[c] Nursing Journal*, **4**, No. 1, 16–17.

Brown, M. M., and Fowler, G. R. (1966), *Psychodynamic Nursing*, W. B[.] Saunders, Philadelphia, Pennsylvania.

Evans, F. M. C. (1971), *Psychosocial Nursing*, Macmillan, New York.

Murray, R. B., and Huelskoetter, M. M. W. (1983), *Psychiatric Mental Health Nursing: Giving Emotional Care*, Prentice-Hall, Englewood Cliffs, New Jersey.

Pasquali, E. A., Alesi, E. G., Arnold, H. M., and De Basio, N. (1981), *Menta[l]*

Health Nursing: A Bio-psycho-cultural Approach, C. V. Mosby, St Louis, Missouri.

Peplau, H. E. (1952), *Interpersonal Relations in Nursing*, G. P. Putnam, New York.

Smith, L. (1981), Problems associated with manic depressive patients, *Nursing (UK)*, **30**, 1307–1309.

Taylor, C. M. (1982), *Mereness' Essentials of Psychiatric Nursing*, 11th edn, C. V. Mosby, St Louis, Missouri.

Topalis, M., and Aguilera, D. C. (1978), *Psychiatric Nursing*, 7th edn, C. V. Mosby, St Louis, Missouri.

Chapter 25

Nursing care of the patient who is suspicious

'The person whose trust is impaired is one who expects bad from every new situation and to whom the kindness and dependability of people must be demonstrated.' (Baldwin, 1955).

INTRODUCTION

Suspicion is a lack of trust in others which is often accompanied by an anxiety, producing anticipation of a response from others or a happening that is feared (Manfreda and Krampitz, 1977). The suspicious person perceives his environment as hostile and his reactions are, therefore, often ones of anger and resentment. He has a general mistrust of others and doubts about everything in general. He constantly questions the motives of others and may confront people with long and involved analyses of their motives. He is secretive and talks in a guarded manner, screening words and protecting thoughts.

Patterns of mistrust and suspicion are common in a number of clinical syndromes; suspicion may be evident in people suffering from paranoid ideation, from deafness or from toxic conditions caused by infection, drugs or alcohol.

Paranoid ideation or behaviours are often rooted in early life experiences of insecurity, loss, pain and disappointment. These feelings are unconsciously denied by the person and ascribed to others in an attempt to provide protection from the pain of these early life experiences.

Most people experience feelings of mistrust on occasions and these feelings may be justifiable. If, however, mistrust is persistent and occurs in most situations, it becomes maladaptive (Evans, 1971). When mistrust develops into delusional thinking, a person may believe that he is being persecuted and act in an impulsive or destructive way, resulting in problems for the community.

PATIENT PROFILE

Rose Patten, aged 61, lives in a large detached house with a wild and overgrown garden. Rose is considered by her neighbours to be an eccentric lady who dresses in the style of yesteryear. She has an air of superiority and little to do with other people. Occasionally, she will engage in the venomous outpouring of words or make cutting and hurtful remarks to people with whom she shares no other formal social interaction.

Despite outward appearances, Rose is considered to be quite wealthy and she has never had the necessity to work. Her constant companions are a collection of dogs, which she takes with regularity to the nearby common.

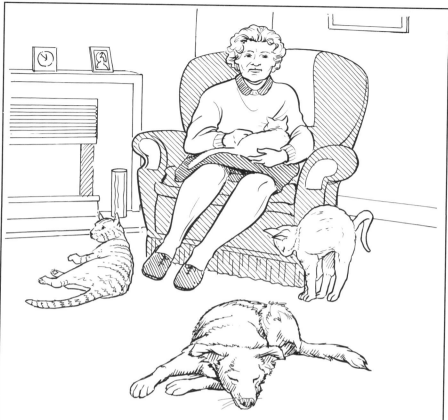

Rose has a long history of mental illness and is well known to the staff of the local psychiatric unit. Regular injections of fluphenazine injection every 3 weeks have enabled Rose to remain in the community for the past 2 years.

The problem arose when the community psychiatric nurse, who had a reasonably good relationship with Rose, left to have a baby. Rose was no longer willing to receive her injections. Although Janet Cook introduced her to the nurse who would be taking over, Rose never answered the door when she called. Over several months the nurse tried again and again to make contact with Rose but, as she was not actually ill, nothing could be done. The consultant was informed. After several months without medication, Rose's feelings of persecution could no longer be contained. After shouting and screaming obscenities at her neighbours, she once more found herself back in hospital. Rose was most upset about being parted from her animals, and Dr Hinsie who had known Rose for many years allowed her to return home, provided that she agreed to receive regular medication from the community nurse.

NURSING ASSESSMENT INTERVIEW

Surname _Patten_   Forenames _Rose Junita_

Name person likes to be called _Sometimes objects to use of 'Rose'_

Address _Meadow View_   Telephone number _____
Ballards Lane   Date of referral/admission _16.2.86_
Willbury
WIL X15

Next-of-kin

Name _Miss I. Stone_   Relationship _Cousin_

Address _Flat 5_
Oakwood
Clare Street, York   Telephone number _—_

Date of birth _7.7.24_   Single/~~married/divorced/widowed~~ _____

General practitioner _Dr S. Kalkman_   Address _Dobbins_
Palmar Avenue
Willbury
WIL 4JJ

Consultant _Dr J. Hinsie_

Status under Mental Health Act _Section 136_

Psychiatric diagnosis _Paranoid state_

History of self-harm or harm towards others _Can be threatening but_
hasn't engaged in actual harm to others

Occupation _Never worked_

Occupational history
As above

Hobbies and interests _Her animals, walking, gardening_

Patient's perceived reason for referral/admission _Blames 'other interested parties'_

Relatives' understanding of patient's problems _—_

NURSING ASSESSMENT INTERVIEW (continued)

Persons of significance in person's life

Family/friends/pets ___ *Four dogs ; seven cats* ___

Spiritual needs

___ *Used to believe she had 'spiritual power'* ___

Problems causing concern at home ___ *Pets* ___

Community services involved/referred ___

Name ___ *Anne Wilkie* ___   Status *Community psychiatric nurse*

Telephone number ___ *0123* ___   Date of referral *17.2.86*

Mental status ___

History of present problems ___ *Has refused medication since Janet Cook left. Neighbour called police because of Rose's behaviour* ___

Previous psychiatric history ___ *History of paranoid ideation over many years* ___

General appearance and behaviour ___ *Eccentric style of dress ; wears many different colours ; in keeping with Rose's usual appearance* ___

Speech and communication patterns ___ *Mutters to self, but rather subdued.* ___

Problems with perception ___ *Does not perceive that she is ill or needs medication* ___

NURSING ASSESSMENT INTERVIEW (continued)

Affective state _Anxious about home and animals_

Disturbances of thinking or judgement _Blames others for inconveniences caused to herself_

Orientation

Person _Fully orientated_

Place

Time

Activities of living

Safety and mobility _Deferred_

Eating and drinking _Deferred_

Elimination

Bladder _No apparent problems_

Bowel

Sleep patterns _Didn't sleep well last night after arriving at 11.00 pm_

Personal needs

General health

Any medical condition for which the person is receiving treatment _No_

Doctor's instructions _To be allowed home on condition that she receives medication_

Areas of concern to patient _Pets_

NURSING ASSESSMENT INTERVIEW (continued)

Problems identified

_____

_____

_____

_____

_____

_____

_____

_____

_____

_____

_____

Date of interview _17.2.86_   Signature _A. Wilkie Smith_

History taken from _Nursing staff in ward_

by _Anne Wilkie Smith_   Designation _Community psychiatric nurse_

Additional information   Date _18.2.86_

Rose is not self-disclosing

USE OF ROY'S ADAPTATION MODEL

Roy's (1980) adaptation model was chosen for Rose's care, as the nurse's main task would be to help Rose to make more positive adaptive responses which would enable her to live harmoniously within the community (see Chapter 7).

PLAN OF NURSING CARE

The plan of nursing care is given in *Table 25.1*.

NURSING INTERVENTION

The first step towards promoting adaptation in the self-concept, role function and interdependence modes was to establish and maintain contact with Rose so that she would consent to receive her medication regularly.

Helping a patient to trust is a difficult and time-consuming process which demands trustworthiness on the nurse's part; the nurse's trustworthiness establishes the extent to which trust is possible in the nurse–patient relationship. Enabling the patient to trust is a slow process, and even the most accepting and consistent nurse may be perceived as untrustworthy by the patient whose previous experiences have led to a lack of trust (Kreigh and Perko, 1983). Initially, a reserved approach to the patient is most likely to succeed. Rebuffs and abusive language have to be accepted by the nurse as part of the patient's illness and not as personal attacks. Sudden outbursts of verbal abuse or accusations provide a primary means of discharging tension for the patient; one of her main defences is to make the first attack on others (Brown and Fowler, 1966).

The nurse's attitude towards the patient is of prime importance. In spite of the fact that the patient is often cold and aloof or superior in manner, the nurse must convey acceptance and treat her with respect. The patient is usually a very insecure person whose domination and sarcasm are attempts to compensate for the inferiority that she feels (Brown and Fowler, 1966). Frequently, she has a particular facility for detecting the nurse's weaknesses and can soon detect the presence of feelings that are not genuine (Murray and Huelskoetter, 1983).

In approaching the patient with basic trust difficulties, the nurse should assess the degree of physical closeness or distance that would be most effective in achieving the goals of adaptation (Parks, 1966). The suspicious person often has difficulty in maintaining contacts with others unless she can keep an emotional distance; therefore, the nurse allowed Rose to set the pace for closeness and involvement.

Because the patient is having difficulties in establishing between what is true and what is not, honesty is an essential component of the relationship. Any misgivings or misunderstandings need to be explained to the patient and the relationship always protected (Murray and Huelskoetter, 1983). Trust is fragile and can be easily broken; therefore, it would be futile to destroy something which takes time, effort and the investment of self (Meize-Grochowski, 1984).

When addressing Rose, the nurse made a particular endeavour to face the patient and to speak clearly, so that the chances of Rose misinterpreting what she said were reduced. Misunderstandings were also reduced by avoiding whispered comments, incomplete explanations or partial messages.

When a patient has difficulty in forming trusting relationships with others, it is important to be as honest and open as possible so that the patient has no reason to be doubtful.

Table 25.1 Adaptive modes, assessments, patient's problems and goals, and nursing orders

Adaptive mode	First-level assessment	Second-level assessment			Patient's problem	Patient's goal	Nursing orders
		Focal stimuli	Contextual stimuli	Residual stimuli			
Basic physiological needs	No obvious needs. Refused medical examination				No problem		
Self-concept		Air of superiority	Superiority is manifested as a defence against feelings of inferiority. Protects self by blaming others	Past life experiences. Very guarded; does not disclose herself to others	Past life experiences. Openness to others severely decreased. Underlying anxiety. Behaves defensively. Has not taken medication	To experience trust. To express feelings related to early experiences. To receive prescribed medication	To encourage the development of trust through the nurse–patient relationship. To protect the relationship. To give medication to promote regulation of cognitive and regulative mechanisms
Role mastery		Accepts role of patient grudgingly		Lacks insight into behaviour	Role perception not based on reality	Increased self-esteem	To show respect and regard for patient. To help her to test reality
Interdependence		Does not mix with others	Perceives others as hostile	? Unsatisfactory role learning	Deficit in positive interaction with others. Tends not to mix. Lacks basic trust	To learn to trust others	To provide a one-to-one relationship but do not pressurise patient into interacting with others if she does not want to

The nurse should not respond to the patient's maladaptive responses, only to the healthy part of her personality. If the nurse approaches the patient with care using appropriate therapeutic interventions, she may become significant to the patient. Adaptation will occur in the self-concept, role function and interdependence modes when the patient learns that people can be trusted and depended on. When the suspicious person begins to feel safe, alterations to suspicious thinking can be explored. The person can be helped to delay expressions of feeling by looking at the *facts* before making a response (Murray and Huelskoetter, 1983). The nurse can help the patient towards adaptation by encouraging her to talk about feelings and events which may have led up to a lack of trust in others.

EVALUATION

The community psychiatric nurse only called on Rose when she was due to receive her fluphenazine because she did not want Rose to question her motives suspiciously if she called at other times. Rose was told to see her general practitioner if she experienced any side effects from the injection.

From the doctor's point of view the nurse's role in giving medication is very important, especially in the control of the patient's positive symptoms, e.g. delusions and hallucinations.

Very often it is the strength of the relationship which exists between the nurse and patient that makes the continuation of medication acceptable and provides a basis for regular support and assessment.

During each visit the nurse tried to increase the amount of time that she spent with Rose, so that Rose would not associate her visits solely with the injection.

Building a relationship with Rose was a very gradual business but there were some indications that Rose was adapting positively.

Initially the nurse was only allowed into the hall to give Rose her injection but, as the months went by, she was invited into other rooms in the house. A person's home territory provides privacy and security. Peripheral areas such as the hall may serve to protect the inner core territory from invasion (Hayter, 1981). It is only when a more trusting relationship has been established that a person will be invited into the core territory.

When evaluating Rose's progress, it was important for the nurse to observe small changes in her behaviour as these provided some measure of goal achievement. Fagin (1967) suggests that, if a nurse fails to notice changes in a patient's behaviour, he or she will continue to interact with the patient as if nothing has occurred. A small change in behaviour may be a considerable step for the patient and, if the nurse fails to observe this, the patient may be discouraged from making further improvements. Movement towards adaptation would then be inhibited.

FACT SHEET: THE SUSPICIOUS PATIENT

The nurse should:

1. Provide a consistent and secure environment.
2. Avoid giving the patient any reason for suspicion.
3. Speak clearly and concisely.
4. Avoid laughing in groups near the patient.

5. Not become involved in arguments.
6. Avoid touching the patient unnecessarily, because of possible mis-interpretations of the social meaning of personal contact.
7. Remember that, when a person dislikes touch because she finds it intrusive, opportunities to reach her will usually be restricted.
8. Provide outlets for aggressive and angry feelings.
9. Allow the patient to experience success.
10. Enable the patient to progress from solitary occupations to activities with others.
11. Help the patient to learn to trust herself.
12. Let the patient see the notes taken in interviews.
13. Recognise the patient's need to test reality (e.g. if she believes that someone is trying to poison her let her observe or assist with the serving of food; the nurse can taste the food, or if necessary, secure an identical portion and eat with the patient).
14. Minimise the patient's access to potentially dangerous articles, since she may manifest problems in the area of safety and may harm herself or others.
15. Remember that the patient's superior attitude meets an emotional need—it builds her self-esteem.

REFERENCES AND FURTHER READING

References

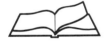

Baldwin, A. L. (1955), cited by Thomas, M. D. (1978), In: *Behavioural Concepts and Nursing Intervention* (eds Carlson, C. E., and Blackwell, B.), J. B. Lippincott, Philadelphia, Pennsylvania.

Brown, M. M., and Fowler, G. R. (1966), *Psychodynamic Nursing*, W. B. Saunders, Philadelphia, Pennsylvania.

Evans, F. M. C. (1971), *Psychosocial Nursing*, Macmillan, New York.

Fagin, C. M. (1987), Psychotherapeutic Nursing, *American Journal of Nursing*, **67**, No. 2, 298–304.

Hayter, J. (1981), Territoriality as a universal need, *Journal of Advanced Nursing*, **6**, 79–85.

Kreigh, H. Z., and Perko, J. E. (1983), *Psychiatric and Mental Health Nursing*, 2nd edn, Reston Publishing, Reston, Virginia.

Manfreda, M. L., and Krampitz, S. D. (1977), *Psychiatric Nursing*, 10th edn, F. A. Davis, Philadelphia, Pennsylvania.

Meize-Grochowski, R. (1984). An analysis of the concept of trust, *Journal of Advanced Nursing*, **9**, 563–572.

Murray, R. B., and Huelskoetter, M. M. W. (1983), *Psychiatric Mental Health Nursing: Giving Emotional Care*, Prentice-Hall, Englewood Cliffs, New Jersey.

Parks, S. L. (1966), Allowing physical distance as a nursing approach, *Perspectives in Psychiatric Care*, **4**, No. 6, 31–35.

Roy, C. (1980), The Roy adaptation model. In: *Conceptual Models for Nursing Practice* (eds Riehl, J. P., and Roy, C.), Appleton Century Crofts, Norwalk, Connecticut.

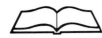

Further reading

Schultz, J. M., and Dark, S. L. (1982), *Manual of Psychiatric Nursing Care Plans*, Little, Brown, Boston, Massachusetts.

Stankiewicz, B. (1964), Guides to nursing intervention in the projective patterns of suspicious patients, *Perspectives in Psychiatric Care*, **2**, No. 1, 39–45.

Stillman, M. J. (1978), Territoriality and personal space, *American Journal of Nursing*, **78**, 1670–1672.

Thomas, M. D. (1978), Trust. In: *Behavioural Concepts and Nursing Intervention* (eds Carlson, C. E., and Blackwell, B.), J. B. Lippincott, Philadelphia, Pennsylvania.

Tousley, M. M. (1984), The paranoid fortress of David J., *Journal of Psychosocial Nursing*, **22**, No. 2, 8–16.

Chapter 26

Nursing care of the patient who is withdrawn

'*The withdrawn person must be sought—he will not seek others.*'
(Topalis and Aquilera, 1978).

INTRODUCTION

Withdrawal is defined as an adaptive or coping behaviour in which a person physically pulls away from or psychologically loses interest in an anxiety-producing situation, a person or a stressful environment (Murray and Huel-skoetter, 1983).

Withdrawal has many forms of expression; it may be expressed by avoidance of contact with others, through short-lived friendship which ends abruptly, through maintaining only superficial interactions with others or through the cynical rejection of other people as worthless (Topalis and Aquilera, 1978).

The person who is withdrawn seems to have built a wall around himself. He is absorbed with his own thoughts and has difficulty in relating to others. His distorted perceptions are not easily shared because of the anxiety engendered by his fear of rejection. The person who uses withdrawal to provide a protection against anxiety may experience increased anxiety and pain as he tries to meet his needs alone. Ironically, his need for human contact is often as great as his fear (Kramer, 1983).

PATIENT PROFILE

Alisia Lowenthal, aged 19, was a quiet girl whose parents divorced when she was 10. Her mother remarried, but Alisia did not get on well with her step-father. She felt that she was never able to please him or to meet the expectations that he had of her.

Her own father whom she idolised was killed in a plane crash only months after the divorce. When she left boarding school, Alisia moved back to Willbury where she had been born and spent her childhood. At first she lived with her parents but later found lodgings with a Mrs Sene whom she had known for years. She regarded Mrs Sene more as a friend and confidant than a landlady.

Dutifully, Alisia spent Christmas in London with her parents but, when she returned to her lodging in Upper Church Street, she seemed even more quiet than usual. She spent a lot of time in her room either curled up on her bed or just sitting staring out of the window. She seemed to be far away, preoccupied and absorbed in her own little world. Once more she had lost her job because she simply failed to turn up or to offer any explanation for her absence.

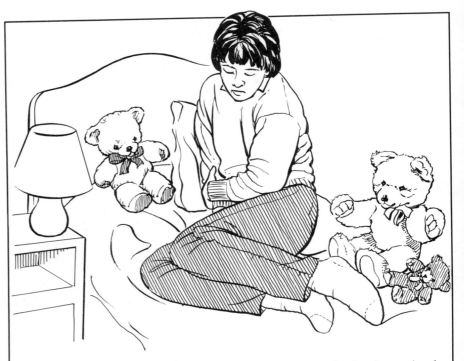

Mrs Sene took Alisia's meals up to her room, but the food remained untouched. Alisia's responses to Mrs Sene's questions were monosyllabic. Her huddled posture and lack of eye contact indicated that she did not want to talk. Most of the time, she buried her face in her hands as if she was trying to shut everything and everybody out. Eventually Mrs Sene decided that Alisia must be ill. She contacted the doctor who subsequently arranged for Alisia to be admitted to a psychiatric unit.

NURSING ASSESSMENT INTERVIEW

Surname __Lowenthal__   Forenames __Alisia Carol__

Name person likes to be called __Alisia__

Address __Hillview__
__Upper Church Street__   Telephone number __3519__
__Willbury__   Date of ~~referral~~/admission __23.9.87__
__WIL 554__

Next-of-kin

Name __Mrs P. Reik__   Relationship __Mother__

Address __31 Penrose Court__
__London__
__W1__   Telephone number __01 — 1194__

Date of birth __22.4.66__   Single/married/divorced/widowed _____

General practitioner __Dr V. Hatton__   Address __Parkway Health Centre__
__Old Barn Road__
__Willbury__
__WIL Q21__

Consultant __Dr J. Hinsie__

Status under Mental Health Act __Informal__

Psychiatric diagnosis __? Schizophrenia__

History of self-harm or harm towards others _____
__No__

Occupation __Unemployed__

Occupational history
__Poor work record — has never managed to hold down__
__a job for more than a few weeks__

Hobbies and interests __All craftwork, collects teddy bears,__
__reading__

Patient's perceived reason for referral/admission __Not expressed__

Relatives' understanding of patient's problems __Mother thinks that Alisia__
__is 'very mixed up'__

NURSING ASSESSMENT INTERVIEW (continued)

Persons of significance in person's life

Family/friends/pets _Not close to mother anymore._
Mrs Sene, friend and landlady

Spiritual needs
Believes in God, but not a regular churchgoer

Problems causing concern at home _Never felt that she had a home since mother's remarriage_

Community services involved/referred

Name _____   Status _____

Telephone number _____   Date of referral _____

Mental status _____

History of present problems _____

Previous psychiatric history _____

General appearance and behaviour _Sits with knees drawn up and head bowed_

Speech and communication patterns _Doesn't initiate conversation. Will answer questions with one-word answers. Averts eyes_

Problems with perception _Has withdrawn into an unreal protective world – doesn't share perceptions yet_

NURSING ASSESSMENT INTERVIEW (continued)

Affective state _Flat mood — doesn't respond positively or negatively_

Disturbances of thinking or judgement _There appears to be disturbances, but again not ready to share thoughts_

Orientation

Person _Deferred, difficult to assess at present_

Place

Time

Activities of living

Safety and mobility _May be oblivious to dangers_

Eating and drinking _Has been leaving food according to Mrs Sene_

Elimination

Bladder _Has been using bathroom at least twice a day_

Bowel

Sleep patterns _Seems to sleep a lot_

Personal needs _Observed to respond to prompting_

General health

Any medical condition for which the person is receiving treatment _Not at present. Had ointment for eczema during the summer_

Doctor's instructions _Encourage relationship building_

Areas of concern to patient _Deferred until rapport can be established_

NURSING ASSESSMENT INTERVIEW (continued)

Problems identified

1. Social withdrawal? Response to anxiety.
2. Impaired social reactions.
3. Lack of interest or awareness of body and appearance

Date of interview _23.9.87_

Signature _P. McIntosh_

History taken from _Mrs Sene_

by _Penny McIntosh_

Designation _Staff nurse_

Additional information

Date _25.9.87_

Incontinent of urine — needs prompting to go to the toilet

USE OF PEPLAU'S DEVELOPMENTAL MODEL

As relationship building was a priority in reaching out to Alisia, Peplau's (1952) developmental model was used to plan her care (see Chapter 7 for an overview of this model).

(a) Orientation phase

During the first phase of Peplau's model the nurse's first task was to establish a relationship with Alisia. Establishing a relationship with a patient who has withdrawn from others requires a great deal of human understanding, sensitivity and intelligence; it requires a nurse who can demonstrate caring as an integral part of nursing. Establishing a relationship with the withdrawn patient is the most important part of the nurse–patient relationship, because what occurs between the nurse and patient at this time can set the pace for subsequent relationships for the patient (Carl, 1963). The nurse must bear in mind that the withdrawn patient does not seek the company of others.

It is the nurse who must act as leader in initiating the relationship and by acting as a surrogate offers the patient the opportunity to develop a more trusting and satisfying relationship than she may have known from past experiences.

The nurse uses the relationship as a vehicle for the purpose of human growth, this being mutually beneficial; through an enabling process the patient is helped to learn that human relationships can be fulfilling and worthwhile.

The withdrawn patient needs more time than usual to learn to place trust in another person. When the nurse initiates contact with Alisia, it must be borne in mind that a demand is being placed on her—a demand for interaction. Therefore, careful consideration needs to be given to the way in which this initial contact takes place, for the way in which the patient is approached will influence the way in which she responds (Parks, 1966).

Parks suggests that one approach which can be useful is for physical distance to be allowed between nurse and patient, particularly when the patient has experienced trust difficulties in past relationships. In considering physical proximity and its possible implications for the patient the nurse may help to reduce or at least not to increase her anxiety. The patient is after all withdrawing as a defence against anxiety. If the nurse is unaware of this and moves towards the patient directly, a lack of understanding and consideration may be clearly communicated to the patient.

Anxiety is an integral part of Peplau's conceptualisation of the person and the nurse must endeavour to reduce the patient's anxiety so that it does not restrict her perceptual field and inhibit learning. If the nurse demonstrates to the patient that the withdrawn behaviour is not perceived as meaningful or important, then the patient's need to defend herself against human relationships and her resultant anxiety is being rejected too (Carl, 1963). Furthermore, the nurse would be failing to meet a basic human requirement—that of territory. Although the personal space surrounding the body is invisible, most people know what it is like to experience discomfort when others invade this space. The withdrawn patient's need for space is even greater. The nurse needs to approach the patient at the level at which she is functioning. If the patient is mute, merely being in the proximity of the patient while respecting her need for distance may help to lessen the gap between the patient's inner subjective world and that of reality. The patient will need time to assess the situation for any threat to herself before she will enable herself to become involved in any

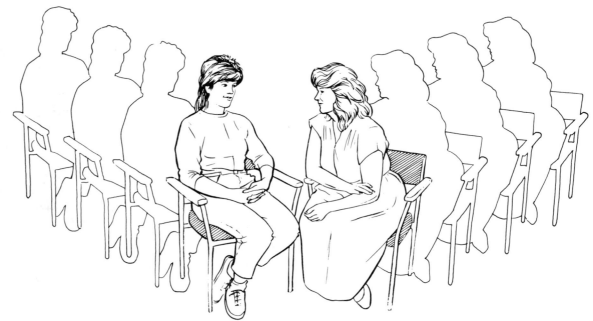

Figure 26.1   The decrease in physical distance as the relationship between the nurse and the patient develops

relationship. A period of orientation thus allows a relationship to be established between the nurse and patient based on mutual trust and set within the dimensions of protracted time and space (*Figure 26.1*).

(b) Identification phase

As the nurse begins to know the patient as a person, the next phase of the relationship can be initiated, that of identification. The nurse works with the patient towards identifying the patient's problems and setting appropriate goals. The goals established at this time may be rather one sided because of the patient's detachment. Nevertheless, the nurse must perceive the patient's needs and determine which goals are appropriate in meeting these needs until such time that the patient is able to clarify her needs and to become involved in problem-solving strategies.

Attempts to pull away the veil which shrouds Alisia's unreal world and to bring her into the world of reality requires that the nurse maintains an interest in the patient. This will mean spending a consistent amount of time with the patient. Sometimes, it is necessary for the nurse to stop and reflect on his or her own behaviour. In a ward full of patients, it is always easier and more immediately gratifying to talk to those patients who respond readily. The nurse's attempts to communicate with the withdrawn patient are demanding on the use of time and self. An attempt must be made to draw Alisia out of herself and yet at the same time without being demanding. The patient must feel free to respond as she wishes and when she is ready to do so. This can mean many one-sided conversations with a patient who responds with short statements and reveals little effect non-verbally in an attempt to maintain her distance (Roberts, 1969). Because of past experiences the patient is often highly sensitive to the attitudes of others, even when these attitudes are not verbalised (Brown and Fowler, 1966). Therefore the nurse's desire to help the patient must be based on genuine motives and on the nurse's own personal qualities of honesty and concern. Anything that interferes with the nurse's ability to know the patient as a person will inhibit the development of trust and prevent the patient from revealing her innermost hopes and fears.

PLAN OF NURSING CARE

(a) Patient's problems
1. Withdraws from others as a response to anxiety.
2. Does not engage in social interactions.
3. Displays a lack of interest in self.

(b) Patient's goals
1. To tolerate the presence of key persons and then others.
2. To exhibit increased involvement with the environment.
3. To receive adequate fluid and food intake.
4. To maintain personal hygiene.
5. To engage in increased activity.
6. To increase contact with the real world of people and objects.
7. To express herself in appropriate activities.

(c) Nursing goals
1. Key nurses to increase time spent with the patient gradually. To increase physical closeness as the patient's behaviour permits.
2. To decrease withdrawal by establishing a non-threatening relationship with the patient.
3. To encourage the patient to eat and drink. If the patient looks blank, remind her that the food is there. Feed only as a last resort; ensure privacy if this is necessary.
4. To encourage the patient to attend to personal hygiene. Place prompters, e.g. soap and flannel, in front of her.
5. To encourage participation in occupational therapy.
6. To provide contact with the physical world through the provision of different textured materials. To use touch as a form of communication if the patient is receptive and if appropriate.
7. To encourage self-expression through painting, drawing, modelling or writing.

(c) Exploitation phase

During exploitation, the working phase of Peplau's model, the nurse acts as a resource person and calls in the appropriate expertise of other members of the multi-disciplinary team to meet any needs of the patient which cannot be met by nursing. This, of course, can only be done when the patient is ready, begins to feel more secure in her relationship with the nurse and will be receptive to additional inputs.

Occupational therapy can help to bring the withdrawn patient into the real world by allowing her to handle and manipulate different materials and textures. The occupational therapist worked towards establishing a relationship with Alisia and enabling her to establish goals within a small relatively non-threatening group. The occupational therapist envisaged that in time Alisia would be able to widen her contacts as she learned to work with and share in activities with other people.

As the nurse–patient relationship developed, the nurse used touch when it seems appropriate to do so. Touching helped to bring Alisia into the physical world of people and objects; it helped her to define herself and to differentiate herself from others, and it enabled her to experience more intensely her own separateness and being (Peplau, 1968). The nurse had to judge carefully when touch could be used positively, as its use could not be therapeutic if forced and unwanted by the patient.

The activities of living no longer seemed important to Alisia and she seemed indifferent at first to meeting her own basic needs. As Alisia would not ask for things for herself, the nurse had to anticipate her needs and to prompt her into carrying out these activities.

(d) Resolution phase

After almost 4 months in hospital, Alisia is now waiting for a place with the Richmond Fellowship. She has been interviewed and accepted for a place in a halfway house for adolescents and young people. Members of the multi disciplinary team feel that this placement will enable Alisia to move toward greater self-understanding, to accept responsibilities and to develop indepen dence in a mutually supportive environment.

As the nurse–patient relationship progressed towards termination, the nurse was able to evaluate the effectiveness of the relationship. Forming a purposeful relationship with Alisia had provided a vehicle for movement towards optimal health.

Through working with Alisia the nurse learned a great deal about the power of non-verbal language in communicating with a person who is dealing with their anxiety through withdrawal. She learned to deal with her own anxiety during long periods of silence and to exercise patience in waiting for Alisia's response.

During the therapeutic process the nurse acted in the roles of leader surrogate, teacher, resource person and counsellor and gradually enabled Alisia to test out relationships with others. Alisia is coming alive, she talks and smiles readily with the nurses and other patients, and she is looking forward to the future.

REFERENCES AND FURTHER READING

References

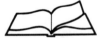

Brown M. M., and Fowler, G. R. (1966), *Psychodynamic Nursing*, W. B. Saunders, Philadelphia, Pennsylvania.

Carl, M. K. (1963), Establishing a relationship with a schizophrenic patient, *Perspectives in Psychiatric Care*, **1**, No. 2, 20–22.

Kramer, A. (1983), Withdrawal, specific behaviours and nursing interventions. In: *Handbook of Psychiatric Mental Health Nursing* (eds Adams, C. G. and Macione, A.), John Wiley, Chichester, West Sussex.

Murray, R. B., and Huelskoetter, M. M. W. (1983), *Psychiatric Mental Health Nursing: Giving Emotional Care*, Prentice-Hall, Englewood Cliffs, New Jersey.

Parks, S. L. (1966), Allowing physical distance as a nursing approach, *Perspectives in Psychiatric Care*, **4**, No. 6, 31–35.

Peplau, H. E. (1952), *Interpersonal Relations in Nursing*, G. P. Putnam, New York.

Peplau, H. E. (1968), Psychotherapeutic strategies, *Perspectives in Psychiatric Care*, **6**, No. 6, 264–270.

Roberts, S. L. (1969), Territoriality: space and the schizophrenic patient, *Perspectives in Psychiatric Care*, **7**, No. 1, 29–33.

Topalis, M., and Aguilera, D. (1978), *Psychiatric Nursing*, 7th edn, C. V. Mosby, St Louis, Missouri.

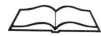

Further reading

Arnold, H. M. (1976), Working with schizophrenic patients: guide to one-to-one relationships, *American Journal of Nursing*, **76**, 941–943.

Blondis, M. N., and Jackson, B. E. (1982), *Non-verbal Communication with Patients*, John Wiley, Chichester, West Sussex.

Davis, A. J. (1984), *Listening and Responding*, C. V. Mosby, St Louis, Missouri.

Golden, M., and Bessant, A. (1985), Social withdrawal, *Nursing (UK)*, **2**, No. 35, 1029–1032.

Jourard, S. M. (1959), How well do you know your patients?, *American Journal of Nursing*, **59**, 1568–1571.

Mason, A., and Pratt, J. W. (1980), Touch, *Nursing Times*, **76**, No. 23, 999–1001.

Paulen, A. (1982), Commit yourself to caring, *Journal of Practical Nursing*, **17**, No. 1, 26–27, 40.

Phillips, B. (1968), Terminating a nurse–patient relationship, *American Journal of Nursing*, **68**, 1941–1943.

Pluckman, M. L. (1968), Space: the silent language, *Nursing Forum*, **7**, No. 4, 386–397.

Rose, L. E. (1983), Understanding mental illness: the experience of families of psychiatric patients, *Journal of Advanced Nursing*, **8**, 507–511.

Schmidt, C. S. (1981), Withdrawal behaviour of schizophrenics: application of Roy's model, *Journal of Psychiatric Nursing and Mental Health Services*, **19**, No. 11, 26–33.

Seymour, R. J., and Dawson, N. J. (1986), The schizophrenic at home, *Journal of Psychiatric Nursing and Mental Health Services*, **24**, No. 1, 28–30.

Teasdale, K. (1986), The withdrawn schizophrenic, *Nursing Times*, **82**, No. 6, 32–34.

Ujhely, G. (1968), *Determinants of the Nurse–Patient Relationship*, Springer, New York.

Chapter 27

Nursing care of the patient who is out of touch with reality

'*The patient who hallucinates has a strong need to believe in the reality of the hallucination.*' (Schwartzman, 1975).

INTRODUCTION

The person who is out of touch with reality may feel estranged from the real world and from himself. He may find it hard to differentiate between what is real and what is not. He may feel that he himself has changed or that his environment is different in some way. He is often a person who is isolated, lonely and misunderstood by others; in his formative years, he may have experienced difficult relationships with his parents.

As a person becomes more and more out of touch with reality, his thought processes become disturbed and he may experience delusions and hallucinations. A delusion is a false belief that cannot be altered by reasoning or evidence to the contrary. A person may believe that his body is changing, that he is dead, that others are out to get him or that his thoughts are being broadcast aloud for others to hear.

Hallucinations are another indication of break with reality. Hallucinations are false sensory perceptions which, unlike normal perceptions, occur in the absence of external stimuli (see boxed section entitled 'Nursing the patient who is out of touch with reality' at the end of this chapter). The hallucinatory process consists of the created perception, the projection of this created perception into the real world and the inability to distinguish between real and created perceptions (Arieti, 1972).

For the person concerned, these experiences are very real; his inner thoughts are conveyed as if they were outer events, giving him the experience of hearing, seeing, smelling, tasting or feeling. He perceives the experiences as if they were coming from the outer environment. Over a period of time, hallucinatory events may replace the relationships that the person once had with real people.

The person who is out of touch with reality often experiences a great deal of underlying anxiety; he may use disguised language as a way of dealing with his lack of social and interpersonal skills (Cook, 1971). When he speaks, he may use words in a highly individual way, making it difficult for others to understand him and increasing his sense of isolation further. The language that a person uses reflects what he is thinking and experiencing. When a person's thought processes are disturbed, this is reflected in his language; there may be a lack of association of ideas or he may invent his own words which have special meanings. Because of painful interpersonal situations in the past, he may now find all relationships threatening and use disguised language to provide a protective mantle.

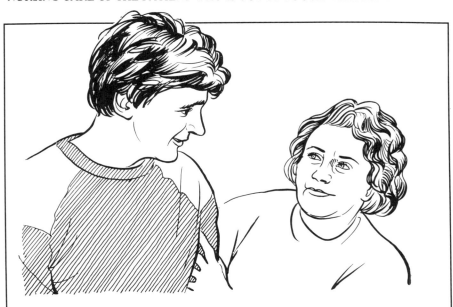

PATIENT PROFILE

Donald Carsen, aged 25, graduated from university with a first-class honours degree and has since been employed as a research assistant in the department of biological science at the university.

The Carsens have always been an isolated family. Having few friends or acquaintances. Mrs Carsen has always believed in keeping themselves to themselves. Mr Carsen is a commercial traveller and spends a great deal of time away from home. Donald has always lived at home except when he was at university; his mother does everything for him.

Donald has two older sisters. Helen, aged 30 and a teacher, is unmarried and no longer lives at home while Martha, aged 34, has been in a psychiatric hospital since the age of 17.

Mrs Carsen visits Martha once a month by herself; she refuses to discuss Martha or to be accompanied on her visits. Mrs Carsen has a sister who has a long history of mental illness. She also is not discussed within the family.

Donald has never been a good mixer, even at university.

The onset of his illness was gradual. One day, he told his mother that he had become invisible. She thought it might have something to do with the nature of his work at the laboratory.

In the meanwhile the head of the biological science department was becoming increasingly concerned about Donald's work. He seems vague and as if he was not really taking in what was said to him. His work lacked accuracy and attention to detail and sometimes Donald was observed to be giggling for no apparent reason.

He was referred to the occupational health department at the university who in turn got in touch with Donald's general practitioner.

Dr Deane was asked to do a domiciliary visit and Donald was admitted to hospital.

On admission, he smiled to himself, frequently nodded his head and was generally uncommunicative.

NURSING ASSESSMENT INTERVIEW

Surname _Cassen_

Forenames _Donald Phillip_

Name person likes to be called _Donald_

Address _12 The Croft_
Willbury Common
WIL YL3

Telephone number _0515_

~~Date of referral~~/admission _15.1.87_

Next-of-kin

Name _Mr and Mrs Cassen_

Relationship _Parents_

Address _As above_

Telephone number _3030_

Date of birth _29.9.61_

General practitioner _Dr G. Perry_

Single/~~married/divorced/widowed~~

Address _The Surgery_
124 Kent Road
Willbury

Consultant _Dr S. Ireland_

Status under Mental Health Act _Informal_

Psychiatric diagnosis _Schizophrenia_

History of self-harm or harm towards others _No_

Occupation _Research assistant_

Occupational history
Fruit picking, petrol pump attendant during
university vacation to supplement grant

Hobbies and interests _Reading, model making, walking,_
swimming.

Patient's perceived reason for referral/admission _Deferred_

Relatives' understanding of patient's problems _'Spends too much time with_
his head in a book' — father's comment

NURSING ASSESSMENT INTERVIEW (continued)

Persons of significance in person's life

Family/friends/pets _Darren Smith — close friend since university_

Spiritual needs

Church of England — does not attend church regularly

Problems causing concern at home _No_

Community services involved/referred

Name _Oscar Smith_ Status _Community psychiatric nurse_

Telephone number _7719_ Date of referral _28.2.86_

Mental status

History of present problems _Became more and more vague and out of touch. Felt like talking to someone who wasn't there_

Previous psychiatric history _None, but Martha suffers from 'a split personality'. My wife won't talk about her and says that visits from myself, Helen or Donald make her very disturbed. I prefer to remember her as she was — she was a beautiful girl_

General appearance and behaviour _Careless dress — stays in one position for a long time without moving_

Speech and communication patterns _Quietly spoken, articulate, uses personalised language_

Problems with perception _Appears to be hallucinated; listens_

NURSING ASSESSMENT INTERVIEW (continued)

Affective state _Giggly_

Disturbances of thinking or judgement _Hallucinations may interfere with judgement_

Orientation

Person _Deferred_

Place

Time

Activities of living

Safety and mobility
Content of hallucination may pose safety threat

Eating and drinking
Not eating much lately but drinks milk

Elimination
Bladder _Deferred - observe_
Bowel

Sleep patterns
Sleeps well; always difficulty in getting up in the mornings

Personal needs
Hygiene and bathing. Wears an upper partial denture

General health

Any medical condition for which the person is receiving treatment
No - there shouldn't be - he's got everything that he needs

Doctor's instructions
Try to build a relationship with the patient

Areas of concern to patient
I shall have to talk to Donald's boss Dr Foley - I hope that it will be possible to keep Donald's job open

NURSING ASSESSMENT INTERVIEW (continued)

Problems identified

Date of interview _15. 1. 87_   Signature _D. Simmons_

History taken from _Mr Carsen_

by _David Simmons_   Designation _Charge nurse_

Additional information   Date _15. 1. 87_

_Mr Carsen will bring in Donald's glasses ;
normally he wears contact lenses_

Table 27.1 Adaptive modes, assessments, patient's problems and goals, and nursing orders

Adaptive mode	First-level assessment	Second-level assessment			Patient's problem	Patient's goal	Nursing orders
		Focal stimuli	Contextual stimuli	Residual stimuli			
Basic physiological needs	Seems unaware of needs	Vague and preoccupied	? Voices interfere with attention span	? Biochemical–genetic factors	Food deficits. Fluid deficits. Elimination deficits	To meet physiological needs, particularly those for food, fluids, personal and elimination hygiene	To ensure adaptation through the physiological mode by supervision and prompting Donald to take food and fluids. To attend to elimination needs and personal hygiene
Self-concept		Little eye contact. Looks down at floor when not 'listening'	Mother addresses her son as Donny rather than Donald	Past experience.	Break with reality. Negative self-concept	To tolerate the presence of the nurse. To experience reality. To develop a positive self-concept	To promote reality adaptation through developing a relationship with Donald
Role mastery		? Unsure of own roles	Mother inhibits separation from herself	Past experience.	Lack of independent role choice	To achieve independent choice of roles	To encourage independence in meeting needs
Interdependence		Seems unaware of presence of others. Distant	Distorted perception	Past experience.	Break with reality—substitutes for interactions with others	To use appropriate verbal language. To express thoughts and feelings. To develop social and interpersonal skills in small group activities	To help Donald to develop interpersonal, social and work skills by joining activity groups when he is ready for them

USE OF ROY'S ADAPTATION MODEL

Roy's (1980) adaptation model was chosen for his nursing care (see Chapter 7).

PLAN OF NURSING CARE

The plan of nursing care is given in *Table 27.1.*

IMPLEMENTATION

The nurse's first priority was to promote Donald's safety. His giggly behaviour and the listening posture that he adopted indicated that he was hallucinated. Impulsive behaviour can occur in response to hallucinatory 'commands', and the nurse was aware that vivid hallucinations can lead to periods of excitement in which the patient may harm himself or others. An environment in which stimuli are reduced can help to prevent such behaviour.

The nurse initiated contact with Donald for short periods only, so that he did not feel threatened or pressurised. The nurse showed respect for Donald's personal space and accepted that developing a relationship with him would take time. The development of this relationship would be an important step in helping the patient adapt through the physiological, self-concept, role mastery and interdependence modes.

Donald was always addressed by name so as to strengthen his identity. He was encouraged to touch others and to manipulate actual objects so as to impress on him that real people and real objects exist. In this way, his sense of touch enabled him to experience a sense of being in the world. It is never easy to communicate with the patient who is out of touch with reality, particularly when the patient uses a language all of his own. This can create anxiety in the nurse but, if the nurse withdraws from the patient, it will only serve to increase his feelings of isolation. Even when the patient seems resistive to attempts to communicate with him, the nurse should make a conscious effort to spend time with him.

Donald used the word 'glung' several times. By asking him what this meant, the nurse did not reinforce the use of his invented words; instead, it communicated a desire to understand him.

If the nurse suggests to the patient that he is understood when he is not, this only contributes to the continued use of individual language; if he assumes that he is understood, then he has no reason to change.

Although the nurse should show a willingness to listen to anything the patient says, responding to anything real that he talks about will help to reinforce reality and to assist him in the process of adaptation. It is usually only when a relationship has been established that the patient will be willing to share information about his hallucinatory experiences. If the patient is challenged about these experiences too soon, he may deny their existence altogether.

The nurse should accept the statements that the patient makes about his hallucinatory experiences but at the same time be careful not to enter his maladaptive processes. The existence of the hallucination is very real to the patient and should not therefore be denied. However, the nurse must make it quite clear to the patient that only *he* hears the voices and that the voices are not audible to others.

There is a method that can be used to help the patient to stop his hallucinatory voices. Donald was instructed to say 'Go away and leave Donald alone.' He was told to say this loudly and clearly and to repeat it several times. He was encouraged

to practise in the nurse's presence so that he would have the confidence to carr
out this procedure when alone (Field, 1985).

Basically the patient must learn to devalue his hallucinations.

If the patient appears to be preoccupied with his voices, then the nurse mu
speak to him in a tone of voice that will catch his attention. The use of clea
uncomplicated sentences are better than non-verbal responses which may be ope
to misinterpretation by the patient.

At first, Donald required supervision in carrying out the activities of daily livin
but he generally responded to prompting. At mealtimes, he would just sit starir
into space. However, if the nurse placed the cutlery in his hands and helped him t
place the first piece of food on his fork, this seemed to prompt him to eat.

EVALUATION

Donald's progress was slow and the nurse was required to adopt the san
therapeutic strategies over and over again. On specified dates, each goal wa
examined in order to determine his movement towards adaptation. He use
more eye contact when interacting with the nurse and in social situations. H
language was more appropriate and he no longer spoke of 'glungs'.

Donald was referred to Oscar Smith, the community psychiatric nurse, soc
after his admission so that Oscar would have the opportunity to establish
relationship with the patient. Donald told Oscar that he had been hearir
voices but that 'they were gone now'. He said that the voices had upset hi
considerably; he had felt confused by two voices that seemed to be constant
arguing about him. The voices made him feel as if he was invisible because the
talked about him as if he was not there.

Donald participated in ward activities but usually needed prompting. H
interactions with other patients were limited. His mother visited the ward ever
day, and sometimes more than once; she seemed to dominate Donald totall

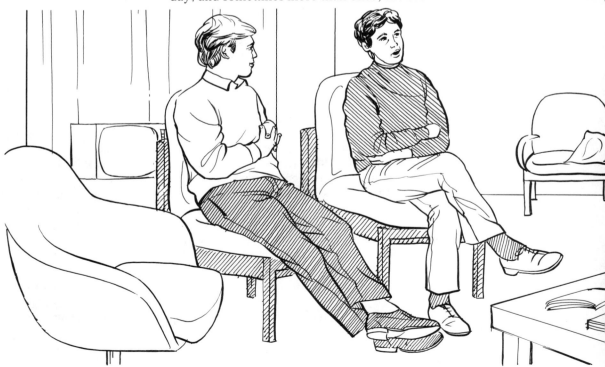

Her need for him seemed to be even greater than his need for her. Dr Deane has tried to discourage Mrs Carsen from visiting so frequently, since her presence has inhibited Donald's participation in organised activities. Mrs Carsen has reluctantly agreed to confine her visits to the evenings.

At the multi-disciplinary meeting, Dr Deane suggested that it would be in the patient's interests if he could be found a hostel placement when he was ready for discharge rather than returning to live at home. The idea of moving into a hostel will probably prove very hard for Donald's mother to accept, but such a move will be essential if he is to gain independence and role mastery as an individual in his own right, and to return to work.

NURSING THE PATIENT WHO IS OUT OF TOUCH WITH REALITY

Hallucinations do not necessarily indicate mental illness and are associated with:

1. Sleep deprivation.
2. Electrolyte imbalance.
3. Starvation.
4. Delirium.
5. Prolonged isolation.
6. Hallucinogenic drugs.
7. Physical exhaustion.
8. Strong emotion.
9. Twilight states, i.e. between sleeping and waking.

FACT SHEET: THE PATIENT WHO IS OUT OF TOUCH WITH REALITY

1. Touch can help to bring the patient back to reality but only if he responds comfortably to being touched.
2. All communications should be simple and related to what is happening in the real world.
3. The patient's identity can be strengthened by calling him by name.
4. The patient's family must not be blamed for his illness. The nurse must focus on their needs as well as those of the patient.
5. The nurse must avoid reinforcing the patient's break with reality.
6. In an excited phase the patient is not responsible for his behaviour. He is at the mercy of his delusions and hallucinations.
7. Try to ascertain whether the patient is experiencing voices that command him to carry out certain actions.
8. Observe and intervene to prevent self-harm or harm to others, patients or staff.
9. Spend time with the patient and show respect for his territorial space.
10. Adopt a non-threatening posture, i.e. arms unfolded.
11. Promote a trusting relationship by showing interest, concern and consistency.
12. Show a willingness to listen to the patient.

REFERENCES AND FURTHER READING

References

Arieti, S. (1972), cited by Field, W. E. (1985), Hearing voices, *Journal of Psychosocial Nursing*, **23**, No. 1, 9–14.

Cook, J. C. (1971), Interpreting and decoding autistic communication, *Perspectives in Psychiatric Care*, **9**, No. 1, 25–28.

Field, W. E. (1985), Hearing voices, *Journal of Psychosocial Nursing*, **23** No. 1, 9–14.

Roy, C. (1980), The Roy adaptation model. In: *Conceptual Models for Nursing Practice* (eds Riehl, J. P., and Roy, C.), Appleton Century Crofts, Norwalk, Connecticut.

Schwartzman, S. T. (1975), The hallucinating patient and nursing intervention, *Journal of Psychiatric Nursing and Mental Health Services*, **14**, No. 6, 23–28, 33–36.

Further reading

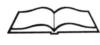

Field, W., and Ruelke, W. (1973), Hallucinations and how to deal with them, *American Journal of Nursing*, **73**, 638–640.

Gerder, C., and Snyder, D. (1970), Language and thought, *Perspectives in Psychiatric Care*, **8**, No. 5, 230–233.

Grace, H. K., and Camilleri, D. (1981), *Mental Health Nursing: A Socio-psychological Approach*, Wm. C. Brown, Dubuque, Iowa.

Gravenkemper, K. H. (1963), In: *Hallucinations in Some Clinical Approaches to Psychiatric Nursing* (eds Burd, S. F., and Marshall, M. A.), Macmillan, New York.

Grosicki, J. P., and Harmonson, M. (1969), Nursing action guide: hallucinations, *Journal of Psychiatric Nursing and Mental Health Services*, **7**, No. 3, 133–135.

Horne, M. (1985), A word in your head, *Nursing Mirror*, **160**, No. 23, 34–35.

Hurteau, M. P. (1963), Disguised language: a clinical nursing problem. In: *Some Clinical Approaches to Psychiatric Nursing* (eds Burd, S. F., and Marshall, M. A.), Macmillan, New York.

Kroah, J. (1974), Strategies for interviewing in language and thought disorders, *Journal of Psychiatric Nursing and Mental Health Services*, **12**, No. 2, 3–9.

Milverton, R. (1985), Institutional neurosis among clients living in the parental home, *Community Psychiatric Nursing Journal*, **5**, No. 1, 11–13.

Pope, B. (1986), *Social Skills Training for Psychiatric Nurses*, Harper and Row, London.

Sugden, J., and Field, R. (1985), Cognitive and thought disorders, *Nursing (UK)*, **2**, No. 34, 999–1003.

Teasdale, K. (1986), Schizophrenia and the family, *Nursing Times*, **82**, No. 7, 41–43.

Chapter 28

Nursing care of the patient who is institutionalised

'Rigid interpersonal behaviour presumes that all people before whom it is enacted are alike in personality. To some extent such interpersonal behaviour can actually provoke a certain uniformity in the behaviour of others.' (Jourard, 1971).

INTRODUCTION

Institutionalisation describes a syndrome of submissiveness, apathy and loss of individuality. The person loses his outside identity, and all its subsequent roles and relationships, and takes on the identity of the institution. He is no longer an individual in his own right; he becomes passive and compliant, and in hospital he conforms to the role of the 'good' patient.

Institutionalisation not only occurs in institutions but also can happen to people living in their own homes. The term is associated with institutions because this is where the condition is mainly observed.

The patient who is institutionalised is often apathetic, lacking in initiative and has no interest in every-day events or in the future. There is often a marked deterioration in personal habits, hygiene and dress. The patient may adopt a characteristic posture, with the head and shoulders down and shuffle about aimlessly. Not all patients exhibit the features of institutionalism in the same way. While one patient may sit around in a chair all day, another may take an active role doing ward work and generally enjoy all the facilities provided by the hospital. The nursing notes often contain remarks such as 'cooperative—gives no trouble'. 'Good worker—helpful in the ward', 'uncommunicative' or 'uncooperative'. These remarks more often reflect the effect that the patient's behaviour has on the staff rather than accurately state the patient's condition.

Barton (1976) has described many factors which have contributed towards the institutionalisation of patients. Most large mental hospitals were built some distance from towns and, for most patients, hospitalisation meant a break from the outside world. In the past, wards have been locked and leave restricted. Some relatives were not given much incentive to visit, being prohibited by the distance and expense. Even if they did visit, the patient's behaviour and that of other patients could be very disturbing and difficult to tolerate.

While some patients worked in the wards and departments, others were not allowed to do anything for themselves. They could not wash or dress without supervision or make their own beds. At mealtimes, tea was served from a large pot with milk and sugar already added; bread was buttered and even spread with jam. Every activity that a patient could carry on for himself on entering the institution was curtailed. Subsequently, this led to enforced idleness.

Authoritarian attitudes were the rule of the day; patients were told where to sit, what to wear and when to have a bath, thereby removing any initiative that they once had. In many institutions, patients were treated harshly, physically assaulted or belittled, humiliated and treated unfeelingly by the staff.

In the overcrowded wards, personal events such as birthdays and anniversaries were forgotten, and there were rarely any places to keep personal possessions such as photographs or other articles of sentimental value.

The ward atmosphere was in many cases dreary and lacking in a homely atmosphere. The drab surroundings communicated to the patient that nothing mattered and contributed to the development of apathy.

Custodial care and interactions placed the patient on unequal terms, thus stunting his growth, reducing his self-esteem and promoting his dependence (Scadden, 1985).

Meals were commonly served in a communal dining room where, despite several sittings, up to 200 patients would be seated at any one time.

Bedtime for many patients would be around 7.00 pm or even earlier, perhaps with the exception of the 'workers' who were able to earn special privileges. Not surprisingly, after an idle day, many patients needed sedatives on top of the tranquillisers that they were already receiving.

After spending some time in a mental hospital, the patients' chances of finding employment or a place to live were diminished. Consequently, many patients never wanted to leave hospital and resigned themselves to their lot.

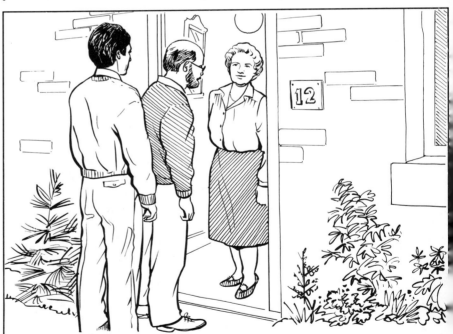

PATIENT PROFILE

Favara Zambroski, aged 61, has spent the last 25 years in a large psychiatric hospital some miles from Wilbury. His parents, now dead, were Polish immigrants; Favara and his twin sister Marie were born soon after they settled in this country.

Most people have forgotten why Favara is in hospital, and Favara regards the hospital as his home. He has shown no symptoms of illness for some years—only the symptoms of years spent in an institution.

Although Favara keeps to himself, he is neither unapproachable nor argumentative. He likes to please the nurses and is regarded by them as a cooperative and willing worker. When he is not working in the industrial therapy unit, Favara likes to keep himself busy by doing odd jobs for the staff. His speciality is cleaning cars. He saves some of the money that he earns and spends the rest on his favourite tobacco.

In spite of the fact that Favara has often said that he does not want to leave the hospital, he has been aware for some time that the hospital is under threat of closure. His fears have been confirmed by items in the local newspaper and through watching a television programme.

Almost a year ago, Favara participated in a behavioural modification programme, and his general appearance and personal grooming have since become more acceptable. He is able to travel into town using public transport and makes the train journey to Bradford each year to spend a holiday with his sister.

Favara has also learned to use the telephone and to cook simple nutritious meals for himself. He has, as far as possible, been prepared to adjust to life outside an institution, a life similar to that enjoyed by other members of the community.

NURSING ASSESSMENT INTERVIEW

Surname _Zambroski_   Forenames _Favara_

Name person likes to be called _Favara_

Address _12 Linden Avenue_   Telephone number _____

Willbury   Date of ~~referral~~/admission _17 . 3 . 61_

Next-of-kin

Name _Mrs M. Bond_   Relationship _Sister_

Address _43 Springfield_

Mill Road

Bradford   Telephone number _—_

Date of birth _14 . 6 . 25_   Single/~~married/divorced/widowed~~ _____

General practitioner _Dr Lever_   Address _60 Links Road_

Willbury

Consultant _Dr H. Kellehear_

Status under Mental Health Act _Informal_

Psychiatric diagnosis _Schizophrenia (reason for admission)_

History of self-harm or harm towards others _None for past 15 years_

Occupation _Factory worker prior to admission_

Occupational history

Hobbies and interests _Television, odd jobs, woodwork,_
keen to do gardening again

Patient's perceived reason for referral/admission _'They put me away_
but I never hurt anyone'

Relatives' understanding of patient's problems _Not known, but sister_
does not want Favara to move nearer to
her permanently

NURSING ASSESSMENT INTERVIEW (continued)

Persons of significance in person's life

Family/friends/pets _Sister — writes to him and sends parcels_

Spiritual needs _Likes to go to Sunday service_

Problems causing concern at home _Not relevant yet_

Community services involved/referred

Name _Clive Pohl_   Status _Community psychiatric nurse_

Telephone number _3121_   Date of referral _1.12.85_

Mental status

History of present problems _No evidence of mental illness now — needs assistance to become independent_

Previous psychiatric history _Disturbed aggressive behaviour on admission (1961); hallucinations and delusions_

General appearance and behaviour _Neat and tidy. Behaves appropriately to situations_

Speech and communication patterns _Quietly spoken; learning to initiate conversation_

Problems with perception _None_

NURSING ASSESSMENT INTERVIEW (continued)

Affective state _Never shows extremes of mood; wants to please_

Disturbances of thinking or judgement _No_

Orientation

Person _No problem_

Place

Time

Activities of living

Safety and mobility

No problems

Eating and drinking

Eats well

Elimination

Bladder _No problems_

Bowel _No problems_

Sleep patterns

Sleeps well

Personal needs

Needs encouragement and approval. Favara is sometimes afraid of doing the wrong thing

General health

Any medical condition for which the person is receiving treatment

_No_

Doctor's instructions

Help Favara to integrate into Linden Avenue

Areas of concern to patient

After some reservations, now looking forward to living at Linden Avenue

NURSING ASSESSMENT INTERVIEW (continued)

Problems identified

Institutionalization has removed ability to live independently – some deficits in knowledge of every-day life. Says that some staff members are like family to him

Date of interview ___4.3.86___   Signature ___Clive Pohl___

History taken from ___Favara___

by ___Clive Pohl___   Designation ___Community psychiatric nurse___

Additional information   Date _____

Favara responds to praise – likes to know that he is doing the right thing

USE OF OREM'S SELF-CARE MODEL

Unfortunately, Favara had to wait some time for a community placement. The hospital authority's plans to purchase a large house and to convert it into bedsitters for ex-patients was thwarted by local residents who objected to the proposal because of fears about a possible depreciation in the value of their own property.

PLAN OF NURSING CARE

The plan of nursing care is given in *Tables 28.1* and *28.2* and in the following sections (a) and (b).

Table 28.1   *Universal self-care requisites and assessments*

Universal self-care requisite	Assessment of self-care abilities
Air	No evidence of ventilatory problems
Food	Eats well
Water Elimination	Adequate intake No evidence of problems
Activity and rest	Acts on own volition. Never complains of sleeping problems
Avoidance of hazards to life and well-being	Sensible regarding safety
Solitude and social interaction	Interacts on own initiation
Being normal	Behaviour within 'normal' limits

Table 28.2   *Developmental and health self-care requisites*

Self care requisites	Patient's problem	Patient's goal	Nursing goal	Type of nursing action
Developmental Effects of illness on human development	Institutionalism has removed ability to live independently	To achieve independent living	To promote independent living	Guiding, educative–supportive
Health deviation Adjustments to ill health	Learning to accept responsibility after years in institution. Some deficits in knowledge necessary for independent living	To accept responsibility for self and others	To promote informed decision making	Guiding, educative–supportive

It took almost 18 months for Favara to be found a place in an already established home where four other patients have been living for over a year. The vacancy was created when one resident decided to move out into her own flat. Dr Kellehear introduced the proposition to Favara gradually. Initially, Favara was very reluctant to accept the idea but, after making a visit to the house with the community psychiatric nurse, he liked the idea of having his own room.

At this stage the nurse's main task was to help Favara to make the transition from the hospital to living in the community. The nurse decided that Orem's (1980) self-care model provided the most suitable framework for Favara's care.

IMPLEMENTATION

The nurse had to enable Favara to engage in those activities necessary to meet his universal self-care needs. From the three nursing systems which Orem describes (see Chapter 7) the supportive education system met Favara's needs most adequately. He was able to learn to perform self-care activities but would be unable to do so without assistance.

The overall aim of nursing was to return the patient to the state in which his self-care activities exceeded those of the nurse. Therefore the nurse was primarily concerned with redressing imbalances in self-care activities.

(a) Patient's goals

1. To reduce his contact with the hospital.
2. To verbalise his fears about discharge.
3. To gain confidence in his ability to live independently.
4. Gradually to establish contacts with others outside the 'family' residence.
5. To approach appropriate agencies should the need arise.

(b) Nursing goals

1. To introduce Favara to the other residents in the house.
2. To provide support as he becomes accepted as a member of the family group.
3. To help him to understand the necessity to adhere to the family budget.
4. To liaise with the occupational therapist who will help Favara prepare for the use of leisure time.
5. To encourage him to take up old hobbies and interests or to establish new ones.
6. To assist him to identify and apply for a course of his own choosing at the college of further education.
7. To discourage him from retaining links with the hospital or staff members.
8. To monitor his integration into the family unit but keep a low profile.
9. To prepare the patient for a gradual reduction in visits without making him feel rejected.
10. To teach him to approach the appropriate agencies should any problems arise, e.g. general practitioner, electricity and gas boards.
11. To help him to identify his particular areas of responsibility in the house.
12. To encourage Favara to make independent decisions.
13. To help him to consider the needs of the other residents as well as his own.
14. To advise him to extinguish cigarettes properly and not to smoke in his room, so as to protect the safety of other residents.

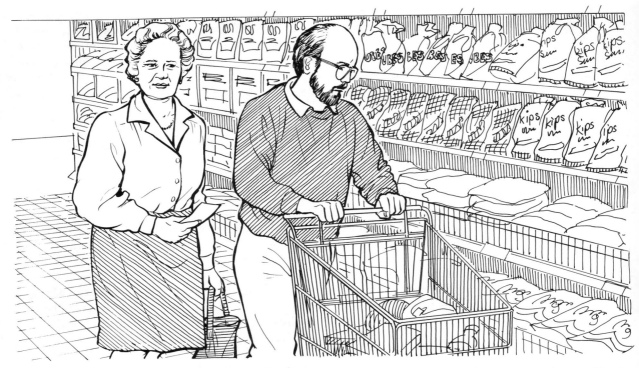

When Favara first visited 12 Linden Avenue with the community psychiatric nurse, only Annie Blant was at home. Pearl Jefferies and James Lacey were at work and Jessica Woodward had gone out for a walk. Annie acted as housekeeper for the others, and in many respects she was like a mother to them. She offered to show Favara around and he seemed to like the bedroom which overlooked the back garden and which would be his.

He was invited to tea on Sunday to meet the other residents. The nurse suggested that he might like to take a small gift, and so he took a nice plant.

The nurse helped Favara to identify his own areas of responsibility within the house, to make independent decisions and yet at the same time to consider the needs and requests of others. Favara said that he would take over the garden and grow flowers and vegetables as there was no one to do this at the present time. Annie requested that he should also help her with the main shopping once a week. Favara said that he was willing to do this.

EVALUATION

A year later, Favara is still enjoying community life. He is more independent, but he dropped out of the carpentry class at the college of further education. He seems to have some sense of belonging and spends most of his time at home. Annie treats him like a son and he usually obeys her without question. Needless to say, there have been disputes and minor disagreements among the residents, but the nurse deliberately plays a low key role, encouraging them to arrive at their own solutions.

During the early days, Favara wanted to go back to the hospital to visit his old friends. Now the hospital has closed and the land sold for redevelopment.

Considering that Favara spent so many years in hospital, he has adapted to community life quite well. Even so, he is quiet and blends into the background.

No one can spend a third of their life in an institution without those years having taken their toll.

REFERENCES AND FURTHER READING

References

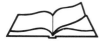

Barton, R. (1976), *Institutional Neurosis*, 3rd edn, John Wright, Bristol.
Jourard, S. M. (1971), *The Transparent Self*, Van Nostrand Reinhold, New York.
Orem, D. E. (1980), *Nursing: Concepts of Practice*, 2nd edn, McGraw-Hill, New York.
Scadden, J. (1985), An ideal typical approach to the study of nurse–patient interactions in psychiatric settings, Unpublished dissertation, submitted for the degree of M.Sc. in Social Research, Department of Sociology, University of Surrey.

Further reading

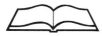

Armitage, P. (1986), The rehabilitation and nursing care of severely disabled psychiatric patients, *International Journal of Nursing Studies*, **23**, No. 2, 112–123.
Barton, R. (1976), *Institutional Neurosis*, 3rd edn, John Wright, Bristol.
Lloyd, R. (1981), Wanted: a change of attitude, *Nursing Mirror*, **153**, No. 11, 32–33.
Meisenhelder, J. B. (1985), Self-esteem: a closer look at clinical intervention, *International Journal of Nursing Studies*, **22**, No. 2, 127–135.
Salmon, P. F. (1983), The long-stay psychiatric patient, *Nursing Times*, **79**, No. 37, 39–40.
Waters, V. (1986), The sound of silence, *Nursing Times*, **82**, No. 23, 40–42.

List of useful addresses

Alateen
61 Dover Street
London
SE1 4YF
Telephone number: 01 403 0888

Self-help groups for young people with parents or other relatives with a drink problem

Alcoholics Anonymous
140a Tachbrook Street
London
SW1V 2NE
Telephone number: 01 834 8202

Will help anyone with a drinking problem

Alcoholics Anonymous Family
  Groups
61 Great Dover Street
London
SE1 4YE
Telephone number: 01 403 0888

Self-help groups for relatives and friends of problem drinkers

Alzheimer's Disease Society
Development Officer
3rd Floor
Bank Buildings
Fulham Broadway
London
SW6
Telephone number: 01 381 3177

Support for sufferers and family. Promotes research and public awareness

Anorexic Aid
The Priory Centre
11 Priory Road
High Wycombe
Buckinghamshire
Telephone number: 0494 21431

Support, advice, self-help groups

Association of Carers
58 New Road
Chatham
Kent
ME4 4OR
Telephone number: 0634 813981/2
(Medway)

Offers opportunities for self-help and counselling to those who lead a restricted life because of need to care for a mentally ill person (and other infirmities)

British Association for Counselling
37A Sheep Street
Rugby
Warwickshire
CV21 3BX
Telephone number: 0788 783 28

Referral service for counselling or any type of problem

British Epilepsy Association
Crowthorne House
New Wokingham Road
Wokingham
Berkshire
RG11 3AY
Telephone number: 034 46 3122

Advises on all aspects of living with epilepsy

Cadett
22 Lansdowne Road
London
W11 3LL
Telephone number: 01 727 9447

Counselling and advice for alcohol and drug problems, glue sniffing, bereavement and depression

Counselling
Alone in London Service
West Lodge
190 Euston Road
London
NW1
Telephone number: 01 387 3010/5470

Advice for young single homeless; age range, 16–25

Cruse
Cruse House
126 Sheen Road
Richmond
Surrey
TW9 1VR
Telephone number: 01 940 4818 or 9047

National organisation for widowed and their children. Counselling service offers help and understanding to widowed whether alone or with children. Practical advice; opportunities for social contact. Has local branches

Depressives Associated
19 Merley Ways
Wimbourne Minster
Dorset
BH21 1QN
Telephone number: 0202 883957

Runs local groups. Acts as a contact

Families Anonymous
88 Caledonian Road
London
N7
Telephone number: 01 278 8805

Can advise people whether there is a self-help group for parents of drug abusers in their area

Good Practices in Mental Health
380–384 Harrow Road
London
W9
Telephone number: 01 289 2034

A voluntary organisation that acts as an information source for health care professionals and others in the field of mental health

Homosexuality
Gay Switchboard
B M Switchboard
London
WC1N 3XX
Telephone number: 01 837 7324

24-hour telephone service, information about groups. Talk over problems on the telephone

The Institute for the Study of Drug
  Dependence
1–4 Hatton Place
Hatton Garden
London
EC1N 8ND

Information service and library. Publishes material about drugs

Lesbian Line
Telephone number: 01 251 6911

Monday and Friday 2–10 pm; Tuesday, Wednesday, Thursday, 7–10 pm. Information and help line.

Mental After-care Association
110 Jermyn Street
London
SW1 6HB

Mental Health Act Commission
Floor 2
Hepburn House
Marsham Street
London
SW1
Telephone number: 01 211 8061

Mind
22 Harley Street
London
W1N 2ED
Telephone number: 01 637 0741

Works to improve services for people who are mentally ill or mentally handicapped. Information, advice, legal and welfare rights services. Group homes, day centres, local groups, publications

Narcotics Anonymous
P.O. Box 246
c/o 47 Milman Street
London
SW10
Telephone number: 01 351 6794

Usually someone there between 2.30 pm and 8 pm each weekday; otherwise an answering machine takes messages. Can give the location of the nearest meeting place or help people with drug problems to start their own self-help group

The National Association of Young People's Counselling and Advisory Services
17–23 Albion Street
Leicester
LE1 6GD

Can put people in touch with local young counselling services. Stamped addressed envelope required

The National Association for Premenstrual Syndrome
23 Upper Park Road
Kingston-upon-Thames
Surrey
KT2 5LB

National Schizophrenic Fellowship
78 Victoria Road
Surbiton
Surrey
KT6 4NS
Telephone number: 01 390 3651

Local support groups. Help and advice for relatives

Open Door Association
447 Pensby Road
Heswall
Wirral
Merseyside
L61 2PQ
Telephone number: 051 648 2022

Self-help group for sufferers of anxiety and agoraphobia. Advice; information

Phobics Society
4 Cheltenham Road
Chorlton-cum-Hardy
Manchester
M21 1ON
Telephone number: 061 881 1937

Publishes material to help people with phobic conditions

Rape Crisis Centre
P.O. Box 69
London
WC1X 9NJ
Telephone number: 01 837 1600

Offers 24-hour service to girls or women who have been raped or sexually assaulted and the opportunity to talk to another woman in confidence. Medical and legal information

Release
Telephone number: 01 603 8654

Advice on legal problems arising from drug misuse. Always someone to answer the phone, but outside normal working hours the operator intercepts calls and gives the caller another number to ring

The Richmond Fellowship
8 Addison Road
London
W14 8DL
Telephone number: 01 603 6373

A charitable foundation concerned with rehabilitation in the field of mental health. Runs halfway houses or therapeutic communities. Accepts people with a wide range of difficulties

Samaritans
3 Hornton Place
London
W8
Telephone number: 01 283 3400

24-hour free confidential help for suicidal or despairing people. Local numbers in telephone directories

Solvent Abuse
Department M50
13–39 Standard Road
London
NW10

The Standing Conference on Drug
  Abuse
1–4 Hatton Place
Hatton Garden
London
EC1N 8ND

National coordinating organisation for services for people with drug problems. Supplies lists of specialist services. Send large stamped addressed envelope with your request for information

Index